The INS and OUTS of
breathing
How we learnt about the body's most vital function

Also by the author

Clinical Exercise Testing

Blood Gases and Acid-Base Physiology

In collaboration

Human Muscle Power

Breathlessness

Hypoxia: Man at Altitude

Hypoxia, Exercise and Altitude

The INS and OUTS of
breathing

How we learnt about the body's most vital function

Dr. Norman L. Jones

The Ins and Outs of Breathing
How We Learnt about the Body's Most Vital Function

iUniverse books may be ordered through booksellers or by contacting:

iUniverse
1663 Liberty Drive
Bloomington, IN 47403
www.iuniverse.com
1-800-Authors (1-800-288-4677)

ISBN: 978-1-4620-3006-4 (sc)
ISBN: 978-1-4620-3004-0 (ebk)

Library of Congress Control Number: 2011910364

Printed in the United States of America

iUniverse rev. date: 01/07/2013

For Graham, Steve and Marty

ACKNOWLEDGEMENTS

To a large extent the book represents my personal odyssey as a clinician, educator and researcher in the field of respiratory medicine. Along the way, I was helped by many teachers, colleagues, friends and family. My first steps were at the Royal Postgraduate Medical School at the Hammersmith Hospital in London: there Charles Fletcher and Moran Campbell were very influential in my career directions. Also at the Hammersmith I was fortunate to count John West, Neil Pride, Arnold Naimark, Ben Burrows and Richard Edwards as colleagues. Moran left there in 1968 to become the founding Chairman at the new medical school at McMaster University in Hamilton, Ontario, and I accompanied him as head of the Cardiorespiratory Unit. In the more than 40 years since then I have been fortunate to work with supportive colleagues. In addition to Moran, these included Kieran Killian, George Heigenhauser, John Sutton and many graduate students. Eric Hultman, Eric Newsholme, and Peter Stewart all gave generously of their expertise during extended visits with us. I am indebted to the Medical Research council of Canada and the Ontario Heart Foundation for thirty years of support.

Through the years it has taken to write the book, I have received loving support from my wife Diana and our three sons, Graham, Stephen and Martin all of whom provided helpful comments and suggestions from their varied viewpoints. Mark Inman and Paul O'Byrne read the manuscript and made many suggestions. I owe a great debt to Dr Anna Lawrence, who volunteered to edit the text, and who corrected many errors and provided countless helpful comments.

McMaster University's Media Production Services brought their considerable talents to bear on the layout and figures and organized all the final production details.

I am grateful to the many copyright holders for permission to reproduce figures, as identified in the Notes section at the end of the book. I have made every effort to contact copyright holders but, for one reason or another, failed in some instances. I apologize in advance for any omissions or errors, which we would be pleased to correct in any future printings of the book.

I

PREFACE

Looking back, I can see the seed of this book has taken 50 years to germinate. In the early 1960s, and living in London, I had just made the career choice to train in chest medicine, I was struggling to understand how the lung worked. Career prospects were not good in the British National Health Scheme, especially for prospective chest physicians, because the Ministry of Health had designated the specialty as one (actually, the only one) in which "negative growth" was planned. The reason for this plan was the dramatic decline in the number of patients with tuberculosis, requiring treatment by so-called tuberculosis officers. Set against depressing clinical future, were the great advances that had been made in the preceding decade in our understanding of how the lungs worked and the new techniques available for the assessment of lung function in health and disease. Also at that time there was a great deal of research going on at several academic centres in the UK. The regular meetings of the Medical Research Society and the Physiological Society were exciting, and offered the opportunity to meet the leaders in respiratory research and those who, like myself, were starting an academic career. I felt extremely fortunate to be working in one of the most productive groups in the UK, at the Royal Postgraduate Medical School at the Hammersmith Hospital. There my mentors were two leaders in the field; my debt to them will be obvious at many points in the book. What will be less obvious is the extent to which they differed; the differences were just as important to me as their individual reputations. There was, on the one hand, Charles Fletcher, son of Sir Walter Morley Fletcher—the first Secretary of the Medical Research Council; educated at Eton and Cambridge; first doctor to administer penicillin; successful director of large epidemiological and clinical research projects; the public face of the medical profession on television; bee-keeper; and severe diabetic.

And, on the other hand, Moran Campbell, proud son of a Yorkshire general practitioner, innovative physiologist and brilliant thinker, who revolutionized oxygen therapy and concepts of breathlessness; author of the seminal *The Respiratory Muscles and the Mechanics of Breathing*, and in his retirement, *Not Always on the Level* (on living with mania and depression); avid cyclist; and notable wit, in the mould of Oscar Wilde. Both Charles and Moran provided me with needed support and direction. In 1968, when Moran was approached to become the founding Chairman of the Department of Medicine at the new Faculty of Health Sciences at McMaster University in Hamilton, Ontario, I also went as Director of the Cardio-respiratory Unit. At the Hammersmith and at McMaster I was helped by many colleagues and students. It can easily be appreciated that many parts of this book might justify a change in the subtitle from "How we learnt…" to "How I learnt…" The autobiographical flavor underscores the fact that it is not meant as a textbook, and hopefully this may widen its appeal.

During my odyssey to understand breathing in all its aspects, what came to dominate my thinking was the inter-connectedness of them all. Not only does breathing respond to support the body's energy demands, it is also affected by changes in many body systems, such as the brain. Changes in breathing, whether too much or too little lead to secondary effects on these systems. In short, breathing is central to the proper functioning of the body and to your quality of life. Then, taking a wider view, the lungs are the only major system in direct contact with the environment, serving to protect the body with a variety of defences, but also taking the brunt of the onslaught, when the air we breathe is toxic.

II

Humanity's learning curve regarding breathing was for centuries slow and gradual, but like everything else there has been a dramatic surge in the past few decades. This book will take you along the curve, with the initial steps being easy to grasp, and the later progress becoming increasingly complex. I hope you will find the journey informative and interesting, even though many of the complexities may leave you struggling, just as they do myself.

Norman Jones
Hamilton
March 2011

INTRODUCTION

As you sit reading this, I may safely bet that up to this second you have been completely unaware of your breathing. Ah, now that I've reminded you, you are able to feel that you are gently drawing air in and allowing it to rebound out, with very little effort. Breathing goes on without us thinking much about it, even if we exercise; our breathing automatically increases, and while we may appreciate the increase, we do not have to do anything consciously in order to "drive" it. However, should anything happen to interfere with the process and make it more difficult, we experience considerable discomfort that brings with it a fear for our lives. Early humans, living in their caves, at some point realized that the breathing movements of the chest were accompanied by other indicators of life, such as warmth and activity; cessation of life was indicated by a lack of breathing, inertia and coldness. Nowadays, we all know breathing is important and that if anything happens to stop it, we survive for very few minutes. We also know, even if not in any detail, that breathing is linked to all body processes which require oxygen and lead to the production of carbon dioxide. One of the most famous researchers of the last century, the Oxford physiologist John Scott Haldane, stated his conviction in 1934 "that the physiology of respiration deals with phenomena which are specifically those of life". Because breathing is perhaps the one physiological process that links all bodily functions, it deserves to be considered "holistically". Also, because the lungs constitute the only organ that is constantly and directly in contact with our environment, the links extend to beyond the confines of the body. A trivial example of the influence of our environment is the increase in breathing that occurs at high altitude. Changes in atmospheric air secondary to air pollution, or more personally to cigarette smoking, are well known to influence breathing and cause ill effects in the respiratory tract—an anatomical region that extends from the nose and mouth through the larynx and airways (bronchi) down to the delicate air sacs (alveoli) where the "exchange" of oxygen and carbon dioxide occurs. There are many causes for diseases affecting the bronchi and alveoli; the episodic bronchial inflammation of asthma affects up to 20% of the population, and chronic bronchitis with destruction of the alveolar walls (emphysema) constitutes what is now known as chronic obstructive pulmonary disease (COPD), the fourth leading cause of death in the USA. Such conditions were thought to be due entirely to the damaging effects of particles and gases breathed into the lungs, as in cigarette smoking, but now we know that there is a complex interaction between them and the body's defences, that includes the individual's genetic make-up. Our newly found understanding allows us to take preventive action to avoid damage to the respiratory system and to treat it when it has occurred.

Breathing is so important to us that phrases to do with breathing are imbedded in the English language; how often do we hear "relax, take a deep breath", "give me some breathing space", "don't worry, you can breathe easy", and the more frightening "I can't breathe in here". Then, there are wider connections to breathing as the most important action in our lives—we are "inspired" to do well, and important aspects of our life act as an "inspiration" for us. Most of the phrases express the links between breathing and our psychological state. Nobel Laureate Dickinson W Richards expressed the importance of breathing to the whole human organism as "truly a strange phenomenon of life, caught midway between the conscious and the unconscious, and peculiarly sensitive to both".

An understanding of breathing and its control has for centuries been a prominent part of

Yoga and other health-related approaches that strengthen links between body, mind and spirit to attain optimal health. This notion has been held since the earliest of times. The Greek word "pneuma" meant both "spirit" and "breath", and the modern German for "breath"—*atmung*—is derived from the ancient Sanskrit *atman*, meaning "spirit". The use of consciously controlled breathing as an aid to meditation has become an important part of so-called "alternative" or "complementary" medicine approaches to healthy living and to living with various illnesses. Thus, there is much to be said for improving our understanding of the process of breathing, its importance to the function of other body systems, and the effects of thoughtful breathing control.

We can become conscious of our breathing for many reasons, from medically insignificant disorders to the life threatening diseases, not only of the lungs, but of virtually any of the major organs, whether affecting the heart, liver or kidneys. Variously described as breathlessness, shortness of breath, being out of breath, and by professionals as dyspnea, the symptom is often considered difficult to explain, even "an enigma". Bearing in mind that it may accompany many illnesses involving the major organs, and not being limited to disorders of lung function, it is not surprising that doctors often are at a loss in trying to explain to their patients what is going on and what to do about it. It is self-evident that its explanation lies in the sphere of "integrative physiology", where the links (integration) between bodily functions lead to a complex interdependence that is difficult to understand. In medical education and research, integrative physiology has lost out during the past two or three decades to more "modern" topics such as molecular biology (genetics), clinical epidemiology (large scale drug trials, "evidence based medicine") and medical economics (affordable health care). It is perhaps unfortunate that these latter-day medical themes have achieved increasing prominence at the expense of physiology, because physiology provides the framework on which they achieve their relevance in health related fields.

People like to talk of things increasing "exponentially"; often the term is undeserved, but when we consider the accumulation of our knowledge of breathing, it seems to fit the bill. For hundreds of years progress was painfully slow, and many long-held theories were nonsensical; during the last century and a half however, knowledge has steadily accelerated to the extent that it is hard to keep up with the many advances being made on a month-by-month basis. The history parallels many aspects of progress in medical knowledge; as Roy Porter has pointed out, the rate at which knowledge is increasing, together with its rapid dissemination in the media and electronic resources, inevitably are accompanied by personal anxiety and public debate.

Whilst not a medical textbook, the present work may help to reduce anxiety and inform debate by dealing with issues that directly or indirectly have to do with breathing. A historical approach is taken to various topics to build a picture of our present-day understanding of breathing in all its aspects. Necessarily, in some parts I will venture into the fields of biochemistry, physics and mathematics. Many concepts related to the physiology of breathing are best understood in very basic physical terms. I hope this fact will not deter readers with little background in these fields, even though for them some sections in the book may not be easy to grasp. However, the main objective of this introduction to the topic of breathing is to gain an understanding of the links between our vital systems and the central role that breathing plays in our wellbeing.

CONTENTS

CHAPTER 1

EARLY BREATHS Warmth and combustion

"By these veins we draw in much spirit for they are the spiracles of our bodies inhaling air to themselves and distributing it to the rest of the body and to the smaller veins, and they cool and afterwards exhale it."

Hippocrates, about 420 BCE (Francis Adams, The genuine works of Hippocrates, 1849)

What can we possibly know about primitive man's understanding of breathing? Very little, coming from the interpretations of cave pictographs and the appearances of primitive graves. From these, we gain an impression of the importance of the chest and heart; hunters knew where to aim arrows in order to kill animals most effectively, and how to protect their chests, both in life as well as the journey into the unknown in death. We may guess that in observing death, they associated the lack of breathing with loss of movement, and rapid loss of body heat. Possibly, the beating of the heart and appreciation of a pulse may have been understood as an accompaniment of life. Also, that death involved the loss of something indefinable, unknowable, that distinguished one person from another, and remained in the memory of their life. Later these observations were elaborated into a concept of the spirit or soul, which might live on after death. Early writings, from as far back as 4.000 years BCE in China and India, incorporated such thoughts, and there is evidence that early Mediterranean medical schools (around 500 BCE) emphasized the importance of the heart and of breathing, and the belief in the heart being the seat of the soul. Nowadays we know almost everything about how and why we breathe; the story of the journey in our understanding is one involving ideas; myths and the need of religions to control our thoughts; advances in science and technology; and the apparent difficulty that men of genius have in earning acceptance of their new ideas. In some ways it resembles both a climb of Everest, and the history of its ascent through the years—beginning with an uncertain goal that becomes clearer; of climbs to increasing altitude separated by plateaus; of improvements in performance that build on experience and improved scientific equipment; and a constant hindrance provided by those who ask "why (on earth) are you doing this. This chapter focuses mainly on the people who began the climb, taking us ever closer to the summit by the end of the 18th century. However, as in all scientific climbs, achieving a summit is illusory, as each generation finds new problems to solve.

THE GREEKS

Hippocrates—in the quotation above—was trying to understand the function of breathing from what he understood about the structure of the respiratory system. His contemporary Plato, on the other hand, took a much more philosophical approach. In the *Timaeus* and the *Republic*, he put forward a quasi-political scheme in which control of body functions was based on a hierarchy of three "souls", whose functions paralleled the roles of three different classes in society as a whole. Thus, the highest, situated in the head, had its counterpart in the philosopher class, and the lowest—in the liver—was identified with the workers; in between,

1

in the heart, was the soul controlling fire and movement, and was related to the warriors. Plato's pupil Aristotle, in the fourth century BCE, elaborated on these principles and began to link bodily processes to organs and to the "elements". In this scheme the four elements were air, fire, earth and water—corresponding to energy, vapors, solids, and fluids; four properties were held to be related to combinations of these primal elements. The four properties were hot (fire/air), cold (earth/water), wet (air/water), and dry (earth/fire). Bodily function was considered in terms of balance between four humors and their related organs—yellow bile/liver (linked to fire), blood/heart (air), black bile/spleen (earth), and phlegm/brain (water).

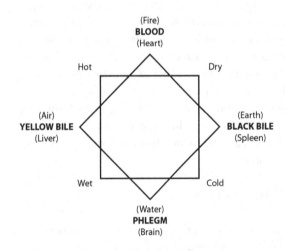

Figure 1 Links between Grecian concepts of elements and humors.

Whilst we may look back on this scheme as fanciful, it is the product of imaginative thought without the benefit of much anatomical understanding (at a time when dissection was discouraged), and lasted more or less intact for hundreds of years. Indeed, it lives on in common usage when someone is described as phlegmatic, sanguine or choleric. It is intriguing that a close

parallel may be drawn between this thinking of the ancient Greeks, and the writings of early Hindu thinkers, many centuries before, who described the necessary balance between *vaya* (air), *pitta* (bile) and *kapha* (phlegm), and their combination to form body tissues, including *rakta* (blood). Also the Hindus expressed the idea that the breath/spirit, or atman, entered the body through the skull.[1] Thus, these two geographically separated groups of thinkers evolved similar concepts related to life-sustaining forces.

Hippocrates, the greatest of the Greek physicians, was who lived on the island of Cos in the fifth century BCE has often been called the "Father of Medicine". Scholars have attempted to separate the myths surrounding his teachings from the evidence left in the remains of the library of the "Hippocratic School of Cos", to collect the "genuine" texts of his teaching. In the texts that have been accepted, on the basis of content and style, to be the work of a single authority, the concepts incorporating the humors are linked also to the seasons, at least partly to explain seasonal differences in the incidence of illnesses. The linkages became those of spring-air-blood, summer-fire-yellow bile, autumn-earth-black bile, and winter-water-phlegm. Medical historians love to harvest the earliest descriptions of their disease-of-interest, however tenuous, from ancient writings, sometimes forgetting that they originate from modern translations of the ancient Ionian dialect. That said, it is clear that Hippocrates understood aspects of breathing and its disorders—In the quotation above, "veins" seems to refer to the bronchi as well blood vessels, and the notion of air being drawn into the body and distributed to the organs would

---

1   in modern German atem= respiration

2

remain until Galen's dissections showed that the vessels contained blood and not air.

The inclusion by the Greeks of the rhythm of the seasons was extended to include the influence of the stars and their position in the sky in ordering effects on the weather and crops, down to the functioning of organs and susceptibility to disease. The interplay between elements and their associated humors was also held to account for what we might nowadays term the psychological type of an individual to explain their behavior. The scheme then can be seen, at a distance of over two millennia as a determined effort to understand the nature of Nature and of "natural laws". It resonates with the recent emphasis on "holistic" approaches to medicine, the cosmic consciousness and the perpetual struggle to understand the unknown—and, to a certain extent, the unknowable.

Among the Greek philosophers, Aristotle's influence was huge, not only because of his own work in embryology and in the classification of animals and plants but also because he was tutor to Alexander the Great. We may guess that his influence led to the establishment in the third century BCE of the Alexandrian school of learning and science, and a medical school, which flourished for three centuries. The Alexandrians began to think in terms of anatomy related to function, as a result of the dissection of animal and human bodies. Dissection of human bodies represented a desecration, but the authorities allowed it on the bodies of criminals, alive or dead; these occurred publicly, and probably were more important as a deterrent than in advancing knowledge. However, the approach to dissection was unsystematic and not based on any clear hypotheses related to function. Drawings dating well into the 13th century CE depict organs

that are misshapen and out of place, and blood vessels and nerves that run bizarre courses.

GALEN

In the second century CE there appeared on the scene a giant figure whose teachings influenced understanding about breathing for longer than anyone else, before or since. Claudius Galen was born in 129 CE in Pergamum, a Greek city on the eastern Aegean coast, now part of Turkey. The Roman Empire was at its most powerful, and Galen traveled widely through it after his initial medical studies, achieving a considerable reputation as a physician to the gladiators. His acute observations of the effects of their injuries allowed him to infer the function of nerves, including the nerves of breathing, and to observe the beating heart and pulsating arteries. He moved to Rome, becoming the physician to the Emperor Marcus Aurelius and the most revered medical teacher in the Empire. He wrote copiously—well over two hundred books have been recognized, and over 80 remain available and have been translated. His translators have been impressed not only by his knowledge but also his apparent arrogance. He believed he knew how and why the organs of the body worked, and each was perfectly designed by God to fulfill its function. He experimented extensively on animals, but mainly to support his theories. Having observed that some gladiators with high neck wounds stopped breathing whilst those with wounds lower in the neck continued to breathe in spite of being paralyzed elsewhere, he correctly inferred the function of the phrenic nerve (a long nerve that travels from the neck down the back of the chest cavity) in controlling the action of the diaphragm. He performed experiments on a newborn litter of pigs, to show that cutting the spinal cord at the level of the second vertebra in the neck stopped breathing, and at the sixth vertebra led to loss of chest

3

movement with preservation of diaphragmatic breathing, thus demonstrating the two muscle groups that drive breathing.

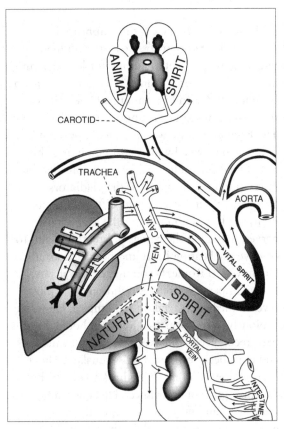

Figure 2 Charles Singer's representation of Galen's view of the lungs and circulation.

Galen's scheme to explain the function of breathing involved three spirits, or "pneuma"—tellingly, the word means "breath" as well as "spirit". The interaction between the three served to maintain all bodily functions. Thus, the most basic pneuma, the "natural spirit", maintained nutrition and growth, and was placed in the liver, receiving nutrition from the gut and distributing it to the body via the right ventricle of the heart. The second pneuma was the "vital spirit", concerned with movement, courage and body heat, was brought in with the air inspired in the lungs, combining with blood in the left heart and supplied to the body via the arteries. Galen was clearly impressed by the considerable force exerted by the beating left ventricle of the heart; blood was pumped into the arteries during contraction, and then flowed back when the heart relaxed; the same process occurred in the veins and right ventricle. The heart's important action was to expand, to draw the pneuma and blood into the ventricle, rather like a valveless bellows which is expanded forcibly before being evacuated; as we all know, this is the opposite action that we recognize now, with contraction (systole) forcing blood into the arteries, followed by relaxation (diastole).The movement of air and blood was conceived as occurring in waves ebbing and flowing. Galen was unable to conceive of the circulation; this crucial concept was to wait for nearly 1500 years, when Harvey performed his experiments and made his imaginative leap. In spite of proposing separate functions for the two ventricles, Galen postulated a connection between the two to "transfer blood and spirit equally from each other by invisible and very small passages". Although he recognized the importance of the valve between the right ventricle and the pulmonary artery leading into the lungs, he misinterpreted its function in trying to explain how these invisible passages worked; thus, "If the mouth of the pulmonary artery always stayed open and Nature had no way of closing it when necessary or of opening it again, the blood could not transfuse through these invisible and delicate pores". Galen's views on physiology remain much more impressive to neurologists than cardiologists and respirologists; his observations on the effects of injuries and experimental section of the spinal cord and nerves allowed him to correctly infer their main functions, whereas his notions on the function of blood, heart and lungs seems ludicrous. Before deriding his scheme,

4

perhaps a reality check would be in order; the medical historian and educator Jacalyn Duffin of Queen's University in Kingston, Canada, suggests to her students that they carry out a thought experiment. "Limit yourself to what Galen knew and the methods of investigation available to him. Then try to refute his theory".

Galen was tied to Greek philosophy, in which all earthly beings and happenings were controlled by outside deities through changes in the four elements. Because the gods are all powerful, this leads naturally to the concept of perfection in all things they create. Galen was obsessed with this thought; all his experiments and observations are used to prove that the body's organs all have a unique function and each is perfectly constructed in order to meet its function. Also, Galen was limited to the available means of investigation of the time—animal dissection and vivisection, and limited dissection of the human body, no means of magnification or measurement of even simple physical properties. Although length, weight, pressure and heat could be perceived, no measurements were available that might have been applied to the study of organ function.

Galen died in 199 CE, and a hundred years later Constantine became Emperor; believing that he owed his many victories to a single Christian God he issued the Edict of Milan, mandating toleration of all Christians and eventually leading to the Holy Roman Empire. Galen's teachings had a special appeal to the early Christian hierarchy, and were adopted as the authoritative texts for medical education for centuries. Charles Singer has pointed out that this was in spite of Galen having little respect for Christianity and rejecting any notion of miracles, saying that God always "works by law, and that it is just for this reason that Natural Law reveals Him". Although Galen's creed was essentially pagan, his monotheistic approach could be incorporated into that of the Christian Church.

The development of a scientific understanding of breathing yields evidence for the aphorism "Steady progress over centuries is not the habit of the human genius". Following Galen, there was remarkably little new understanding for many centuries; this was a period of Scholasticism, when everything that can be known was known, and because all earthly activity was under the control of God, there was no need for original investigation, and certainly no need for dissection. The soul of man belonged to God; the body was corruptible and unworthy of study. Any advance in knowledge was achieved by the application of logic to irrefutable axioms; for the first 1500 years CE, Galen's views were the axioms of physiology. The mood was "anti-scientific", and led, for example to the sack of Alexandria with destruction of the great library there at the end of the fourth century. It was a period in which the Church held all the trump cards, and anyone who questioned religious dogma or advocated scientific investigation of Church-supported beliefs, was almost certain to incur incredible penalties. Roger Bacon (1214-1294) was imprisoned by the Church for 13 years for his scientific ideas, and Galileo was made to recant his ideas about planetary movements, as late as the sixteenth century.

THE RENAISSANCE

In the early Middle Ages, Arabic scholars flourished, and intellectual leadership was taken on by Arabic speaking scholars in the second half of the first millennium CE. They translated the Greek texts and Galen's works, and they traveled to Spain and the kingdom of Sicily to spread their knowledge ever closer to the Roman Empire; their influence can be traced to the teachers at the first medical school at Salerno, just south of Naples. Although Arabic writers were influential, their understanding of the physiology and anatomy of breathing remained based in Galen. Some criticized Galen; Ibn an-Nafis of Damascus wrote in about 1250 that Galen's invisible connections between the right and left ventricle did not exist, that blood was heated and refined in the right ventricle and then passed into the lungs; a small part of the blood then passed into the pulmonary vein and left ventricle where it was mixed with air to produce vital spirit. Thus, he was close to divining the lung circulation, but his ideas were lost; his writings were discovered by an Egyptian physician in 1924.

The High Middle Ages saw a reduction in the church's influence, together with the artistic and cultural activity of the Renaissance, and the founding of Universities in the twelfth (Paris, Bologna, Oxford and Montpelier) and thirteenth centuries (Cambridge, Padua and Naples). The cultural and social importance of science was gaining sway; the investigation of causes of death led to a gradual lifting of prohibitions against dissection. The result was a great increase in the quality of anatomical teaching, beginning with the Bolognese scholar Mondino, working in the Salerno medical school and in Bologna (he authored *The Anothomia* of 1316). Many Renaissance artists began dissecting the human body; the drawings of Leonardo in the latter half of the 15th century represent a great advance in the accuracy of anatomical drawing. It seems likely that the "Reformer of Anatomy" Vesalius (1514-64) recognized the importance of professional artistry, for his 1543 masterpiece *De Humani Corporis Fabrica* (On the Fabric of the Human Body) is exquisitely illustrated by woodcuts that used Leonardo's technique. Although a work on anatomy and keeping to the Galenic tradition, Vesalius clearly had

problems with the physiological implications of his careful studies of the heart. Not finding any possible passages through the very muscular septum between the two ventricles, he questioned God's wisdom in causing blood to "sweat" through invisible pores. Vesalius was born in Brussels and had a peripatetic student life, ending at the University of Padua, where he graduated in Medicine and was immediately appointed professor of Anatomy at the age of 23. He fell foul of several establishment figures in Medicine, both for his criticisms of Galen and for his questioning of God's wisdom. However, his influence on the "young Turks" of the age, such as Servetus and Harvey, was immense. The time for a paradigm shift had arrived; the year in which the *Fabrica* was published, 1543, coincided with the publication of *The Revolution of the Heavenly Orbits* by Nicolas Copernicus, in which Ptolomeic astronomy was comprehensively dismantled, marking the beginning of the Scientific Revolution.

Vesalius' book, completed when he was only 28, was one of the first textbooks to be printed with the new mechanical printing process, ensuring a widespread distribution and numerous re-printings that continued well into the 18th century. Coming to the lungs, he described the air passages and noted that the lungs collapsed when the chest cavity was opened; in a dog, he removed a rib without damaging the pleural membrane that lines the inner surface of the chest wall, so that he could observe the expansion of the underlying lung. Although a lack of magnification kept him from correctly inferring the function of the lung circulation, it seems likely that Harvey, arriving in Padua some years later, was influenced both by the anatomical detail and the results of the experiments, in developing his ideas for investigating the form and purpose of the body's blood flow.

The next step was taken by Michael Servetus, who was born Miguel Serveto, in Spain at Villanova di Xixena—at times he used the pseudonym Michael Villanovanus, in the vain hope that his seditious tracts would not be ascribed to him. Working in Paris in the 1530s, he was helped by Vesalius in demonstrating dissections at the medical school. He was an intellectual giant, publishing works on theology, geography, medicine and astrology, but as a thinker he was more radical than might be thought prudent. His greatest work, containing the first description of the pulmonary circulation, was titled *Christianismi Restituto*, or "Christianity Restored", and contained *De Trinitatis Erroribus*, or "On the Errors of the Trinity", in which he portrayed the history of Jesus as superior to the Church's dogma regarding the Holy Trinity. It seems that he hoped to restore Christianity to its simpler beginnings. He has been seen as the founder of the Unitarian Church, but was denounced by Calvin, captured and tried in April 1553. He escaped from prison, but was foolhardy enough as to visit Geneva, Calvin's stronghold, in August. Ironically he was recognized during his obligatory attendance at Church on Sunday, and immediately arrested. Sentenced to death on October 27th he was promptly burnt at the stake, together with as many copies of his book as could be found.

One of the five surviving copies of Servetus' book is held by the library of the Royal College of Physicians in London. In 1964, as I was writing my thesis on pulmonary gas exchange for the postgraduate MD degree I was able to hold in my hands a book that someone must have hidden away 500 years before, in defiance of the Church's judgment on Servetus' theology. Calling on my rudimentary high school Latin I translated page 170—"Therefore the communication is not through the centre of the heart, as is commonly thought, but by an elaborate device the blood is driven from the right heart ventricle through the pulmonary duct; in a long course through the lungs the blood is mixed and made yellow and passes into the vein…the mixture of air and blood suitable for the formation of the vital spirit is drawn onward to the left ventricle of the heart by diastole". A strange and sad footnote to the life of Servetus is that during the 1941 occupation, the Germans ordered the destruction of a beautiful statue to Servetus in Annemasse, a few miles from Geneva.

THE EARLY ITALIAN UNIVERSITIES

In the years following Servetus' account, there appeared several publications that have been held to describe the circulation, but the consensus is that its full physiological implications were not realized until Harvey published *de Motu Cordis* in 1628.

William Harvey was born in Folkestone on the coast of the English Channel in 1578, and entered Cambridge in 1593 on a scholarship that stipulated he was "to study subjects pertinent to Medicine" . He graduated BA in 1597, and in 1598 enrolled in the faculty of medicine in Padua as a pupil of the great anatomist Fabricius. Fabricius had previously organized the building of the first anatomical theatre, a wooden structure with steep sides, that allowed students to stand on an elevated series of narrow balconies and view the dissection below; the pit of the theatre was accessible through a concealed door, through which the cadaver was brought, or rapidly removed if necessary. Fabricius had made a study of the valves in the veins of the leg, although their function had to await Harvey's demonstration. Also in Padua at the time was Galileo, who taught physics and mathematics

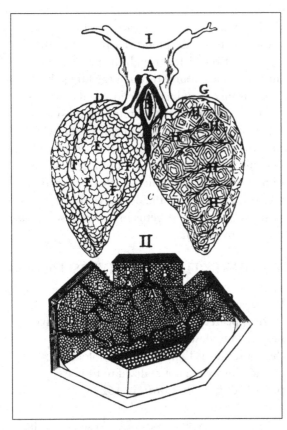

Figure 3 Lung structure shown in Malpighi's *De Pulmonibus*

the beat of the heart." With commendable restraint he did not publish his theory of the circulation until 12 years later, when his great work *Exercitatio Anatomica de Motu Cordis et Sanguinis in Animalibus* (An anatomical dissertation on the movement of the heart and blood in animals) was printed in Frankfurt. The book described physiological experiments in humans and dogs, and applied mathematical logic to the measurements. Some evidence of the circulation had been present for centuries; venous blood flow was stopped by a bandage to the upper arm before blood-letting, and a tight ligature applied to stop arterial flow before amputation. Harvey, with a series of simple studies of the perceived flow in veins and the action of their valves (illustrating the studies with a figure from a book by his teacher Fabricius), and of the arterial pulse, made the imaginative leap to "confirm that the blood passes through the lungs and heart by the force of the ventricles, and is driven thence and sent forth to all parts of the body. There it makes its way into the veins and pores of the flesh…then from the lesser to the greater veins…and finally into the right auricle of the heart."

Understanding the function of the valves that Fabricius had demonstrated in veins, he realized that blood did not ebb and flow in the arteries and veins, but went in one direction only. He estimated the capacity of the left ventricle at two ounces; with a pulse rate of 72 times in a minute, the left ventricle would throw into the aorta the equivalent of three times the body weight of a heavy man every hour. The blood flows "in such quantity, in one direction, by the arteries, and in the other direction by the veins, as cannot possibly be sullied by the ingested food. It is therefore necessary to conclude the blood in the animals is impelled in a circle, and is in a state of ceaseless movement". Here we have a monumental advance in thinking applied to organ function; it was made without Harvey

and had already shown the importance of measurements of mass, distance, time (with a pendulum) and heat (with an early thermometer). Harvey clearly took the new scientific concepts and measurements on board, applying them to a study of blood flow; after graduating in Medicine in 1602 he left Padua to settle in London, later being appointed physician at St. Bartholomew's Hospital. In his lecture notes of 1616 appears the following, "It is plain from the structure of the heart that the blood is passed continuously through the lungs to the aorta as by two clacks of a water bellows to raise water. It is shown by the application of a ligature that the passage of the blood is constantly in a circle, and is brought about by being able to see the connections between arteries and veins either in the lungs or body tissues, and without an understanding of metabolism or gas exchange; he realizes that he has not explained the function of the lungs and their blood flow, whether to cool blood or transfer vital spirit into the body, and still feels it necessary to acknowledge a debt to "Galen, that divine man, the Father of Physicians". Later, in various places in his writing he notes "life and respiration are convertible terms, for there is no life without breathing, and no breathing without life", and linking breathing to combustion—"air is necessary to a candle and to fire". However, Harvey did as much to demolish the Galenic view of breathing, as Galileo did in refuting Aristotelian astronomy.

The microscope was invented around 1600 and underwent gradual development by Galileo and others, coming into use in Italy around 1625. In the late 1650s Marcello Malpighi became Professor of Theoretical Medicine in Pisa, becoming great friends with Giovanni Borelli, who held the chair of Mathematics there. They worked together to make the University of Pisa a centre of natural sciences, parting when Borelli returned to his alma mater in Messina. The two corresponded, and in 1662 Malpighi wrote two letters to Borelli (*De pulmonibus*) in which he described the microscopic appearances of the air sacs and capillaries in the lung, terming the arrangement "una rete mirabilis" (a wonderful network). He described the bronchial air passages dividing and progressively subdividing to end in "an almost infinite number of vesicles full of air". We know now that "almost infinite" amounts to some 300 million alveoli in the human lung. His technique of inflation and drying remains to this day the standard method of preparing lungs in order to observe alveolar structure. In his second letter he describes studies of the blood flowing through the lungs of a living frog with each heart beat in tiny vessels coursing among the "vesicles" (alveoli). Later he described the movement of "globules of fat, of a definite outline, reddish in colour…a likeness to a rosary of red coral"; these globules were the red blood corpuscles, actually already described by the Dutch microscopist Johannes van Swammerdam, and later accurately measured by Anthon Leeuwenhoek in 1674. The latter reported his observations in a letter to the Royal Society in London, reflecting a new trend in publishing science; Malpighi also sent many such letters, benefiting from editorial review and peer comments, as well as getting others to pay for publication.

THE "OXFORD GROUP"

Although it appears that Italian academics in the 17th century moved around almost as much as those in the USA today, in that time Padua was the centre of new ideas in breathing. Harvey reaped the benefit of the anatomical tradition of Vesalius and Fabricius, appreciated the mathematics and physics of Galileo, and probably learnt the value of new methods of measurement applied to physiology by Sanctorius, who was also at Padua. But there was resistance towards accepting these new fangled notions "to the movement of the heart [that] was only to be comprehended by God". The University of Paris officially denied the existence of the circulation for more than 50 years following the publication of *de Motu Cordis*. In England, Harvey complained that his clinical practice declined because of his avant-garde views, but one would not have guessed this from his progressive rise up the ranks in the Royal College of Physicians. In 1643 he was nominated by the King (Charles 1), with whom he had developed a close friendship, to the post of Warden at Merton College at Oxford, where he found himself in close contact with five of his

9

most fervent supporters who were themselves observing and experimenting with great enthusiasm. Oxford thus replaced Padua as the center of research into the function of breathing through the second half of the 17th century.

The most senior of the Oxford Group was Thomas Willis, a renowned physician who later became Professor of Natural Philosophy at Christ Church College, Oxford. He was the author of the massive and influential *Practice of Physick* in which "rational pharmaceutics" was advocated, perhaps the forerunner of present day "evidence-based medicine". In this book he showed himself both up-to-date and forward thinking—"it is not for nothing that the Blood-vessels that are anywhere in the Lungs do curiously wait upon those of the air and every where insinuate and intimately mingle themselves". He also realized the problems of breathing at altitude. However, his main research was into the blood vessels of the brain, for which he has since been known for discovering the "Circle of Willis", the main arterial network at the base of the brain. He was helped in his research by Richard Lower, also at Christ Church, who was a highly respected Oxford physician, and the first to demonstrate blood transfusion. Lower identified the lungs as the site of "arterialization" of venous blood. In a letter to Robert Boyle in 1664, Lower writes—"the arterial blood owes its red color to a mixture of air in the lungs and … the venous blood owes its dark color to loss of air during its passage through the body". He was able to show by ligaturing the trachea of a dog that this prevented the change in color, and he also debunked the idea that the heart had anything to do with heat transfer in the body. Lower stoutly defended Harvey—"One perhaps may be surprised at the fact that after Harvey the distinguished Descartes… (is) in doubt if the heart causes its own movement, or if it is not rather put into motion by the blood".

The discipline of chemistry was slowly advancing, but its practitioners had few tools. They described appearances (whether solid, liquid, powder, gas, etc), examined the effects of added water, heat and flame, and recorded changes in colour, touch and taste. The observations were interpreted so as to confirm previous beliefs, and few were able to identify changes that did not fit received wisdom. However, Lower was one of the few to beak this mould. At the time, nitre (potassium nitrate) was already in use in gunpowder and fireworks; it could be burned in the absence of air to yield a gas that supported combustion. Lower had the idea that a similar gas was a constituent of atmospheric air, which he called "spiritus nitro-aereus" or "nitro-aërial particles".

The Anglo-Irish aristocrat Robert Boyle, son of the first Earl of Cork ("a ferocious and successful land-grabber of Elizabethan times") and the acknowledged father of chemistry, was Richard Lower's mentor. With the help of Robert Hooke, the son of a humble curate who was also at Christ Church, and a genius at designing and making chemical and physical apparatus, Boyle ran an experimental laboratory that examined the properties of air. They first investigated its pressure; Galileo was aware that a property of the atmosphere was weight, and his pupil Evangelista Torricelli devised a method of measuring atmospheric pressure. He filled a closed glass tube with mercury and inverted it, placing the open end in a container full of mercury; a space appeared at the upper closed end, since called the Torricellian vacuum. In a letter to Cardinal Michelangelo Ricci in 1644 he reported that the height of the mercury above the level in the container—i.e. the pressure supporting the column of mercury—was "a cubit and a quarter and an inch besides". He realized that there would be objections to the concept of a vacuum "abhorred by Nature", but advanced arguments and other experiments in support of his theory, and concluded "we live at the bottom of an ocean of air". Atmospheric pressure has since then been measured in terms of millimeters of mercury (mm Hg or, by the classicists, Torr).

Boyle and Hooke devised apparatus to extend Torricelli's observations, and showed that sound was not transmitted and a flame was extinguished in a vacuum; Boyle derived his Law from the measurements they made.[2] They found that a mouse was unable to live in a chamber in which wood had been burnt, or another animal had breathed, showing that some part of air was essential for both life and combustion.[3]
Also, using their vacuum pump, they showed that a gas was released from blood.

John Mayow was perhaps the most precocious of the Oxford group; at the age of 25 he published the results of experiments in his book *de Respiratione* and he died at the age of 35. He measured changes in volume that occurred as a candle burnt out, and a mouse died in closed chambers, and found them to be about the same; also "let any animal (mouse) be enclosed in a glass vessel along with a lamp (candle)…we shall soon see the lamp go out and the animal will not

long survive the fatal torch", because "the air…is in part deprived of its nitro-aerial particles"; finally "by the breathing of animals, is reduced in volume by 1/14th". In hindsight, we can say that Mayow showed that only part of the air was required for combustion and life, and that part, called by him "nitro-aerial" we now call oxygen; also, that he was lucky. I say this because in combustion, the same volume of carbon dioxide is produced as the oxygen used—the total volume should be the same, yet he measured a 7% reduction. The reason may have been a reduction in temperature when the candle went out, with a fall in water vapour and absorption of carbon dioxide by the water in the chamber. He did not recognize that carbon dioxide was produced by combustion and living processes.

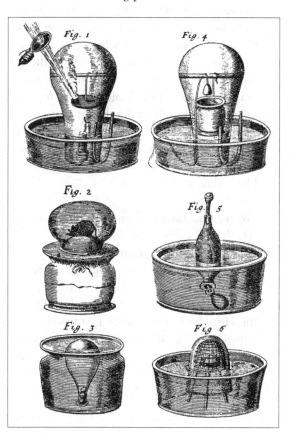

Figure 4 John Mayow's experiments

2   Boyle's Law states that for a gas at constant temperature the product of pressure and volume is a constant; a doubling of pressure leads to a halving of volume, etc. The implications for breathing at altitude and depth are obvious, and many physiological measurements use the equation to standardize for changes in atmospheric pressure.

3   This observation had been made by Leonardo da Vinci 200 years before, but forgotten.

PRESSURE

This may be as good a place as any to deal with the vexing question of pressure which features in many sections of the book. It's vexing, or confusing, because many different units are used in its measurement. There have been attempts to standardize to a single unit, the Pascal (Pa), defined as the pressure exerted by a force equal to 1 Newton acting on an area of 1 square meter; 1000 Pa is termed a kilopascal (kPa). However, it is difficult to get scientists to change their habits. Different units continue to be used by convention, largely because of the different methods by which pressure has been measured, or because the size of the numbers can become cumbersome. Pressure may be important in absolute terms, for instance at altitude or depth, but more often it is pressure differences that are being measured, acting to move gases and liquids in the body in such functions as breathing, blood flow and diffusion.

We are surrounded by ambient pressure which varies with altitude, weather conditions, and temperature. Usually measured with a mercury (Hg) barometer in millimeters, thus mmHg (= 133.2 Pa). The standard pressure at sea-level is 760 mmHg .This is also termed 1 Atmosphere (Atm), a unit used in diving and to measure the amount of gas in a cylinder, because the numbers can be astronomical in any other unit (1 A = 101.32 kPa).

Blood pressure is measured in mmHg above ambient. An arterial pressure of 100 mmHg, would be 860 mmHg in absolute terms, but what is important is the pressure relative to ambient pressure, sometimes termed gauge pressure.

The pressure of respired gases such as oxygen is measured in mmHg, and usually termed a "partial" pressure. "Partial" refers to the effective pressure exerted by the gas alone. For example oxygen constitutes 20.93% of dry air, and thus exerts a pressure of 760 x 0.2093= 160 mmHg (21.3 kPa). This unit is also used for gas pressure (eg. O_2 and CO_2) in blood.

Because it's difficult (and dangerous) to measure air pressure in the lungs with mercury, a water filled manometer was used for the purpose, and even though electronic pressure transducers are used now, the unit remains the centimeter of water, cm H_2O (= 98.07Pa). The unit usually is not absolute, but relative to atmospheric pressure. For example, the pressure in the thorax during inspiration might be – 10 cmH_2O; in absolute terms this represents the difference between the atmosphere at 980 cm H_2O and in the thorax of 970 cm H_2O. It's the pressure difference that moves air into the lung.

Like Lower, Mayow interpreted his results in terms of "nitro-aërial particles" , which "when introduced into the mass of blood by the action of the lungs…produce a very marked fermentation such as is required for animal life". He felt this theory also accounted for the change in the colour of blood during its passage through the lungs, because of the following experiment—"If spirit of nitre (dilute nitric acid) is poured upon a liquid saturated with volatile salt and sulphur, such as the spirit of hartshorn impregnated with its own oil (a source of ammonium carbonate), a very marked effervescence and a very ruddy scarlet colour will be produced in the liquid, and yet this florid colour changes into a dark purple when the liquid ceases to effervesce".

17TH CENTURY SCIENTIFIC SOCIETIES

The Oxford Group clearly benefited from discussions and interactions; like any successful scientific group, each one of its members seemed to bring his own particular expertise, and together they formed an important part of the fledgling Royal Society. Two earlier scientific societies in Italy (the Accademia dei Lincei in Rome and the Accademia del Cimento in Florence) lasted for only a few decades at the beginning of the 17th century. The Royal Society in London and the Academie Royale des Sciences in Paris, both founded in the 1660s, remain the pre-eminent scientific bodies in their respective countries to this day—there is no greater national accolade than for a scientist to be elected FRS (Fellow of the Royal Society).

The Royal Society probably benefited from the social changes that accompanied the end of the (English) Civil War. Boyle's collaborator, Robert Hooke, left Oxford to become the Royal Society's curator of experiments (Boyle's experimental output in Oxford fell after Hooke left). Hooke drew up the statutes of the Society in 1663—what today would be termed its Mission Statement. Its "business…is to improve the knowledge of natural things, and all useful Arts, Manufactures, Mechanick practices, Engynes and Inventions by Experiment—(not meddling with Divinity, Metaphysics, Morals, Politics, Grammar, Rhetorick, or Logicks)". Rules were set regarding the form and length of oral presentations at the Society's meetings, setting a tradition that is maintained to this day. Although established under Royal Charter, the Society received no funds from King or State; members were charged a shilling per week. Their ideals were lofty, but possibly because of them the intellectual snobs of the day were very critical—they were lampooned in *Gulliver's Travels*. Hooke went from strength to strength, showing himself to have few equals, before or since, in experimental physiology. Notably he showed that the act of breathing was not necessary for blood to be arterialized in the lungs, as long as they were supplied with fresh air. He showed an acute perception of combustion—"it is made by a substance inherent, and mixt with the Air". In spite of his achievements, his ideas did not catch on; it seems that he was so in advance of his time that most of his fellow scientists were unable to grasp and profit from them. Also he made an implacable enemy of Isaac Newton, who refused the presidency of the Royal Society while Hooke remained a Fellow.

It remains a puzzle that these brilliant thinkers, all working on more or less the same topic and in close contact with one another, could not take the next step. There was a long hiatus— almost 100 years—during which little advance was made. Perhaps it was due to the fact that by 1703 they were all dead, but also they were unable to devise a testable concept and their analytical methods were too primitive. Boyle

13

himself realized that although the evidence suggested that there were particles in the air that were necessary for life, there was no "positive proof of ... a volatile nitre abounding in the air"; in fact he wrote an essay with the sad title *"On the Unsuccessfulness of Experiments"*. It was not until Joseph Black had exploded the "phlogiston" theory in 1754, that the next real advance was made.

THE "PHLOGISTON THEORY" OF COMBUSTION

New concepts in medical science not infrequently set the subject back, at least for a time. Why the eminent chemist, and Physician to the King of Prussia, Georg Ernst Stahl in 1684 elaborated the phlogiston theory of combustion and breathing, instead of developing a chemical theory consistent with the previous advances, will presumably never be known. He held that heat produced in the body was purely frictional, as the blood passed through the small vessels, and the chest movements were required merely to move the blood. He wrote "It is wholly clear", "it is quite evident", that nothing is added to the blood as it comes into contact with air in the lungs. He argued that "phlogiston" (from the Greek word for inflammable) was something that all combustible substances contained. When the substance was burned, the phlogiston was released into the air, but in such small quantities that it could not be detected, leaving the dephlogisticated ashes behind. Of course, this theory implies that loss of phlogiston should be accompanied by a fall in weight, whereas Boyle had shown that metals gain weight when subjected to very high temperatures; Stahl explained this away by stating that phlogiston was replaced by a hypothetical "heat substance" that had negative weight.

Carl Wilhelm Scheele was born (1742) in Pomerania, a part of Sweden that shifted from time to time between that country and Germany; his native tongue was German. He grew up in a poor family, but was very bright and as a teenager became apprenticed to a pharmacist in Gothenburg. He read widely in Chemistry, and repeated many classic experiments by devising his own equipment and making careful measurements. He produced oxygen in several ways, including heating mercuric oxide and potassium nitrate, and observed that a candle burnt more brightly and for longer than in the same volume of air. In 1774 he wrote to Lavoisier, asking him to subject silver carbonate to heating with a burning glass (Scheele could not afford one). Scheele predicted that two gases would be produced—one that could be absorbed by lime water (which was carbon dioxide) to leave dephlogisticated air (later named oxygen)—"I would be infinitely obliged if you would know the result of this experiment"—he ended. A few years later, in 1777, he published his main work, Über Luft und Feuer, in which he interpreted his results in terms of phlogiston, proposing that both fire and light were due to the combination of phlogiston and dephlogisticated air. Scheele declined many offers of academic positions, remaining a small-town pharmacist, and dying of tuberculosis at the age of 44.[4]

The Phlogiston Theory is now seen as an aberration in the development of theories regarding breathing and combustion, but at the time it afforded plausible explanations of these processes, of the refinement of metals from their ores, and of the action of acids.

---

4 In his short life, Scheele was extraordinarily productive: In addition to oxygen, he discovered many organic acids, including lactic acid, and three elements—manganese, barium and chlorine.

Although it assumed questionable concepts such as negative weight, we need to remember that this was the age of alchemy. Its basis is similar to the concepts of "pneuma" and "vital spirit" of centuries before: phlogiston was the principle inherent in Fire, still considered one of the elements. Although mentioned briefly above, for the sake of our story it is worth elaborating the concept a little more, if only to clarify how it was finally rejected. Thus, materials that burned in air were held to be rich in phlogiston, and gave up their phlogiston to air during burning; similarly venous blood contained phlogiston which was expelled to air during breathing, as air became more and more phlogisticated it lost its capacity to support life and combustion. The explanation for the effects of burning a metallic ore to obtain the metal can be expressed in the following reaction—

Metallic ore (calx) + Phlogiston in Charcoal → Metal + Fixed Air

Similarly, the process of calcination can be expressed by—

Metal + Air → Calx + Phlogiston

Interestingly, the reaction which led eventually to the overthrow of the theory, was the production of mercury from its red oxide, an unusual reaction since it occurs at very high temperature without the need for charcoal (carbon)

Red oxide (calx) + Air → Mercury - Phlogiston

—the end result being the production of "dephlogisticated" air.

The Scotsman Joseph Black was born in Bordeaux in 1728 and entered the medical school at Glasgow University at the age of 16. He became so fascinated by chemistry that his final year thesis was on a chemical topic—*De Humere Acido a Cibis Orto et Magnesia Alba*. It was presented to the Edinburgh faculty on the 11th June, 1754, and published two years later (*Experiments upon Magnesia alba, Quicklime and some other Alkaline Substances*). It made his reputation, and gained him an academic appointment at Glasgow; he was Professor of Chemistry there and later at Edinburgh for more than 40 years. In some of his most important experiments he showed that chalk lost weight and gave off a gas when incinerated, and by passing it through lime water, showed that the same gas was given off when any mild alkaline carbonate was treated with hydrochloric acid. He also showed that the same gas was present in expired air, and he termed the gas "fixed air". We know it as carbon dioxide. By careful weighing Black showed that gains and losses in weight accompanying burning or acid treatment were the opposite to those predicted by the phlogiston concept.

PRIESTLEY, SCHEELE AND LAVOISIER; OXYGEN

The discovery of oxygen has from time to time been a contentious issue, with the contenders being Priestley, Scheele and Lavoisier. However, both Priestley and Scheele were so bound to the phlogiston theory, that they could only interpret their experimental results in its terms; it was left to Lavoisier to repeat their work and name the "dephlogisticated air" they had found, "oxygen" (from the Greek for "acid forming"). Both Priestley and Lavoisier prepared oxygen at about the same time by subjecting red oxide of mercury to intense heat; this compound had been known to ancient alchemists as a source of quicksilver (mercury).

Joseph Priestley was born in 1733, in Yorkshire of devout parents, and graduated from a clerical college to become a non-conformist minister. He gave poor sermons and his religious views did not meet with the approval of all his parishioners; this, and the fact that he had learnt several languages, led to him taking a position as a languages teacher at Warrington Academy. He attended meetings of the Royal Society and after writing a book on the history of electricity was made a Fellow, even though he had no scientific training or experience. The lure of a better salary led to him becoming a minister of a free church in Leeds, and he moved to a house near a local brewery. The large amounts of Black's "fixed air" produced during the brewing process provided the intellectual motivation to get involved in experimentation. Thus he was free of preconceived notions, but had to develop his own apparatus and experimental approaches. He persuaded the brewers to let him experiment in their vats; he found the "fixed air" to lie in a layer about a foot deep above the liquor; it was clearly heavier than air; candles went out in it, and mice died; if he poured water from one glass to another in it, the water became filled with bubbles and tasted nice—he had invented soda water! Hoping that it might cure scurvy, he was asked to accompany Captain Cook on a long voyage to the South Pacific. However, because he dissented from the beliefs of the Church of England the invitation was withdrawn. Soda water, although found to be a pleasant drink, proved inferior to "sweetwort and cabbage preserved in vinegar" as a preventive for scurvy. Another job change saw him become librarian to Lord Shelburne, which gave him more time to pursue his experiments. In 1774 he published his results in the acclaimed *Experiments and Observations on Different Kinds of Air*, revealing himself to be a brilliant scientist and thinker, as well as an engaging writer. Priestley used a burning glass to convert mercuric oxide

to mercury and oxygen; by careful weighing he showed that there was a loss in weight associated with the production of the gas, in which a flame burned very brightly and a mouse survived twice as long as in air. He breathed it himself—" I fancied that my breath felt peculiarly light"—and foresaw that it held promise medically. He notes "Who can tell but that, in time, this pure air may become a fashionable article in luxury. Hitherto only two mice and myself have had the privilege of breathing it". Initially he misinterpreted the results of his experiments, believing that the evolved gas was "nitrous air" which he had produced a few years before; this gas, known nowadays as "laughing gas" or nitrous oxide, has the property of supporting combustion and life. Priestley used the reduction in volume when it was mixed with air, as a test of air quality—the "nitrous air test"; the idea behind this test was clearly linked to the "nitro-aërial particles" of Lower and Mayow a century before.

When applying the nitrous air test to the gas produced from the burning of mercuric oxide he was misled by a small difference in volume change during the reaction. However, in a communication to Royal Society in the Spring of 1775, he describes how he reflected on the difference "upon my pillow" leading the next morning to additional experiments that confirmed the fact that he had "procured air…between five and six times as good as the best common air that I have ever met with". He found that "dephlogisticated air" (that supported combustion) could be reformed from the "fixed air" (which did not), by placing a sprig of mint in it. The "mouse and candle tests" showed that that combustion and life could be continued, whereas both the candle went out and the mouse died when placed in "fixed air". In this way Priestley had stumbled on photosynthesis by plants. In 1776 he published

"*Observations on Respiration*" in which he related changes in the colour of blood to the composition of the gas it was mixed with. He wrote "the brightest red blood became perfectly black in any kind of air that was unfit for respiration, as in fixed air, inflammable air, nitrous air, or phlogisticated air; and after becoming black in the last of these kinds of air, it regained its red colour upon again being exposed to common air, or dephlogisticated air".

Priestley gained many honors, including several from France that he had to decline for political reasons. Also, his religious views and his support of the French revolutionaries prevented him gaining advancement in England, even leading a mob in Birmingham to burn his house. Finally, in 1794, because of the continuing war between Britain and France he and his family left to settle in Pennsylvania. While they escaped to America, Lavoisier was executed in Paris.

Antoine Laurent Lavoisier, responsible for a Scientific Revolution at least as important as that of Copernicus, with terrible irony met his fate in the course of the great political Revolution in France. Born in 1743, he showed himself to be an innovative genius when at age 22 he entered a competition, sponsored by l'Academie des Sciences, for a proposal to improve street lighting in Paris. The prize was won by a group of professional engineers, but Lavoisier's plan was so original that the judges awarded him a special medal. Like several other elite scientists before him and since, he was fortunate to have an exceptional research assistant—his wife Marie-Anne Paulze; they married when she was 14. She became an able experimenter, kept meticulous notes, drew diagrams and pictures of the major experiments that showed her to be an accomplished artist, and translated scientific papers from English.

After reading of all Lavoisier's accomplishments and completed projects, one is left to wonder how he was able to carry out the experiments that finally destroyed the phlogiston theory. The experiments made use of the technological improvements in furnaces, glass retorts for heating substances and collecting gases, and in accurate weighing methods. The previous 50 years had also seen improved communication between scientists, with the formation of the major scientific societies and their publications (Proceedings). Lavoisier repeated many of Priestley's and Scheele's experiments, and by 1777 he was able to firmly conclude that the formation of a calx when a metal was heated in air was due to the combination of the metal with a part of the air that he termed "eminently respirable". Further experiments in which he burnt mercury in air led to the conclusion "that atmospheric air is composed of two elastic fluids of different and opposite qualities"—one that supported life and combustion which he called

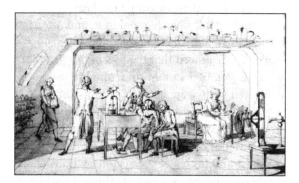

Figure 5 Marie-Ann Lavoisier's sketch of her husband's experiment on gas exchange during exercise - Séguin pedaling a treadle.

oxygen and one that was inert, called "mephitic air" and later azote (in English—nitrogen). He calculated the proportions in air to be 16% oxygen and 84% nitrogen. This erroneous conclusion (dry air contains approximately 21% and 78% respectively) is a reflection of the difficulty in making the measurements and standardizing the conditions, for example, to eliminate water vapour. However, most of the measurements he carried out proved to be extremely precise. With his friend, the renowned physicist and mathematician Pierre-Simon de Laplace , he devised experiments to study changes in weight that occurred during the burning of metals in closed retorts; no change occurred. This finding led to the inference that any increase in the weight of a metal as it changed into its calx was accompanied by an equal reduction in the weight of air in the retort; also he deduced that "matter can neither be created nor destroyed"—known now as the Law of Conservation of Mass. Lavoisier then realized that the loss of oxygen during burning and the increase in weight as a metal turned into the calx, meant that the calx was an oxide. In the case of carbon, the product of burning was the oxide of carbon. Lavoisier and Laplace next constructed a calorimeter; surrounding a closed chamber by ice they measured the heat generated by burning charcoal in it, and after placing small animals (mainly guinea pigs) inside. They showed that the loss of oxygen that accompanied both combustion and life was associated with a similar heat production. Both processes were equivalent in terms of heat production, oxygen consumption and the production of carbon dioxide and water. Lavoisier and his colleague Séguin (who was the subject for the experiment) showed that heat production and oxygen consumption increased during exercise; in their paper *Premier mémoire sur la respiration des animaux* they conclude "In respiration, as in combustion, the atmospheric air supplies the oxygen and the caloric; but since, in respiration it is the substance itself of the animal, the blood which supplies the combustible, if animals were not replacing usually by food what they lose by respiration, the lamp would be short of oil, and the animal

perish, just as the lamp goes out when it lacks nourishment". The link between breathing and the body's metabolism is clear, and enduring; but there is the ghost of phlogiston in "caloric", something associated with life and comparable to the light of a flame. The concept of "caloric" was destined not to survive the work that was to come in the following century, which established the chemical nature of metabolism, and there was also uncertainty regarding where heat production occurred, whether in the lungs, blood or tissues. Nevertheless, the fact remains that Lavoisier had accomplished a paradigm shift and revolutionized chemistry completely. Gone were the old, largely meaningless chemical names, that could now be replaced by constituent elements; for example, "calx" was replaced by "oxide". Many scientists—including Priestley—held on to the phlogiston concept; in his case, one has to wonder whether sour grapes were the reason, because it seems likely that he felt Lavoisier gave him too little credit. After all, he had come to Paris to tell him of his experiments with mercuric oxide (just as Scheele had sent him a letter suggesting a crucial experiment), and had pointed out a flaw in Lavoisier's reasoning in his initial presentation to l'Academie at Easter 1775 (the "Easter Memoir"). The correction was made in November, without acknowledgement.

Someone else who surprisingly held on to phlogiston theory was the Honourable Henry Cavendish, an extremely eccentric, but very productive and wealthy English aristocrat—it was said that he left his house only when he attended meetings of the Royal Society. His most brilliant idea became the germ of what would become the Periodic Table; the germ was the concept of *equivalence*. He measured how much hydrogen was produced by the action of acids on different metals. For example 24 parts of iron, compared to 28 of zinc and 50 of

18

tin evolved one part of hydrogen; the numbers compare to the respective atomic weights of 26, 30 and 50 of more modern times. The eminent psychiatrist Oliver Sacks recommends the biography of Cavendish written by George Wilson in 1851, commenting "it may be the fullest account we are ever likely to have of the life and mind of an autistic genius."

The first paper Cavendish gave to the Royal Society, in 1766, was entitled "*On Factitious Air*". By factitious he meant manufactured; he had made an inflammable gas by the action of strong acids on metals; he called it "inflammable air", and a few years later Lavoisier renamed it hydrogen (in Greek—water maker). Cavendish went on to show that the only product of the reaction between "inflammable air" and "dephlogisticated air" was water, and by careful adjustment of the combining volumes, showed their proportions to be two to one (i.e. he had "discovered" H_2O). To maintain the phlogiston theory, it had to be modified so that—

Water = dephlogisticated air + phlogiston

because nothing else was produced.

Lavoisier saw things differently; he repeated Cavendish's experiments and concluded that water was the oxide of hydrogen. Thus was the phlogiston theory finally laid to rest, and chemistry set on a new course; Lavoisier had firmly established the dominant role of oxygen in all of the processes critical to life, although where the body's combustive processes took place remained to be established. The new direction he identified had been signposted by his predecessors, of whom Boyle (with Hooke, Lower and Mayow), Black, Priestley and Scheele, and Cavendish were the foremost. All deserved Nobel prizes, whose foundation was to await another century.

Lavoisier's tragic death was related to his "day job": he was a farmer-general, one of a group (Ferme Générale) who paid a fee that allowed it to collect taxes. Although there was no evidence that he profited unduly, the revolutionary Convention decided in 1793 that all those that had signed the most recent contract with the old government should be tried. In spite of his achievements and reputation he was arrested and tried by a revolutionary tribunal on May 8, 1794. No one in power spoke for him and he was found guilty, together with 27 others, including his father-in-law, of conspiring with the enemies of France. Execution by guillotine took place the same day in the Place de la Révolution (now Concorde)' and his friend and first biographer Joseph Lagrande observed that it "took but a moment to cut off that head which a hundred years would be unable to replace". His reputation remained unsullied; his life was celebrated in a glittering ceremony in Paris, less than two years later, and all the leading chemists of the day lauded his achievements, as they still do to this day.

We are now on the threshold of the 19th century and there is one more prodigy that comes on the scene to advance our knowledge of breathing several steps further. Humphry Davy was born in Cornwall and in his teens had already read Lavoisier's book *Traite Elementaire de Chimie* published less than ten years before in 1789. He was taken on as assistant to a local surgeon-apothecary who allowed him to experiment as much as he wished. The result was a paper in Dr Thomas Beddoe's journal *Contributions to Physical and Medical Knowledge, principally from the West of England*. Published in 1797, when Davy was only 19, it described the identification of oxygen and carbon dioxide liberated when blood was subjected to a vacuum pump. Dr Beddoes was interested in the medical uses of oxygen and other gases, going so far as to raise the funds for one of the first institutes that combined medical care with research—the Medical Pneumatic Institute near Bristol in the West of England. Beddoes invited Davy to become its Superintendent of the Laboratory—at the age of 20! It is apparent that he had the hallmarks of an exceptional director of research, comparable to those of two centuries later; he took advantage of new technology and quickly amassed an impressive stack of equipment. He persuaded Dr Beddoes to build a huge electric battery (based on Alessandro Volta's discovery of 1795) in order to study the chemical changes induced in solutions by currents, producing hydrogen and oxygen from water, discovering sodium and potassium, and generating light through incandescence of heated platinum and by producing arcs between rods of carbon. Davy tested many original ideas and was not put off by criticism, which merely led to more experiments or a reinterpretation of data; he asked much of his assistant Michael Faraday: and like all respiratory physiologists of the 20th century, he experimented on himself and his friends. In common with a few of (the best!) modern physiological geniuses he was exuberantly enthusiastic, impetuous and constantly treading the knife edge between safety and danger.

20

Davy purified nitrous oxide and tested its effects—Joseph Priestley and Samuel Taylor Coleridge were subjects in the project—demonstrating its intoxicating properties, and predicting that "as nitrous oxide…appears capable of destroying physical pain, it may probably be used with advantage during surgical operations"' though it would be almost 50 years before this suggestion was acted upon. In 1800 Davy published *Researches, Chemical and Philosophical, chiefly concerning Nitrous Oxide, or Dephlogisticated Nitrous Air, and its Respiration*, in which these studies

were described. They caused a sensation and established his reputation. In the book is a figure showing a "Mercurial Air-holder and Breathing Machine"; this consisted of a counterbalanced metal bell suspended in a tank of mercury, which could contain a gas and allow measurement of the volume changes as a subject breathed into and from it. This would now be called a spirometer, and the design is strikingly similar to spirometers that I encountered when beginning my training in the 1960's—except that mercury was replaced by water. In one experiment we can see the beginning of pulmonary function measurements; Davy filled the spirometer with hydrogen and "respired 102 cubic inches of hydrogene apparently pure, for rather less than half a minute, making in this time seven quick respirations". H e then analyzed the gas in the bell, and from the dilution of hydrogen was able to calculate the amount of gas remaining in the lungs following a complete expiration

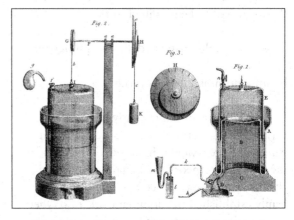

Figure 6 Humphry Davy's "Mercurial air-holder and breathing machine"

(the residual volume), correcting the volume for changes in temperature. This volume was 37.5 cubic inches (614 ml); he realized this seemed rather low, but explained "my chest is narrow, measuring in circumference but 29 inches". Inert gas dilution remains to this day a staple method for measuring residual volume, though it was not used clinically until the 1930s. Among many other inventions was the Miners' Safety Lamp, which used Davy's finding that the heat of a flame could be separated from its light by a cooled wire mesh; as well as giving light, it also provided warning of the two deadly gases encountered by miners—methane or "fire-damp" and carbon dioxide or "choke-damp". Davy was inundated by many awards, including a knighthood at the age of 34, but this marked the end of his productive years. He was extremely popular, and he enjoyed a life outside science; there is some argument regarding the cause of his death in 1829—whether following a long struggle against the ravages of syphilis, or as a result of an incautious number of breaths of his favourite gas, nitrous oxide ("laughing gas"). He may have been the first frequent user of this intoxicant, but was certainly not the last; generations of anesthetists ("just testing!"), and impecunious medical students (dropping in to the delivery wards when no one was around), have enjoyed its rapid inebriating hit.

Although the details remained to be discovered, by the end of the 18th century, it was known that breathing was the inspiration of atmospheric air through the windpipe (trachea) and into a branching system of airways (bronchi), to reach the air sacs (alveoli). Oxygen into entered blood, and carbon dioxide was removed. The process of gas exchange was essential to life and movement, being increased by muscular activity, and ceased with death. The mechanisms linking heat production to the uptake of oxygen were debated extensively through the 18th century, but the most popular theory seems to have been that combustion occurred in the lungs and the heat that was generated warmed the heart, and through the circulation, the rest of the body. It would be many years before respiratory gas exchange became linked to the

chemical reactions of the living body's internal combustion engine. The gradual development of the chemical basis of heat production is the focus for the next chapter.

CHAPTER 2

THE NEED TO BREATHE Combustion equals respiration

"Dans les champs d'observation le hazard ne favorise que les esprits preparés. Where observation is concerned, chance favours only the prepared mind."

Louis Pasteur made his oft-quoted aphorism at the inauguration of the Faculty of Science at the University of Lille, in December, 1854. The 19th century saw a huge increase in our understanding of the essential life-sustaining processes of breathing, which support cellular respiration both by supplying oxygen and removing CO_2. The advances came as part of the scientific revolution, in which experimentation by brilliant thinkers was crucial. The present chapter tracks the path taken in our understanding of the chemical processes that require oxygen and generate CO_2.

By the end of the 18th century, Lavoisier had made his meticulous experiments to demonstrate that the process of combustion was equivalent to the process of respiration in an animal, with loss of oxygen and production of carbon dioxide. He took Priestley's concept regarding the chemical basis of life processes, and placed it on a firmer theoretical basis through measurements of heat, oxygen and carbon dioxide. The living body sustained combustion processes that were equivalent to the combustion occurring in a flame; oxygen is used, heat is liberated and CO_2 is produced. He has justly been described as the "father of quantitative physiology", for his influence can be seen clearly in the work of the physiologists that followed him.

In the 19th through to the 20th century, an acceleration of knowledge regarding the physiology of breathing occurred in two phases—the first related to advances in physics and chemistry that accompanied the Industrial Revolution, and the second gained impetus from two world wars, related to a need to understand what happened at great heights and depths. The story to now has been quite straightforward in terms of individual contributions to understanding, often made by "amateur" or part-time scientists, but the 19th century was a time of great expansion in university-based research, in laboratories that were well equipped with "state of the art" technology, and a proliferation of scientific journals and meetings that immeasurably increased the dissemination of experimental results and discussion between scientists. French and German chemists were initially pre-eminent, but into the 20th century Scandinavian, British and North American scientists were driving forces in physiology. Early on, many philosophical battles were waged between the scientists, who wished to establish a purely mechanical (chemical and physical) basis for biology, and religious leaders who hoped to retain concepts of divine control and design that were outside human comprehension, and expressed in the Old Testament.

Before tracing the development of chemical theories of combustion, we should remember that for a long time there was a great debate about where it took place. Well before there was any understanding of the processes involved in heat production, its linkage to breathing and the action of the heart placed them in the heart and lungs. In the 2nd century Galen asserted that the *spiritus vitalis* resided in the heart, from whence heat was distributed to the rest of the body. This view went virtually unchallenged, partly for reasons of religion, until the end of the 16ᵗʰ century, when Harvey described the circulation. However, the real point of departure from the Galenic view came in the 17ᵗʰ century, with the experimental studies of Boyle and his Oxford colleagues into the constituents of air and the changes that occurred when substances were burnt and animals breathed. Then in the late 18ᵗʰ century, Joseph Priestley carried out a modification of John Mayow's experiments. He found that when a burning candle and a mouse were placed together in an air-filled sealed jar, they died in a shorter time than if they were placed separately in the same jar. Both the candle and the mouse required the same component in air in order to survive. A few years later Lavoisier was to identify the primary role that oxygen played in both combustion and respiration, and usher in the modern era of chemistry.

COMBUSTION—CENTRALLY IN THE LUNGS OR DISTALLY IN THE CELLS OF TISSUES?

The extremely influential German chemist Baron Justus von Liebig, was born in 1803 and began studying chemistry by helping in his father's paint shop in Darmstadt; his academic successes led to his appointment as professor of chemistry in Giessen. There he established a laboratory that soon gained an international reputation; a contemporary print shows it to be crowded with students and visiting scientists. A man of many ideas, he exploited his studies of meat extract, building a huge factory in Uruguay, where 200,000 head of cattle a year were processed into "Liebig's Extract of Meat". When it came to the question of where combustion could be taking place in the body, von Liebig was less farsighted; in his 1842 textbook of physiology, he theorized that because entry of oxygen and

release of carbon dioxide occurred in blood and the lungs, these would also be the sites of chemical combustion. However, a few years before, in 1837, the Berlin chemist and physicist Heinrich Gustav Magnus had made quantitative analyses of the gases released from both arterial and venous blood from horses, when samples were exposed to a Torricellian vacuum. He identified carbon dioxide, oxygen and nitrogen, and showed that all blood contained at least twice as much CO_2 as O_2, and very little nitrogen. He found higher amounts of O_2 and less CO_2 in arterial blood than venous, and argued that chemical combustion therefore had to take place between the two blood compartments, ie. in the tissues. However, because he merely shook blood samples with atmospheric air, and because his methods were relatively crude, many scientists derided this discovery, being unable to conceive that combustion could take place anywhere other than in the lungs. The general realization that chemical reactions took place in the cells of the body tissues had to wait for Pasteur to perform his experiments on fermentation.

Louis Pasteur's biochemical discoveries were as revolutionary as those of his contemporary Darwin in the field of evolution. His father was a tanner in the Jura region of France, who used chemical processes that had evolved practically, without an understanding of their chemical basis. Louis was born in 1822, and struggled through his academic training in chemistry, obtaining his diploma at Besançon in 1842. However, he was determined to make chemistry his career and worked towards his doctorate as a laboratory assistant. His first scientific success came in his mid-twenties when he followed up an observation made previously—that two organic substances, with the same chemical and physical properties, could have different effects on polarized light (stereochemistry), with one form rotating it to the right (dextro-rotatory, d-form) , and the other to the left (laevo-rotatory, l-form)[1]. Equal mixtures of the two forms (racemic mixtures, dl-form) had no effect on polarized light, the one cancelling the other. The chemical that he studied was tartaric acid, a bi-product of wine-making. He found that the crystals of the two forms had slightly different faceting under the microscope, and then observed that a mould contaminating a solution of both forms broke down only the "right-handed" one; the mould was specifically using only this optical form as a growth factor. Pasteur, with his "prepared mind" saw that this meant that the mould was a living organism, capable of complex chemical reactions. Because the effects on polarized light were observed in solutions as well as crystals, they were due to differences in the way the same atoms were arranged in the molecules. The metabolic specificity of the d- and l-forms different carbon compounds is seen also in glucose; although the l-form can be produced chemically, only the d-form can be metabolized by living organisms.

By the early 19th century, France had become a pre-eminent producer of wine, but the methods were based on the experience of the wine-maker. Wine making was more of an art than science, and when something went wrong, as when fermentations went sour, the effects were economically disastrous. One of his students asked Pasteur to investigate his father's failure to produce alcohol from the fermentation of beet sugar. Pasteur first found that failed batches contained lactic acid, in contrast to ethanol in successful brews. Next he examined the sediment under a microscope; whereas successful batches contained living yeast, the failed batches contained none; instead, he found "other globules, much smaller than yeast". He concluded that the two types of fermentation were due to two different living cells, and supported this conclusion by taking minute amounts of the two sediments and showing that the respective chemical reactions also occurred in the laboratory. He felt that the chemical processes of fermentation were linked to the living state of the cell—"all true fermentations are accompanied by the formation, development and increase of living cells". Thus, Pasteur made an imaginative leap to first conclude that living cells had the ability to transform—we would now say metabolize—a variety of organic compounds. The processes were unique to a given organism and essential for their growth and survival.

Baron von Liebig, on the other hand, refused to believe a living cell was required in fermentation processes; furthermore he asserted that he had tried to repeat Pasteur's observations, and had failed to show that fermentation by yeast was always linked to its growth. Thus began one of the more acrimonious of scientific debates. Von Liebig derided Pasteur's vision of "an act of life", favoring his own theory—that ferments (catalysts) speeded up reactions by donating "atomic vibrations".

Pasteur made another experimental observation that is often forgotten, but which predated the findings of others, that metabolic processes in cells were different according to whether oxygen was present. He observed that much less sugar—in fact about 1/20th—was broken down by yeast cells in the presence of oxygen, than when the cells were deprived of the gas. He had discovered the difference between aerobic and anaerobic glucose metabolism, showing that aerobic metabolism is more efficient.

---

1   Many organic molecules exhibit this property, including glucose and lactic acid

CHEMICAL REACTIONS

The main problems facing the early respiratory physiologists were related to the lack of rational conceptual schemes that allowed them to link body processes to the chemical changes associated with combustion, fermentation, heat production, oxygen extraction from the air and carbon dioxide evolution. Lavoisier had made a giant leap by showing that these processes could be dealt with quantitatively, by introducing the concept of elements combining in consistent amounts, and by demonstrating the Law of Conservation of Mass, a chemical balance sheet could be drawn up. Lavoisier demonstrated quantitatively that the process of respiration was the biological equivalent of chemical combustion. Chemicals were "burned" in the body associated with oxygen consumption and the production of carbon dioxide. New concepts were required to explain where the life-giving combustion was taking place; such concepts arose from improvements in microscopy which showed a fine structure unique to each organ, made up of cells. This paved the way to understanding the biology of cellular processes, and thence to the physiological meaning that such processes had to breathing, and to the "holistic" integration between breathing and the processes going on throughout the body. Developments in all these fields went on in parallel, but may best be considered in terms of separate topics, such as metabolism and biochemistry, the carriage of oxygen and carbon dioxide by the circulation, and the structure and function of the lungs.

From the point of view of chemistry, Lavoisier introduced a revolutionary concept when he separated chemical mixtures from compounds—formed by combination between elements in strict proportions. He classified compounds as acids (combination of oxygen and non-metals), bases (oxygen in combination with metals), and salts (combinations of acids and bases). Humphry Davy used Volta's battery to show that the passage of currents through salts led to migration of acids to one electrode (negative) and bases to the other (positive). Both Lavoisier and Davy went farther than merely advancing concepts, they accurately quantified them.

DALTON'S ATOMIC THEORY

John Dalton was the son of a Quaker weaver and teacher who lived in Manchester, and is yet another in our builders of breathing who made exceptional contributions without having a conventional chemistry education(it has to be said, though, that he was exceptionally gifted when it came to brain power; he became a schoolteacher at the age of 12). Dalton was interested in the properties of gases, and particularly the nitrogen-oxygen gases found by Priestley. On the basis of simple measurements—temperature, pressure and gas concentrations, together with an intuitive interpretation of previous work, he advanced the Atomic Theory in 1803. Dalton's advanced the idea that his "ultimate particles" of a gas combined in unique proportions, and he devised a notation that he used to describe them. Thus, for the nitrogen-oxygen gases he denoted nitrous oxide as N_2O, nitric oxide as NO and nitrogen peroxide as NO_2, to demonstrate the relative proportions of nitrogen and oxygen as 1:2, 1:1 and 2:1 respectively. In 1802 his paper "On the expansion of elastic fluids" he showed that the pressure of a mixture of gases, such as for example atmospheric air, equaled the sum of the pressures exerted by each individual gas. This "Dalton's Law of Partial Pressures" allowed calculation of the proportions of individual gases to the total (measured) pressure. It also led to the conclusion that the absorption of gases by liquids, for example of oxygen by blood, was determined by their partial pressure and influenced by temperature. He was the first to point out that water vapour was always present as a component gas of the atmosphere, its content being a function of temperature.[2]

Dalton's ideas concerning the amount of gas dissolved in a liquid led to the definition of absorption coefficients.[3] His concepts regarding the movement of gases between the gas and liquid phases were expanded by Thomas Graham, who was professor of Chemistry at the Anderson Institution in Edinburgh. Realizing that gaseous diffusion was an important feature in the exchange of respired gases, he measured the rates at which gases of differing molecular weights moved through porous plugs of plaster and disks of platinum containing fine holes. He incorporated the properties of gases already described by Davy and Dalton to develop what came to be known in 1830 as Graham's Law of Diffusion. This stated that gases diffused at rates that were proportional to the square root of their density; much later this law was a key component of quantitative descriptions of gas exchange in the lungs.

26   The combination of elements (atoms) in different proportions, and why certain elements

would combine and others would not, was solved in 1852, when the concept of valency was introduced by Edward Frankland. Valency expressed the capacity of an atom to combine with others, in terms of proportionality; thus, in relation to hydrogen the compounds HCl, H_2O, H_3N and H_4C (hydrochloric acid, water, ammonia and methane, respectively) the valencies of Cl (chlorine), O_2 (oxygen), N_2 (nitrogen) and C (carbon) were 1, 2, 3 and 4 respectively. Frankland pictured the concept in structural terms, in which each atom possessed a number (valency) of bonds, shown as lines connecting atoms; thus carbon had 4 bonds that could combine with 4 hydrogen atoms (1 bond each) to form methane—

$$\begin{matrix} & \text{H} & \\ & | & \\ \text{H} - & \text{C} & - \text{H} \\ & | & \\ & \text{H} & \end{matrix}$$

And would combine with two atoms of oxygen (valency 2) to form carbon dioxide with two double bonds—

$$\text{O} = \text{C} = \text{O}$$

The property of carbon to form compounds with single, double and even treble bonds allows the formation of many different combinations, especially with hydrogen, oxygen and nitrogen.

This structural "modeling" opened the way for organic chemistry; whereas chemistry initially was concerned with minerals found in the earth, the new chemistry was more concerned with compounds built up by plants and animals. The change in focus was of

2   The pressure that water vapour exerts in air that is in contact with a water surface is dependent on its temperature, increasing from 5 mm Hg(or 0.6% of total pressure) at 0°C, to 47mm Hg (6.2%) at 37°C, and 760 mm Hg (100%) at 100 °C. These pressures and contents represent 100% of water saturation at these temperatures; out of contact with a water surface, eg. in a desert, the amounts are less—air is less than 100% saturated. As dry air is brought into the lungs, its water content increases and its pressure reaches 47 mm Hg in the alveoli. Consequently, considerable amounts of water may be lost from the lungs in dry environments.

3   The volume of a gas that dissolves in a unit volume of a liquid, at standard temperature and pressure.

great industrial importance because of the production of textiles, dyes and foods. Organic compounds, fats and oils, sugars and other vegetable compounds such as organic acids and alcohols, could be analyzed and the constituent elements—carbon, hydrogen, oxygen and nitrogen could be measured. The key element in organic chemistry is carbon, because of its ability to form double bonds; Michael Faraday made the crucial discovery of benzene (C_6H_6) in 1825; the chemical structure in valency form is

$$-\overset{|}{\underset{H}{C}}=\overset{|}{\underset{H}{C}}-\overset{|}{\underset{H}{C}}=\overset{|}{\underset{H}{C}}-\overset{|}{\underset{H}{C}}=\overset{|}{\underset{H}{C}}-$$

The three double bonds confer a huge capacity to form other compounds by freeing up the bonds to attach other molecules in "side chains".

LONG CHAINS OF CARBON: FATTY ACIDS

The key observations that established the structure of fats were made by a contemporary of Lavoisier, but who lived twice as long, surviving the Revolution and dying in 1889 in his 103rd year. Michel-Eugène Chevreul was born in Angers into a medical family, but moved to Paris at an early age to work in the National Museum of Natural History. He was a talented organic chemist who was also interested in the

perception of colour, leading him to develop dyes for the Gobelin tapestry factory. He is best known for his work on animal fats, described in his book *Reserches chimiques sur les corps gras d'origine animal,* published in 1823. Using simple techniques he heated fat with acids, he showed that animal fats were composed of long hydrocarbon chains that he called fatty acids, attached to glycerol in the proportion of 3 fatty acids to 1 glycerol, leading to their designation as triglycerides.

Analytical chemistry in the early 19th century revealed that that a wide variety of naturally occurring substances were made up of chains of carbon atoms with attached hydrogen atoms. The length of the chain determined their physical properties; very short chains occurred in volatile liquids and longer chains occurred in oils, waxes and fats. In animal fats the building blocks were acidic, ending in a -COOH group, and called fatty acids, and they all contained an even number of carbon atoms. As the number of carbons varied from 8 to almost 30, they were termed long chain fatty acids. Those containing double bonds were termed unsaturated, in contrast to those in which all the carbon bonds were saturated, the 4 bonds of each carbon being linked to 2 carbons and 2 hydrogens by single bonds. One of the most common animal fatty acids is palmitic acid, which contains 16 carbon atoms; at one end is a methyl group -CH_3 and at the other a carboxyl group -COOH; in between are 14 CH_2 groups, making

27

$C_{15}H_{31}COOH$. A more informative way of writing this is $CH_3(CH_2)_{14}COOH$.

As Chevreul established, in animals fats exist mainly in combination with glycerol, as triglycerides—

Glycerol   3 Fatty Acids

In this form, fatty acids are neutral, rather than acidic, and stored as globules of oil in fat cells (adipose tissue), liver and muscle. Triglycerides are found also in blood as tiny fat particles (chylomicrons), together with "free" fatty acids loosely associated with the plasma protein, albumin. Before triglycerides can be used as fuel, the fatty acids have to be split off from their combination with glycerol. This process occurs at the various storage cites—mainly adipose tissue, liver and muscle, and also in the walls of capillaries. The fatty acids are transported to tissues, where they are oxidized to CO_2 and water. For palmitic acid the reaction is represented by

$$C_{15}H_{31}COOH + 23O_2 \rightarrow 16CO_2 + 16H_2O$$

Although this much was known by the end of the 19th century, it was not until well into the 20th, that this process, lipolysis, was fully understood. A reasonable guess might be that that –CH_2 groups are successively split off from the chain and oxidized. However, in 1905 the German biochemist Franz Knoop, studied fatty acids of different lengths that he "labeled" by attaching a phenyl group to the end carbon (COOH) group.[4] When these fatty acid compounds were fed to dogs, only a 2C-phenyl compound appeared in urine; Knoop deduced that the fatty acid was progressively split into two carbon portions at the second (β) C from the carboxyl (COOH) end of the molecule. Since the naturally occurring fatty acids all have an even number of carbon atoms, this means that fatty acids can be completely broken down into 2C units. However, it also means that fatty acid breakdown is accompanied by the formation of acetic acid (CH_3COOH), and very little acetic acid is normally detectable. What <u>are</u> detectable, notably in states of starvation and diabetes, are 4-C compounds such as acetoacetate; in these situations carbohydrates are not available. To cut a very long story short, these findings showed that normal fat breakdown normally takes place hand in hand with carbohydrate metabolism . Knoop himself postulated that no acetic acid could be normally found because it was very rapidly dealt with, but it was not until 40 years after Knoop's experiments that Albert Lehninger established that the acetic acid produced in β-oxidation is attached to co-enzyme A (CoA), followed by entry into the Krebs (citric acid) cycle as acetyl CoA (see below).

RINGS OF GLUCOSE, CHAINS OF GLYCOGEN

A further brilliant advance in the structure of organic compounds was made by the German chemist August Kekulé in 1865; apparently whilst riding on top of a London double-decker bus, he day-dreamed of atoms whirling

4   As the phenyl group could not be broken down in the body, it remained attached to the end group, acting as a label for it.

in circles and had the inspirational idea that carbon atoms could combine in a ring; a related apocryphal tale has it that he dreamed of carbon atoms turning into six snakes in a circle, with each biting the next one's tail), thus discovering the benzene "ring"—

The concept paved the way for further advances in understanding metabolic processes. The glucose molecule, described in biochemical notation as $C_6H_{12}O_6$, could be viewed as a 6-carbon benzene ring, in which one of the carbon atoms is replaced by O, with the spare bonds being taken up by OH groups.

Again, a conceptual model allowed the structural composition of an organic compound to be understood well enough for it to be applied to biological and, later, physiological problems. Also,

ring structures such as glucose can be modified by changing the position of side chains, leading to variations in structure among compounds that have the same constituents. Thus began the field of structural or spatial chemistry that has been of such importance in the past 50 years.

ENZYMES

The Swedish chemist Jöns Jakob Berzelius was one of the great chemical thinkers of the mid 19th century. In addition to introducing modern chemical notation, by representing elements by the initial of their Latin or Greek name, he saw that the (organic) fermentation process had features in common to the purely chemical (inorganic) processes in which simple chemicals such as acids and metals could speed up a reaction without being used up in the reaction. In 1835 he pointed out that in a similar way that metals such as gold and platinum act to speed up the conversion of hydrogen peroxide into water and oxygen, fermentation of sugar into ethanol by yeast obeyed the law of conservation of matter, and would also be more acceptable in living systems than an acid or metal. He wrote—"We have here a new force, belonging to both inorganic and organic Nature, for bringing about chemical reactivity through the action of certain materials, simple as well as complex, solid as well as liquid. They accomplish this … without a necessary change of their own components…". This thought ushered in the concept of "the enzyme theory of life", in which all chemical reactions occurring in the body are controlled by the activity of specific enzymes.

Whereas Pasteur limited his research to micro-organisms, Berzelius was interested in animal muscle; as early as 1807 he had found an acid in the muscles of hunted stags and later showed that it was identical to that formed during the

29

souring of milk—lactic acid. He also felt that the highest amount of acid was found in stags which had defied the hunter the longest. This finding did not receive much attention in the next few decades, until methods were developed to study isolated (mainly frog) muscle. The muscle could be stimulated to contract and the blood could be changed in composition and flow. Such studies showed that blood could be replaced by a salt solution, without affecting muscle, as long as the solution contained oxygen. Although muscle could be made to contract in the absence of oxygen, it then fatigued more rapidly and produced more lactic acid and carbon dioxide than when oxygen was present.

In addition to understanding that chemical reactions provided the underpinning for all body functions, the convertibility of all forms of energy, as expressed in the First and Second Laws of Thermodynamics, gained acceptance. Justus von Liebig wrote in his textbook *Animal Chemistry*—"The contraction of muscles produces heat; but the force necessary for the contraction has manifested itself through the organs of motion in which it has been excited by chemical changes. The ultimate cause of the heat produced is therefore to be found in the chemical changes". The parallel between tissue metabolism and combustion was still being drawn. However, whereas both require oxygen and produce carbon dioxide and water, the energy release of combustion produces heat only, in contrast to metabolic processes where energy is used for muscle contraction, nerve conduction, liver function and all the myriad living processes on which we depend. In the debate between Liebig and Pasteur, it is possible to say that both were right and both wrong, because eventually, in 1897—after both their deaths , Eduard Buchner obtained a soluble substance, by subjecting yeast to a great pressure, which was active even in the

absence of any yeast cells.[5] By that time, in 1878, Wilhelm Friedrich Kuhne had introduced the term "enzyme" for these soluble ferments; he defined an enzyme as a substance that speeded up the rate of a specific reaction many thousand fold, and without being changed by the reaction. We will leave further discussion regarding the importance of enzymes for a later chapter on maximal exercise, where the rates of different reactions under control of enzymes impose limits to the use of fuels.

Full understanding of the reactions involved was built on a basic framework that included both the chemical composition of metabolic fuels and careful analytical experiments that related chemistry to physiology. Quantitative chemistry allowed amounts of fuels used for metabolism to be related to the amounts of oxygen used and CO_2 produced. The energy released from the metabolism of the fuels is transferred to form the versatile molecule adenosine triphosphate (ATP), which powers all the cellular functions in the body.

THE IMPORTANCE OF GLUCOSE AS A FUEL

Glucose cannot be held in high concentration anywhere in the body, because in solution it acts osmotically to draw water across cell

---

5   Eduard Buchner trained as a chemist, but one vacation went to work in the microbiology laboratory of his older brother Hans in Munich, who was trying to develop a preservative for a yeast extract. One preservative was sucrose, and Eduard observed a constant stream of bubbles from the preparation; he realized that the extract of the crushed yeast was splitting sucrose into glucose and fructose, and then turning the glucose into ethanol and carbon dioxide. By showing that soluble enzymes played important roles in cells, more complex than had been previously realized, Buchner paved the way for modern biochemistry. He was awarded the Nobel Prize for chemistry in 1907.

membranes; it is stored as insoluble glycogen granules, mainly in the liver and muscle. The great French physiologist Claude Bernard was the first to show that muscle contained glycogen in 1859, and the German biochemist O. Nasse identified glycogen as the source of lactic acid and carbon dioxide in 1869. Glucose is first split off from glycogen and transported to tissues, where it undergoes progressive breakdown, a process termed glycolysis.

GLYCOLYSIS

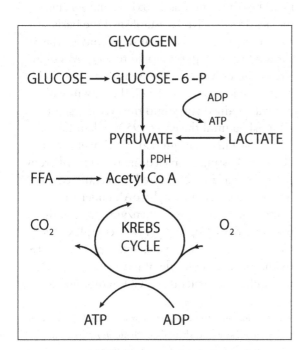

Figure 7 Pathways of energy metabolism

Between 1910 and 1930 the breakdown of glycogen and glucose in and muscle became recognized as occurring in a series of steps, several of which were associated with the formation of sugar-phosphate compounds, finally ending in pyruvic acid, from which lactic acid was formed. The major players in these advances were Gustav Georg Embden, the professor of biochemistry at Frankfurt, and Otto

Myerhof, who was a lowly assistant at the Physiological Institute at Kiel University at the time he was awarded the 1922 Nobel Prize. The chain of chemical events that occurs in the breakdown of glycogen/glucose to pyruvic acid is known as the "Embden-Myerhof pathway". The process of glycolysis, whereby glycogen is broken down to lactic acid, is rapid and does not require oxygen—it is "anaerobic"; it is the major source of energy during an all-out sprint, but it carries the distinct drawbacks that it is energetically inefficient; glycogen is soon used up and because lactic acid is a strong acid, muscle stops working if too much of it accumulates there.[6] It has to move out of muscle into the bloodstream, where an increase in acidity stimulates breathing; the resulting blowing off of CO_2 helps to reduce the acidity. However, we have all experienced the feeling of breathlessness that accompanies a brisk climb of a few flights of stairs. To continue climbing, we have to slow up; we notice that after 2 or 3 minutes our breathing eases—we have "got our second wind", indicating that lactate production has stopped and pyruvate is being broken down "aerobically. Our breathing settles down because less CO_2 is being evolved.

THE CITRIC ACID OR KREBS CYCLE

One of my student colleagues used to boast that he had passed a series of biochemistry exams, knowing only the "Krebs Cycle"; such was its importance in the metabolic function of all

31

---

6   The reaction (glucose to lactic acid) may be written as $C6H12O6 \rightarrow 2CH3CHOHCOO- + H+$; an acid such as lactic acid (LaH) splits into a negatively charged anion (La-) and positively charged hydrogen ion (H+), and the hydrogen ion can then react with bicarbonate (HCO3-) to form carbonic acid (H2CO3) leading to release of CO2. This reaction can be written as— $H+ + HCO3- \rightarrow H2 CO3 \rightarrow H2O + CO2$

body systems that any question could be turned into a detailed exposition of all its intricacies. Hans Adolph Krebs was born in Hildesheim, close to Hanover in northern Germany, and in 1918 enrolled in medical school, first at Göttingen, transferring to Freibourg and finally to Munich where he obtained his degree in 1923. During this peripatetic education he was influenced by several great scientists, including Franz Knoop in Freibourg, who had discovered the biochemical pathway of fat oxidation. These influences led to the notion that medical research could benefit from the application of modern biochemistry. Accordingly he became an assistant to the famous Otto Warburg at the Kaiser Wilhelm Institute for Biology at Brlin-Dahlen. Warburg was a pioneer in the biochemistry of enzymes and in the use of tissue slices for the study of metabolism. Krebs decided to study the way liver formed urea from ammonia and CO_2—the reaction ($2NH_3$ + CO_2 ↔ NH_2CONH_2 +H_2O) does not happen spontaneously, and Krebs had the intuitive leap that it occurred in a cycle involving three amino-acids—the first incorporated one CO_2 and an ammonia molecule to form the second, which in turn incorporated another ammonia to form the third, that in turn released urea to become the first again. It was the first "metabolic cycle"—the ornithine cycle, and it earned him instant recognition in the international biochemistry community in 1933, and the 1953 Nobel Prize. At the time the work was published he was supported in Warburg's laboratory by what we would now call "soft money", which ran out; accordingly he went to Freiburg, and began the research that was to result in one of the greatest biochemical innovations of the century. However, on April 1st 1933, Hitler's anti-Semitic programme was put in place and on April 12th Krebs received "notification of immediate removal from office"; on June 20th he arrived in England almost penniless and without a job,

but with the equipment he needed to carry on. Frederick Gowland Hopkins, now knighted and President of the Royal Society, who had mentioned in glowing terms the Ornithine Cycle in his Presidential Address, learnt of his plight and arranged for him to work at Cambridge; by July 7th he was already back at work on his next cycle, which had as its aim the elucidation of the mechanism whereby pyruvic acid was oxidized to CO_2. He studied pigeon muscle, and built on the work of the Austro-American Albert Szent-Györgi, who had identified the role of the mitochondrion in muscle oxidation.[7] During the next 5 years Krebs established the basis of a cycle in which 8 chemical steps convert the 3 carbon atoms in pyruvic acid to CO_2. Although Krebs had established the steps that occur in his "Citric Acid Cycle" by 1937, the way in which pyruvate gained entry into the cycle was not established until the early 1950s, when Lester J Reed and his colleagues at the University of Texas at Austin, unraveled the reaction whereby pyruvate was first converted to acetate (carried by co-enzyme A as acetyl-CoA), under the control of a very complex enzyme system, the pyruvate dehydrogenase (PDH) complex. Acetyl-CoA then enters the Cycle, and is progressively oxidized; each molecule of pyruvate uses 3 O_2 molecules and generates 3 CO_2 molecules. As

---

7   The mitochondrion (plural—mitochondria) is a structure in the muscle cell where these chemical reactions are organized; it is often referred to as the powerhouse of the cell, and "the world's tiniest rotary motor". Among its many functions, the most important is to link oxygen to the production of ATP from ADP, by a complex series of enzymes that form "the electron transport chain". In their evolutionary history, they started out as single celled organisms (bacteria) that invaded primitive cells incapable of aerobic metabolism, and remained ever since. This evolutionary invasion has an important outcome; the mitochondrion is unique amongst cellular structures in having its own genetic code, completely separate from the human genome.

glycolysis produces 2 molecules of pyruvate from each glucose molecule derived from glycogen, the complete oxidation of one molecule of glucose generates 6 molecules of CO_2, whilst using 6 molecules of O_2; as an equal amount of O_2 is used as CO_2 is produced. Thus, by the end of the 19th century there was at least a nascent understanding of the biochemical processes essential to life, of aerobic (oxygen requiring) and anaerobic (in the absence of oxygen) processes. The cellular oxidation of glycogen is associated with oxygen consumption and the formation of carbon dioxide, and requires enzymes for the reactions to take place sufficiently rapidly. Importantly, the quantitative relationships between the metabolic fuels and the oxygen used and CO_2 produced in cellular "combustion" had been established. Three main processes had emerged—

1.Anaerobic glycolysis, in which glucose molecules were broken down to lactic acid without requiring oxygen, but leading to CO_2 evolution through the reaction of H^+ with bicarbonate (HCO_3^-)—

$$C_6H_{12}O_6 \rightarrow 2CH_3CHOHCOO^- + H^+$$

$$H^+ + HCO_3^- \rightarrow H_2O + CO_2$$

2. Aerobic glycolysis, in which glucose is broken down to CO_2 and water—

$$C_6H_{12}O_6 + 6O_2 \rightarrow 6CO_2 + 6H_2O$$

3. Fatty acid oxidation—for example

$$C_{11}H_{23}COOH + 17O_2 \rightarrow 12CO_2 + 12H_2O$$

These reactions do not take us far into how they are linked to the liberation of energy that may be used to power cellular functions. It was not until the mid 20th century that these

oxidations were linked to so-called "high energy phosphates"—a topic we shall leave for a later chapter on exercise.

Before leaving these reaction between the combustion of metabolic fuels and the accompanying use of oxygen and production of CO_2, let me emphasize the important differences between them. First, reaction (1), whilst not requiring O_2, leaves us with an acid to deal with, leading to CO_2 being evolved. Second, in relation to O_2 consumption, less CO_2 is produced in reaction (3) than reaction (2); 30% less, in fact (12/17). Both these facts have implications for breathing, especially in exercise. Finally, there are implications that arise from the fact that the two main sources of energy, glucose and free fatty acids, have to be stored, because otherwise we would run out of them very quickly. Neither can be stockpiled through increases in concentration because glucose exerts an osmotic effect, tending to draw water from tissues, and fatty acids are acid and cannot be allowed to become very concentrated.[8] Glucose is stored in liver and muscle as the inert branching molecule, glycogen. Fatty acids are stored in combination with glycerol on a 3-to-1 basis, as triglycerides in adipose tissue and muscle. Finally, the fact that "fats are burned in the flame of carbohydrates" has implications for the rate at which these fuels are metabolized, especially during exercise, when they are needed rapidly and often abruptly.

The 20th century saw the concepts broadened and the links between fuel combustion and energy release clarified. The coordination between

---

8   Osmosis is the process whereby water moves through a semi-permeable membrane such as a cell wall which separates solutions of substances such as glucose having different strengths, the direction of water movement being from the lower to the higher concentration.

metabolic processes and the support systems of breathing and the circulation became revealed in all its glory. We will consider these aspects in the chapter on breathing during exercise, but the beginnings of concepts related to physiological coordination involved studies that examined the part played by blood. Specifically, what we needed to know was how blood supplied tissues with oxygen and removed carbon dioxide from them, and the processes that enabled this "gas exchange" to occur between the internal metabolism and external environment.

CHAPTER 3

LUNG STRUCTURE AND THE FUNCTION OF BREATHING

"And therefore, O students, study mathematics and do not build without foundations."

Leonardo da Vinci, Notebooks, 1508-18.

In spite of dissection and animal vivisection, the early observers had difficulty in understanding what they were seeing in the lungs; illustrations in their books seem to imply that they were unable to draw what they saw, and perhaps they were impelled to portray the contents of the chest in accordance with Galen's view of lung function. To our eyes, both the science and the art appear very "primitive". The first time Art came to the rescue of Science was in the early years of the 16th century, when Leonardo made numerous drawings to illustrate both the anatomy and the workings of the lungs and chest. The structure of the bronchial tree is beautifully laid out, but even Leonardo had to show communications that brought air and blood together in the heart. One has the impression that this was against his better judgment, because he wrote that "the air… cannot enter the heart unless there is an outlet. Therefore two passages are necessary. When the lung exhausts air …a passage sends air into the concavity of the heart…and a second passage through which air issues from the heart and returns together with other air…" Here we clearly see that Leonardo was most interested in what structure told him about the function of the lungs, rather than their anatomy alone.

There were no such constraints on the Flemish artist Jan Stephan when he made woodcuts to illustrate *De Humani Corporis Fabrica* of

Andreas Vesalius, published in 1543. The branching of the bronchi and blood vessels, as seen by the naked eye, are accurately depicted, but it took another 100 years before Marcello Malpighi brought the lens and a primitive microscope to reveal the finer structure.

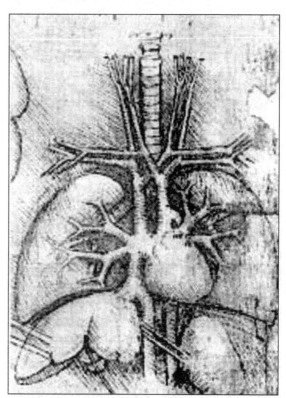

Figure 8 Leonardo's drawing of thoracic anatomy, showing non-existent connections between blood vessels, and between blood vessels and airways

THE AIRWAYS

In the three centuries that followed Vesalius, only minor details were added regarding the irregular branching system known as the bronchial "tree". In 1661 Malpighi depicted the branching of the bronchi both conceptually and from his observation of the frog lung.

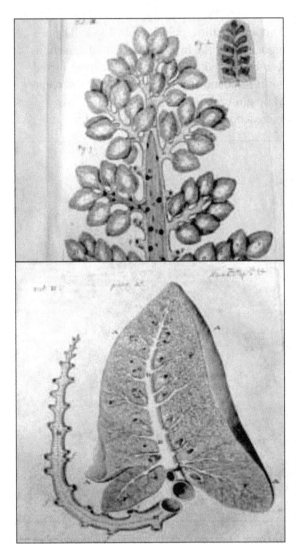

Figure 9 Malpighi's drawings of airway branching and lung structure

It took 200 years to make much of an improvement on Malpighi's description. In Henry Gray's *Anatomy- Descriptive and Surgical* of 1858 we can see the meticulous drawings of Dr. H.V. Carter, "late demonstrator of Anatomy at St.

George's Hospital". These show only the first five or six "generations" of bronchi; their walls contain cartilage in the form of bands that partially circle the tubes; in the case of the trachea, these leave the posterior third without firm support, but in the bronchi cartilage provided support round the whole circumference, and especially at the branch points.

In the mid-19th century, the airways attracted anatomists with a bent for measurement and relationships between structure and function; and, if we are talking nationalities, the credit clearly goes to the Swiss. Christoph Theodor Aeby began his career in anatomy at the University of Basel, later becoming professor at Berne. Throughout his career he made careful measurements of the structural differences between species, and their functional implications. He amassed a large collection of animal skeletons, the basis for his studies that, unusually for the time, sought to apply mathematical principles to variations in form, that might be explained in terms of function. His most famous work, published in 1880, presented measurements made on wax or metal casts made of the human bronchial tree from which he argued that bronchi were mainly side branches from a single main airway. Later workers drew a different inference—that the airways showed irregular dichotomous branching—successive branching into two more-or-less equal sized bronchi. Also in Berne, though in the department of physiology and a few decades later, Fritz Rohrer also measured length and caliber of airways down to a diameter of 1.5 mm using calibrated probes, mainly to learn more about airflow in bronchi and the factors that determined resistance to the flow of air to the alveoli. Rohrer's doctoral thesis in 1915 is acknowledged to be a classic, because it presented morphometric data from which a mathematical equation was derived to

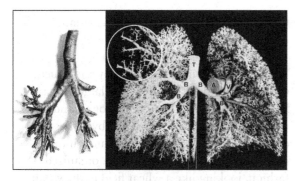

Figure 10 Theodor Aeby's bronchial casts, made of metal in the 1870s (left), contrast with Weibel's resin preparation (from Weibel, 1984) (right).

describe flow resistance in the lung. H also drew attention to the volume of the airways, which translates functionally into a volume that is breathed in but does not reach the alveoli and thus does not take part in gas exchange. This portion of the inspired air is known as the "anatomical respiratory dead space"—constituting about 1/3 of a normal resting breath, but of course a much smaller proportion of larger breaths, as in exercise. The Swiss dominance in airway morphometry was continued some 50 years later by a collaboration between an anatomist and a mathematician. Ewald Weibel, who in 1966 was to become the professor in Aeby's former department in Berne, met Domingo Gomez in 1959, when he went to work in New York's Bellevue Hospital, which for decades had been a centre of cardiac and pulmonary investigation. Gomez was a Cuban who had fled the Castro regime from the fledgling Heart Institute in Havana; in his mid-fifties, he was already a prolific medical researcher who brought mathematical insight into anatomical and physiological problems. Together, Weibel and Gomez made an analysis of airway caliber related to the successive "generations" of bronchi. They estimated that on average there are 23 generations of airways. Although each successive branch was associated with a reduction in diameter, there was a

gradual increase in the <u>total</u> cross sectional area of the airways. This arrangement was described as resembling a trumpet with a wide bell, and it indicated that flow resistance was greatest in the large airways and progressively fell with successive generations. Then they showed that the regular reduction in airway diameter went on as far as the 15th generation, after which the airways increased in size as they branched. This zone corresponded physiologically to a point where the flow of fresh air virtually ceases, and further movement of oxygen into the gas exchanging region takes place by molecular diffusion; the airways at this distance into the lung are termed respiratory bronchioles, and they lead into alveolar ducts and thence into alveoli. This work of Weibel and Gomez was

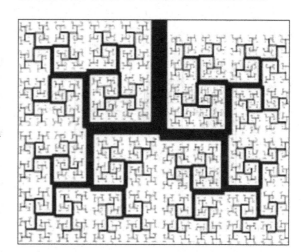

Figure 11 Mandelbrot's fractal model of airway branching

published during the early 1960s; since then other "models" have been proposed for the branching of airways, including those based on fractal geometry, but theirs remains a landmark in understanding what determines the flow of air into the normal lung.

A novel way of describing the branching of the airways was presented by Benoit Mandelbrot in his *The Fractal Geometry of Nature*, published in 1982. Mandelbrot, the "Father of Fractal Geometry" was born in Warsaw; his family fled the Nazis in 1936, and he received most of his early education in Paris, where he received his PhD in Mathematical Science in 1952. He spent 32 years on the research staff of the IBM Thomas J Watson Research Center in Yorktown Heights, New York. In his own words—"I coined the word fractal in 1978 from the Latin *fractus*, which describes a broken stone—broken up and irregular. Fractals are geometrical shapes that, contrary to those of Euclid, are not regular at all' First, they are irregular all over. Second, they have the same degree of irregularity on all scales. A fractal object looks the same when examined from far away or nearby—it is self-similar".

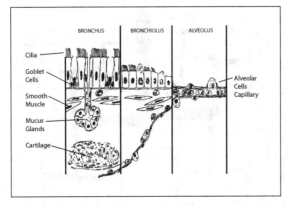

Figure 12 Diagram to show the changing structure of bronchi, from central bronchi (surface cilia, mucous glands and cartilage) to terminal bronchioles (thin without cilia)

This last property epitomizes the airways; take a small section of the bronchial tree and you cannot tell which generation it is without an indication of the scale. Each branch is proportionally similar, in terms of its length and area, anywhere in the tree. Mandelbrot made the intuitive leap that this arrangement was associated with an optimal distribution of airways within a given lung volume;

functionally, the arrangement is associated with optimal distribution of airflow.

With improvements in microscopy, the structure of the bronchi was revealed. The large airways have a ciliated endothelium, mucous glands in their walls, and are supported by circles of cartilage. Cilia are microscopic hairs on the inner lining cells which beat in an organized fashion, looking like a wheat field in the wind; they move particles up the airway to be removed by coughing and swallowing. Mucus helps this process. Finally the cartilage support stops the bronchi from collapsing when subjected to the pressure changes during breathing and coughing.

ALVEOLI, AND THEIR VENTILATION AND BLOOD FLOW

Writing in 1662 to his friend Giovanni Alfonso Borelli, Marcello Malpighi described how the small airways ended in air sacs which had capillaries in their walls—"an almost infinite number of vesicles full of air…but they are found more clearly and easily in the inflated lung after it has been dried" (this remains a standard technique for examining lung structure). Malpighi also observed red cells moving through the capillaries in the living frog. The Oxford physician Thomas Willis confirmed Malpighi's observations in 1684, writing "the bronchial pipes lead into the utter cavities, viz. the numerous little Bladders discovered by Malpighius". Later, in his massive *Practice of Physick* he observes "we may conjecture that it is not for nothing that the blood-vessels that are any where in the lungs do curiously wait upon those of the air and every where insinuate and intimately mingle themselves". Bearing in mind that this was written before much was understood regarding lung function and the purpose of breathing, we may look at this statement as an intuitive understanding of the importance of close matching of alveolar ventilation to capillary blood flow (later known as "V/Q" matching) for gas exchange. In his book Willis provides a drawing of the "little bladders", resembling a bunch of grapes, that is clearly more imaginative than realistic, not surprising in view of the fact that he lacked the necessary magnification to see alveolar structure. The lack of adequate magnification remained a problem well into the 19th century, by which time the basic building blocks of tissues—the cells—could be recognized. Henry Gray in his 1858 *Anatomy* does not provide a drawing, limiting his description to "The air-cells are small, polyhedral, alveolar recesses, separated from each other by thin septa, and communicating freely with intercellular passages. They...vary from 1/200th to 1/70th of an inch in diameter; being largest on the surface...and at the apex (of the lung)". The observation of the largest alveoli at the top of the lung was not explained until 100 years later, as we shall see. The network of capillaries (Malpighi's "rete mirabilis") was also accurately described as running in the fine walls or septa of the alveoli, but there was much controversy regarding what lined the alveoli. Well into the middle of the 20th century there were some anatomists, who argued that perhaps the capillaries ran "uncovered" in the airspaces, thus keeping the distance and barrier between air and blood at a minimum. However, they did not consider the difficulty that this arrangement would lead to in keeping the alveoli free of the liquid that would flood from the capillaries.

These arguments were not resolved until the electron microscope was brought to bear on the controversy, and techniques were developed to fix the delicate tissue so that it could be examined in an undistorted way. Whilst the electron microscope was invented in 1939, it was not until 1950 that the fixation problems were surmounted by George Palade of the

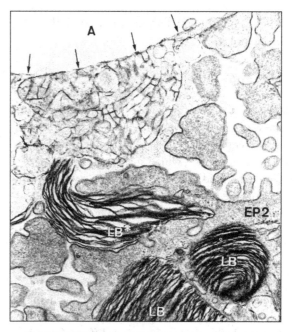

Figure 13 Webel's photomicrograph of type 2 (EP2) alveolar cells containing lamellar bodies (LB), the source of the alveolar (A) surface-active layer (arrowed)

Rockefeller Institute in New York. The new methods allowed Frank Low of Louisiana State University in New Orleans in 1952 to publish his findings on the air-blood interface, clearly showing that the alveolae were lined by the epithelium, or outer layer, of a very thin alveolar cell, later known as the type 1 cell, which had an inner "basement" membrane. The same general structure was seen in the walls of capillaries, which were covered by an endothelium, or inner layer, that had its own basement membrane; the two basement membranes were fused in alveolar walls, but separated by a potential space in septa away from, or in the corners of alveoli. The functional importance of this arrangement was discovered later: the fused basement membranes provided an excellent barrier to the movement of fluid from the capillaries into alveoli; fluid accumulation occurred first in the alveolar angles

39

and around the smallest airways (terminal bronchioles).[1]

The early electron microscope studies revealed two types of cell lining the alveoli; in addition to the type 1 cell that provided the cellular lining to the wall, a second type of cell was described with a different structure. The type 2 cell contained "lamellar bodies", which suggested that they secreted a fluid product. This product was shown to have the property of reducing surface tension forces, thus helping to keep alveoli open. Ewald Weibel and Joan Gil succeeded in demonstrating this final lining layer to the alveoli in 1977: they showed it to contain fatty acid (phospholipid) molecules arranged in a parallel border that allowed alveoli to resist collapse. . As this lining is only one molecule thick, we can ignore any effect it might have as a barrier to gas diffusion, but it is important in reducing the tissue surface tension (it is a "surfactant").The functional importance of the alveolar lining layer or surfactant we will leave to a later chapter which will describe the respiratory distress syndrome, a condition that occurs in premature infants who are unable to synthesize it.

40

The electron microscope was also used to re-examine estimates made by the light microscope of the number of alveoli and their surface area—an important dimension when we think about the lungs' capacity for gas diffusion. A variety of geometric and statistical methods were applied to show that estimates of the number of alveoli were similar, at about 300 million in the adult lung, but not surprisingly, estimates of the surface area were much larger than previous values of about 75 square meters; in fact, Weibel's new estimates were about 130m² (a tennis court has an area of 250 m²). The increase may be explained by Lewis Fry Richardson's "coast of Britain" effect. Richardson pointed out that the length of Britain's coastline from measurements made on maps depended on the scale of the map; the length is largest in maps of the smallest scale, because these reveal all the irregularities of the coastline; basically, it's a measurement that will always be indeterminate and dependent on scale. Because the resolving power of the electron microscope is so much greater than the light microscope, the measuring scale is much less, and the calculated surface area so much greater; the higher value is clearly the more functionally appropriate, because we want to know how easy it is for molecules of O_2 and CO_2 to pass between the capillary blood and alveolar air, i.e. the capacity for gas diffusion between the two sites. With the help of mathematically sophisticated colleagues, Weibel derived the variables that determined oxygen diffusion. In addition to alveolar surface area these included the volume of blood in capillaries (about 200 ml only), and the thickness of the alveolar-capillary membrane (about 1 μm, or 1 thousandth of a millimeter). Combined with the known rate of reaction between oxygen and hemoglobin an overall rate of 200 milliliters of oxygen could be transferred per minute, *per millimeter of mercury (mmHg) difference in pressure*. As the average pressure difference may be as much as 50 mmHg, this implies a large reserve capacity for oxygen diffusion (at least 2-fold), but it may still be possible for diffusion to limit oxygen transfer in some situations, such as very high oxygen requirements in athletes, and at very high altitudes, where the oxygen pressure difference becomes small. Weibel's interest in the structural dimensions of gas exchange, led him to investigate differences between mammalian species; he wanted to know the functional

1   Pressure in the capillaries is higher than in alveoli, tending to push water and plasma out; in health the small amount that leaks out is reabsorbed by lymphatics. Where capillary pressure increases, as in heart failure, water accumulates to cause pulmonary oedema.

implications of the differences between, say, a pigmy mouse and a horse. Working with the Harvard biologist C Richard Taylor, a leading expert in animals' capacity to exercise, he found that both maximum oxygen uptake and the diffusing capacity for oxygen (calculated from microscopic measurements on lungs) were related to body mass, and that there was again an apparent two-fold spare capacity available in the lungs. However, the very "athletic" species, such as racehorses and antelopes, as in human athletes, had much less spare capacity than their less athletic relatives. We will return to this monumental study in Chapter 7. But for now, we will consider the processes involved in moving oxygen into the body, and removing carbon dioxide.

CHAPTER 4

BREATHING OXYGEN INTO, AND CARBON DIOXIDE OUT OF BLOOD

"It is not for nothing that the Blood-vessels that are anywhere in the Lungs do curiously wait upon those of the air and every where insinuate and intimately mingle themselves".

Thomas Willis, Practice of Physick, 1685

This is the second time I have cited this quotation, reflecting the deep impression it made when I first came upon it. Dr Willis, the son of a Wiltshire farmer, was made Sedleian Professor of Natural Philosophy at Oxford at the age of 21. Realizing that that fortune might be added to fame by moving to London, he did so six years later, to acquire the largest and most fashionable practice in the city. Although he is best known for many achievements in neurology, including the first description of the vascular Circle of Willis at the base of the brain, his hugely influential *Practice* contains many innovative ideas in physiology and clinical medicine. In the passage quoted above, he reasoned that the function of the lungs depended on a close matching between the air filled alveoli and blood filled capillaries. It is not too much of a stretch to say that he anticipated the rigorous treatment of 300 years later which quantified the effects ventilation-perfusion ("V/Q") ratios on the effectiveness of pulmonary gas exchange.

MEASURING THE PRESSURES OF OXYGEN, NITROGEN AND CARBON DIOXIDE

Our understanding of gas exchange in the lungs, began with the insight of Evangelista Torricelli, who in the 17th century realized that pressure was exerted by the atmosphere, and then proceeded to measure it. In 1794, John Dalton showed that individual gases in a gaseous mixture such as air exerted a pressure that was in proportion to the fraction of the atmosphere that they occupied—their fractional concentration. In an atmosphere in which the pressure was 760 millimeters of mercury (mm Hg), oxygen—comprising 21%—exerted a pressure of 160 mm Hg (760 x 0.21), nitrogen (78%) one of 592 mm Hg, and carbon dioxide (less than 0.1%) less than 1 mm Hg. Thomas Graham went a step further in 1829, when he presented his Law; he found that gases diffuse at a rate dependent on pressure differences, but eventually the pressures of each gas would equalize. Thus the stage was set for understanding how oxygen moved into blood and CO_2 left blood, but the relationships between pressures and amounts of gases in fluids were more complex, depending on their solubility; very little nitrogen was contained in blood, compared to oxygen, in spite of its greater pressure.

The German chemist Gustav Magnus was the first to measure the blood gases. In 1845 he observed that blood could carry sufficient oxygen to support oxygen supply to body tissues where combustion took place, and CO_2 was added to venous blood, to be carried back to the lungs and eliminated by breathing. It was left to another German chemist, Lothar Meyer, to show that the gases existed in blood in chemically bound forms. Initially a student of medicine, he worked in the laboratory of Robert Wilhelm Eberhard Bunsen in Heidelberg and there wrote his thesis *Die Gase des Blutes* in 1857.[1] Meyer used boiling in a vacuum to liberate gases in blood, followed by measured absorption of oxygen and CO_2. He calculated the absorption coefficients for the gases in blood and discovered that the absorption of oxygen increased with pressure only to a certain point, above which uptake became very small; the findings were not consistent with simple diffusion and absorption according to Graham's Law. Meyer realized that this could be an important factor allowing oxygen to be taken up at the higher pressures in the lung and speedily unloaded in the tissues. He also saw the implication of the finding for living at high altitudes.

Lothar Meyer dedicated his dissertation to Carl Friedrich Wilhelm Ludwig, Germany's leading physiologist of the time. Carl Ludwig obtained his medical degree in Marburg, but was suspended from the medical school because in attempting to introduce liberal reforms in Germany he openly supported the ideals of the French Revolution. Although his academic brilliance was recognized, he was unable to obtain an academic position in Germany; he became professor of physiology in Zurich, and later in Vienna. However, in 1865 he was appointed professor in Leipzig, where he developed the foremost laboratory for medical physiology; Leipzig University grew to be the hub of German scientific research. Ludwig recognized the importance of Lothar Meyer's studies, and he set out to

improve methods for blood gas analysis. As doyen of German physiology he had only one serious rival, who became an implacable opponent in an acrimonious scientific debate during the last quarter of the century. Eduard Friedrich Wilhelm Pflüger also obtained his medical degree in Marburg, and had been similarly rebellious, but otherwise differed from Ludwig in the way he wielded academic power. Becoming professor of physiology at the University of Bonn in 1859, he undertook research in many aspects of human physiology and founded an influential scientific journal which uniquely bears his name to this day—the *Pflügers Archiv für die gesammte Physiologie des Menschen und der Tiere*. The title reflects the extent of his intended influence over "the whole Physiology of Men and Animals", and he used its pages to criticize scientists with views divergent to his own. Pflüger was a master of scientific method; his laboratory developed improved methods for the extraction of gases from blood and their analysis. Between them Ludwig and Pflüger produced a series of gas pumps, tonometers for equilibrating bubbles with the gases in blood and thus measure their pressures, and equipment to measure small volumes accurately.

A realization of the importance of oxygen consumption in sustaining cell metabolism, together with improved analytical techniques stimulated interest in measurements of oxygen uptake and carbon dioxide production, and their linkage to breathing. One of Pflüger's disciples, Nathan Zuntz, made extensive studies between 1870 and the end of the century, into the changes associated with food ingestion (demonstrating the increase in metabolism that occurred after eating and intravenously-administered foodstuffs). A portable apparatus allowed him to measure the volume of breathing—or ventilation, and the

1   Lothar Meyer later became professor of chemistry in Karlsruhe and eventually in Tübingen. Independently of Mendelèjeff, who had also worked in Bunsen's laboratory, he described an arrangement of the elements in a natural system (The Periodic Table) that is usually associated with Mendelèjeff's name. This independent finding was recognized formally when they jointly were awarded the Royal Society's Copley Medal in 1887.

concentrations of expired gases during many activities. The method was hardly improved upon until miniaturization and electronics was brought to bear in the 1960's. We will return to the linkages between metabolism and breathing when considering breathing during exercise.

Ludwig interpreted the results of his blood gas contents as evidence of combustion occurring in the blood and in the lung tissue. The finding of lower carbon dioxide and higher oxygen pressures in arterial blood than in gas from the lung, suggested an active secretion of oxygen inwards and carbon dioxide outwards. Pflüger, with his improved methods and measurements made on urine as well as blood from many sites, showed conclusively that the exchange of gases between the tissues and blood and between blood and lungs could be explained by diffusion, through pressure differences between these compartments. In his view there was no evidence for a secretion of oxygen by lung cells, and the body's chemical

combustion took place in the peripheral tissues; living cells governed their oxygen consumption, but did not influence the content of oxygen in blood. One would think this would have been the end of this debate, but in fact it continued well into the 20th century; the greatest of British respiratory physiologists, John Scott Haldane, went to his grave in 1936 still wrongly maintaining that active secretion of oxygen took place in the lungs. This belief was founded in experiments he had carried out in 1896, in which arterial PO_2 was estimated at 185 mmHg—well above its pressure in the atmosphere. It took the systematic and meticulous measurements of the Danish physiologists August and Marie Krogh to finally settle the question, and end what had come to be known as the "Great Copenhagen-Oxford Debate" between the Kroghs and Haldane, conclusively won by Copenhagen. Haldane was reluctant to accept defeat, and although he accepted the Kroghs' findings, continued to maintain that secretion occurred when the lungs were subjected to stress, as in altitude. Haldane excepted, there was universal acceptance from 1920 onwards, that oxygen moves into the blood and then into the tissues by diffusion, down pressure differences or "gradients". The same basic mechanism drives carbon dioxide out of the tissues and eventually into expired air. But Lothar Meyer had found that the amounts of the two gases carried in blood could not be accounted for by their solubility alone; chemical combinations had to be involved. Which brings us to hemoglobin and the red blood cells.

OXYGEN IN BLOOD

Oxygen is carried in blood by a marvelous iron containing compound—hemoglobin; as a first step in thinking about it, a few words to justify "marvelous". As organisms evolved in complexity, and especially as they moved out of the sea, and as air also evolved from having no

44

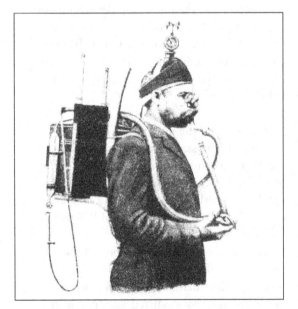

Figure 14 Nathan Zuntz demonstrating his more-or-less portable apparatus for measuring oxygen uptake during activity

oxygen to containing 21% of the stuff, so too did respiratory pigments evolve. These combined with oxygen and carried it to cells for their metabolic processes. Some contained copper, the *hemocyanins*, blue pigments found in mollusks, but most contained iron, including hemoglobin. Now, lots of chemicals are able to combine with oxygen, in oxidation reactions, but the problem is that once they have combined, it's difficult to get them to give the oxygen back; hemoglobin does not become oxidized, but takes up oxygen avidly in the lungs and gives it up just as readily in the tissues. In some primitive animals it merely exists in solution in the plasma of blood, but in higher animals it is carried in the red cells, or corpuscles; this arrangement allows them to have higher concentrations of hemoglobin in their blood. Thus, while sea water, and cell-free plasma, only carry about 0.5 ml oxygen in a 100 ml solution, human blood carries about 20 ml, a forty-fold increase; interestingly this makes the amount in blood roughly the same as in the air. Not only that, but blood takes up oxygen many times faster than plasma, which is just as well, because blood is only in close contact with air in the lungs for 1-2 seconds. The unraveling of the mystery that was hemoglobin is just as fascinating as the gradual comprehension of other breathing mysteries that we have already considered.

HEMOGLOBIN

Vincenzo Antonio Menghini, a Bolognese physician wrote in 1746 that he had burnt blood to obtain a red powder that was attracted to a magnet, correctly inferring that it contained iron. Berzelius in the following century confirmed the finding, and chemically split the blood pigment into two components, a protein (globulin) and a red compound containing iron oxide (heme); it was the start of iron therapy for anemia. A large step forward in discovering its chemical composition was made by the

brilliant German chemist Felix Hoppe-Seyler. After qualifying in medicine at Leipzig, he was professor of physiology in Berlin and then professor of applied chemistry in Strasbourg. When he was appointed in 1861, that city had recently been annexed from the French, and large amounts of money were lavished on the University, leading to it becoming a centre of scientific research. Hoppe-Seyler benefited from these politically motivated changes, and was able to build a laboratory equipped with the most up-to-date instruments. He developed his interest in blood after hearing that miners dying of carbon monoxide poisoning had been found to have very pink blood in their hearts (the pink colour was carboxyhemoglobin, formed by carbon monoxide combining with hemoglobin, thereby displacing oxygen). It was Hoppe-Seyler who called the blood pigment "hemoglobin" in 1862, obtained it in crystalline form to aid its further study (it was the first protein to be crystallized), and established its chemical formula and molecular weight. He studied solutions of hemoglobin in a spectroscope, that had recently been invented by Bunsen and Kirchoff, and found that light of specific wavelengths was absorbed, thus discovering the absorption spectra of the oxygenated and de-oxygenated forms.[2] Using this technique, he was able to show that the hemoglobin found in many animals was remarkably similar. Not only did Hoppe-Seyler characterize the hemoglobin molecule, but he also opened up the whole field of spectroscopy in biological chemistry,

---

2 In the latter half of the 20th century, oxymeters were developed; by shining light through the skin of an ear lobe or finger tip and quantifying absorption at two wavelengths corresponding to oxygenated and deoxygenated hemoglobin, the % occupied by each form (the % saturation) was instantly measured. Nowadays no one goes through a serious medical procedure or is admitted to hospital without this routine measure.

leading to the identification of many enzymes and other chemicals involved in energy transfer. Hoppe-Seyler's findings were extended by meticulous analytical methods employed by Carl Gustav von Hüfner, a student of both Bunsen and Ludwig and Hoppe-Seyler's successor in Tübingen. Using a complex technique in which he first displaced oxygen from hemoglobin with carbon monoxide, he calculated that 1 gram of hemoglobin combined with 1.34 ml of oxygen; using chemical analysis he determined that hemoglobin was composed of 0.342% iron. Assuming that each molecule of hemoglobin combined with one molecule of oxygen, he calculated the same capacity, of 1.34 ml/g. This means that a healthy human with a hemoglobin content of 15g/100ml of blood, has an oxygen carrying capacity of 1.34 x 15, or 20 ml/100ml. This work was confirmed by many in succeeding years, but modified very little, and thus established the oxygen carrying <u>capacity</u> of human blood; any amount of oxygen below capacity is expressed as a percentage of the capacity and termed its saturation ($SO_2\%$). The main variable that determines blood oxygen saturation is the pressure of oxygen (PO_2).

THE OXYGEN "DISSOCIATION" CURVE

An interest into man's capacity to exist at high altitudes, led the man later known as "the father of aviation medicine", to measure oxygen content in animals subjected to partial vacuums. Paul Bert was a French physician who after studying under "the founder of clinical physiology"—Claude Bernard—at the Sorbonne, became his successor as professor of physiology. Bert was involved in early balloon ascents, some of which famously met with tragic ends. He measured the oxygen <u>content</u> of arterial blood samples and related them to the ambient <u>pressure</u>; in 1872 he was the first to publish graphs relating the two variables,

pressure and content or saturation, later termed the *oxygen dissociation curve*. This demonstrated that as pressure falls from the sea level atmospheric pressure, there is initially little fall in oxygen saturation, but then there is a dramatic fall.

Bert's measurements were quite crude, but they were improved upon by the Danish physiologist Christian Bohr only in 1891. At the age of 31, Bohr had become professor of physiology at the University of Copenhagen in 1886, following graduate studies with Ludwig in Leipzig. With his two famous pupils, August Krogh and Karl Hasselbalch he made many contributions to exercise physiology and the processes of lung gas exchange. In contrast to the children of famous scientists who struggle to achieve the high expectations placed on them, Bohr's son Niels gained the Nobel Prize for physics in 1922; Niels' son Aage won the Prize in 1975.

In 1885, Christian Bohr confirmed Lothar Meyer's findings with accurate measurements; he showed that the dissociation curve of a weak solution of hemoglobin was hyperbolic, rising sharply to reach a flat plateau where it was fully saturated. Later Bohr, Krogh and Hasselbalch studied whole blood, revealing in 1904 that the shape was actually S-shaped, or sigmoid. To describe the curve, we may start at a high oxygen pressure and work our way down and to the left (fig 16). The pressure of oxygen in dry air at sea level amounts to 21% of an atmosphere (760 millimeters of mercury) or about 160 mm Hg; once in the airways water vapour makes its pressure felt (47 mm Hg), reducing the oxygen pressure to about 150 mm Hg (21% of 760 – 47). In the alveoli, carbon dioxide appears and oxygen is taken up, and at the end of this exchange the oxygen pressure is down to 100 mm Hg; at this pressure in blood the amount of oxygen bound amounts to about 97% of hemoglobin's capacity—it is "97% saturated". The upper part of the curve is almost flat, so that a reduction in pressure to 60 mm Hg still leaves blood about 90% saturated; however, this is at the upper bend of the S-shape, or "knee" of the curve; a further fall of 40 mm Hg to 20 mm Hg is accompanied by a dramatic release of oxygen, leaving the hemoglobin only 30% saturated. Bohr realized the physiological implications of this finding—that oxygen is avidly taken up in the lungs and readily given up in the tissues. Also that reductions in O_2 pressure that occur with altitude have little effect the amount of O_2 in blood below 12,000 feet, but above 15,000 feet critical falls in O_2 content may occur.

Christian Bohr's group also showed that the curve was not physiologically constant; its position could be shifted according to the concurrent pressure of carbon dioxide, being shifted to the right by high carbon dioxide pressure, and conversely to the left by low "PCO_2"; this has since been known as the "Bohr effect" although more generously should be known as the "Bohr-Krogh-Hasselbalch effect". In addition to the shape of the curve, the Bohr effect also aided oxygen uptake in the lungs where PCO_2 is relatively low, and oxygen release in the tissues where PCO_2 is high. The findings provided proof of the mechanism postulated by Georg Gabriel Stokes, who in 1864 had found by spectroscopy that blood shaken with CO_2 became partially deoxygenated.

Christian Bohr's description of the oxyhemoglobin dissociation curve evoked interest, especially in Britain, in the physiology departments of Oxford and Cambridge, where traditions of research in respiratory physiology and in the properties of hemoglobin began, and where they exist to this day. In the early part of the 20th century there was a close collaboration

between the two laboratories and their principal investigators, JS Haldane in Oxford and Joseph Barcroft in Cambridge.

John Scott Haldane was born into an aristocratic Scottish family, the Haldanes of Gleneagles: he qualified in medicine in 1884 in Edinburgh and moved to Oxford in 1887,

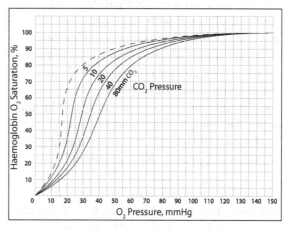

Figure 15 The oxygen dissociation (hemoglobin saturation vs. pressure) curve published by Bohr, Krogh and Hasselbalch in 1904, showing the effect of CO2 pressure (from zero on the left to 80 mmHg on the right)

becoming a lecturer in physiology and quickly developing a reputation for his research in the physiology of altitude and of work at depths— both diving and in mining. One of his great interests was on the effects of carbon monoxide, both related to mining and on its effects on the oxyhemoglobin dissociation curve. He introduced many technological innovations in gas and blood gas analysis, devising the Haldane apparatus—in which small volumes of gas could be subjected to oxygen absorption by pyrogallol and carbon dioxide absorption by potassium hydroxide, the "gold standard" method of gas analysis. In 1905, with his long-time colleague John Gillies Priestley, he published a simple method for sampling average alveolar gas from the gas exchanging regions of the lung. Haldane's experiments always had a strong practical rationale. He also showed a legendary ability to walk the tightrope between high risk and safety (in studies of great pressures, or breathing carbon monoxide, for example), setting a standard for the generations of respiratory physiologists that came later. For reasons that must have their parallel in the novels of CP Snow, with their Byzantine university politics, Haldane was not appointed Professor of Physiology at Oxford when it fell vacant in 1905, on the retirement of Sir John Burdon-Sanderson. This must have been hard to take, because Sir John was his uncle and he had named his son after him (John Burdon Sanderson Haldane). He was up against a formidable opponent, the neurophysiologist

Charles Sherrington, but in the event neither was successful, the post going to Francis Gotch. Then, when Gotch died in 1913, Sherrington and Haldane re-applied and the former was successful. This resulted in Haldane resigning from his position as Reader, and he left the department to continue his research in a makeshift laboratory in his garden shed. There he called on the long suffering members of his family to act as subjects—notably his son Jack.[3]

JS Haldane's counterpart at Cambridge was Joseph Barcroft, who graduated in physiology and biochemistry at Cambridge in 1896,

and spent the rest of his long career in the physiology department there; he was made its Director in 1925. He began with studies of oxygen uptake and carbon dioxide production in an isolated tissue, the salivary gland of the dog, demonstrating increases in metabolism during secretion of saliva. The studies required meticulous gas analysis in small blood samples, leading him to contact Haldane, and in 1902 they published a paper jointly on their method, which employed methods to liberate oxygen and carbon dioxide from whole blood, followed by quantitative analysis of the evolved gases, in samples as small as 1 ml. Barcroft was a lifelong admirer of Bohr, although when it came to theories of oxygen secretion in the lung, he realized that August Krogh had got it right, and he parted company with the concept held by Bohr and Haldane. Barcroft explored the problems related to the shape of the dissociation curve and the controversy over oxygen secretion, and after some years of painstaking but often frustrating work, he was able to ascribe them to differences in methods, and in particular to the conditions, such as temperature and acidity that existed in the sample at the time of analysis. Barcroft's papers, unlike most of those that we read today, do not shy away from telling it like it is—"It was clear that we had found our way into the morass in which our predecessors had already floundered so hopelessly, and our newer and more certain methods instead of saving us from their embarrassments had only made the uncertainty of our position more certain".

However, the meticulous work eventually led to standardization of methods, and the important finding that the curve was shifted to the right by both temperature and acidity—adding these two factors to the effect of increasing carbon dioxide pressure.[4] We are now in a position to

3   JBS Haldane took part in his father's experiments from the age of 4, and carried on his work, and tradition, in diving physiology through the second World War, when safe methods of escape from submarines were needed. Later, he made great contributions to genetics and many other aspects of human biology; he became a staunch Marxist, writing regularly for the British communist newspaper the Daily Worker, eventually becoming its editorial board chairman.

18 A final factor was added in 1967, independently by

summarize why hemoglobin is such a wonderful protein- the *essenza mirabile*- its characteristics promote uptake of oxygen in the lungs where oxygen pressure is high and PCO_2, temperature and acidity are low, compared to the tissues (where PO_2 is low, but PCO_2, temperature and acidity are high) when oxygen is released. Barcroft realized the huge importance of hemoglobin's characteristics to human adaptability to different environments and stresses- "But for its existence, man might never have attained any activity which the lobster does not possess, or had he done so, it would have been in the body as minute as a fly."

THE STRUCTURE OF HEMOGLOBIN

Hemoglobin is the best understood complex protein, not least because it was the first to be crystallized and have its chemical composition established (Hoppe-Seyler), and to be analyzed spectroscopically (von Hüfner and Stokes); the two main parts of the molecule, the iron-containing haem and the large protein globulin, were thereby recognized. Then its structure was worked out by a string of future Nobel Laureates- Hans Fischer succeeded in synthesizing a haem molecule identical to that obtained from hemoglobin in 1927; Linus Pauling worked out the secondary (atomic) structure of haem and the helical arrangement of the peptide chains of the globulin part; finally,

the quaternary (3-dimensional) structure that accounts for hemoglobin's marvelous properties was revealed by the X-ray crystallographic studies of Max Ferdinand Perutz and his colleagues at the University of Cambridge in 1959. These three were awarded the Nobel Prize in 1930, 1954 and 1962, respectively; their work had great implications in biological science, especially for the mechanisms of enzyme activity, and ran parallel to the elucidation of DNAs structure.

Hemoglobin's functional characteristics are explained by its structure. It contains four haem molecules, each of which contains an iron atom in its ferrous (Fe^{2+}) form; each haem is embedded in a long folded peptide chain, the whole assuming an almost spherical form. The chains are identical in composition but differ in their amino acid sequencing, leading to different bonding between them, and thus to changes in the angles between them. This is the secret behind the S-shape of the dissociation curve.

Four different types of hemoglobin peptide chains are recognized (α, β, γ and δ) which are capable of conferring different dissociation curves, but the normal adult type contains two α and two β chains.[5]

In 1970, Perutz showed that as deoxygenated hemoglobin takes on oxygen, the first binding sites are in the heme of the α chain; in so doing hydrogen bonds are broken to increase the affinity of the β chains for oxygen: the hemoglobin changes from a "tight" to a "relaxed" state. Associated with

---

Reinhold and Ruth Benesch at Columbia University in New York City, and Alfred Chanutin and Richard Curnish at the University of Virginia; the organic phosphate 2,3-diphosphoglycerate (2,3-DPG) formed from glucose becomes attached to the hemoglobin molecule, making itless able to take up oxygen.. Specific enzymes in the red cell control 2,3-DPG concentration, influenced by chronic changes in oxygen content (such as at altitude and in anemia) and the acidity of blood (such as in diabetes).

---

5 For example, the hemoglobin found before birth (fetal type) contains two α and two δ chains, associated with a curve that aids loading of oxygen at low oxygen pressure. It is replaced with the adult type soon after birth.

this change is an increase in the acid strength of hemoglobin as it takes up more hydrogen ions (oxyhemoglobin is a stronger acid than deoxyhemoglobin). Finally the hemoglobin becomes fully oxygenated when about 97% of the oxygen carrying sites have become filled. When oxyhemoglobin reaches the tissues, where oxygen pressure is low and acidity high, the processes reverse; oxygen is rapidly released, and hydrogen ions are "buffered" by the weaker acid of the deoxygenated form.

Before leaving hemoglobin we will mention myoglobin, the oxygen carrying pigment present in muscle. As long ago as 1678, Lorenzini noted that there was a great variation in the redness of muscles in the rabbit, and Kühne, who made several contributions to the discovery of hemoglobin, in 1865 showed that differences in colour were not due to blood; he washed blood out of muscle and found a hemoglobin-like pigment remained in the actual muscle fibres. A lot more work led to the discovery that the pigment consisted of a heme molecule buried in a single α chain, and it was named myoglobin; its dissociation curve was shown to be much steeper than hemoglobin. Myoglobin reaches its oxygen capacity at low oxygen pressure; whereas hemoglobin is only 20% saturated at an oxygen pressure of 20 mm Hg, myoglobin is 90% saturated at the same pressure. Because of this characteristic it mops up oxygen very avidly and rapidly (at least ten times as fast as hemoglobin), acting to increase the oxygen content of tissues, such as muscle, even when PO_2 is low. Myoglobin thus acts as a store for oxygen in muscle, making it available at times when its consumption exceeds its supply, for example at the start of heavy exercise.

The characteristics of the oxyhemoglobin dissociation curve become very important in situations where oxygen is in short supply and oxygen requirements are high; the climbing of high mountains obviously couples these two factors, so we will leave further discussion of the curve for later, when destination Everest will force us to think more about it.

BLOOD CARBON DIOXIDE

Traditionally, the supply of oxygen to tissues has assumed a dominant role in the maintenance of function, but a case may be made for the importance of carbon dioxide. Because it is a gas that is produced by metabolism, the balance between metabolism and breathing is crucial to the amount existing in the body. Also as carbon dioxide acts as an acid when dissolved in water, there are many potential effects of both increasing and lowering its pressure in blood, from brain blood flow, through kidney function to the activity of nerves, muscles and even the enzymes involved in biochemical reactions. This makes the carriage of carbon dioxide by blood an important topic; the mechanisms that have evolved allow man to lead a far more active life than primitive organisms.

Although Boyle and Lower had shown that roughly equal amounts of oxygen were used and carbon dioxide produced during combustion and respiration, it was Lavoisier and his colleague Séguin who demonstrated and quantified the finding in man. Then, Lothar Meyer showed that equal amounts of oxygen were taken up and carbon dioxide given off as blood passed from the venous to the arterial side of the lungs. The amount of both gases was much greater than expected from their solubility in water, indicating that both were carried in combination. Furthermore, it became clear that blood carried at least twice as much carbon dioxide as oxygen, but there was much argument through the 19th century as to how it was carried; how much in the red blood cells, plasma, and in simple solution.

Gustav Magnus in 1837 thought CO_2 was carried in free solution, but twenty years later Lothar Meyer found that only part of the CO_2 was released when blood was subjected to a vacuum, the rest requiring treatment with acid. It was left to Nathan Zuntz to show in 1867 that red blood cells contained a lot of CO_2 and that plasma obtained from whole blood samples equilibrated with CO_2 at a given pressure contained more CO_2 than plasma alone which had been exposed to CO_2; thus, the red cells helped to carry more CO_2 not only combined with hemoglobin, but also because the red cells allowed more to be carried in plasma. Zuntz was a disciple of Pflüger, for many years acting as his assistant in Bonn; he was an extremely able experimenter in physiology, devising a portable apparatus capable of measuring oxygen uptake during exercise. He was the first to make such measurements at altitude and during sport activity; both these topics will feature in later chapters.

CARBON DIOXIDE, CARBONIC ACID AND BICARBONATE[6]

It was not until 1921 that the Danish chemist Carl Faurholt, professor in the College of Pharmacy in Copenhagen discovered that when CO_2 enters water it forms carbonic acid (H_2CO_3), or bicarbonate ion (HCO_3^-), depending on the ionic conditions—

$$CO_2 + H_2O \rightarrow H_2CO_3$$

or
$$CO_2 + OH^- \rightarrow HCO_3^-$$

Faurholt also established that the reaction was slow, and also that when the first reaction

occurred only about 1/1000 of the CO_2 appeared as H_2CO_3. His findings were picked up by physiologists who had to explain how such a slow reaction, known as the hydration of CO_2, could possibly deal with all the CO_2 produced by metabolism so that it could be transported to the lungs. Oscar Michael Henriques, a young physician working in the state Serum Institute in Copenhagen measured the rate at which CO_2 escaped from serum alone and from serum containing red cells. In 1924 he reported that half the CO_2 was liberated in 2 minutes from serum, but in only 5 seconds from samples containing red cells, and he concluded that CO_2 must be carried in blood in a similar way to O_2, bound loosely to hemoglobin. However, others theorized that the dramatic increase in rate must indicate a catalyst was present in the red cell, and in 1932 two Cambridge chemists, Norman Urquhart Meldrum and Francis John Worsley Roughton, demonstrated its presence, naming it carbonic anhydrase. Roughton, a direct descendent of William Harvey, had already worked in Joseph Barcroft's laboratory on the rate at which O_2 combined with hemoglobin, finding it incredibly fast. Two other Cambridge chemists, David Keilin and Taddeus Mann went on to establish the enzyme's structure, showing in 1940 that an atom of zinc was essential for its function, and that its action could be inhibited by sulphonamides. Although carbonic anhydrase is absent in plasma, it was subsequently found in a variety of tissues where rapid CO_2 exchange occurred—such as the stomach, kidney and muscle capillaries. Roughton calculated that the carbonic anhydrase in red cells accelerated the hydration of CO_2 about 13,000 times; the increase can be shown in the elementary experiment of dropping a minute amount of blood into soda water and watching the stream of bubbles come from it.

---

6   A colleague recently remarked that some students wondered why it is bicarbonate, and I don't know. It should be hydrogen carbonate: perhaps it is just laziness, it doesn't have anything to do with 2.

THE CO$_2$ "DISSOCIATION" CURVE

A final experiment needs to be mentioned before we put the story of CO$_2$ transport together. Johanne Ostenfeld Christiansen was a young Danish trainee who in 1909 went from Copenhagen to work towards her thesis in JS Haldane's laboratory in Oxford; she found herself working with the two dominant physiologists there, Haldane himself and Claude Gordon Douglas, an expert in exercise physiology. Under their direction she measured the relationship between the amount of CO$_2$ and its pressure in blood, its "dissociation curve".

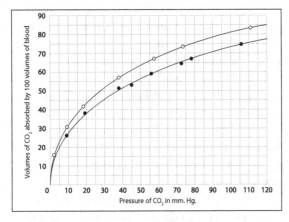

Figure 16 The 1914 graph of Christiansen, showing a greater amount of CO2 is carried in deoxygenated (upper curve) compared to oxygenated blood (Haldane's blood).

Although the technical difficulties inherent in these measurements was appreciable, she was able to show that oxygenated blood carried less CO$_2$ than the deoxygenated form, at any given pressure; the effect was large enough to account for much of the CO$_2$ leaving blood as it flowed from the venous to arterial side of the lungs. The paper describing the results was published in 1914, with Christiansen as first author; ever since, the effect has been known as the Christiansen-Douglas-Haldane (C-D-H) effect, but also, more commonly as "the Haldane effect". When Johanne Christiansen came to defend her thesis in Copenhagen, she was criticized by the senior examiner for being the first author on the paper, and it has been taken as a measure of Haldane's chivalry and generosity; this may be true, although in those days the Journal of Physiology required authors to appear in alphabetical order.[7]

CARBON DIOXIDE TRANSPORT.

We are now ready to put the story of CO$_2$ transport together; let's start with blood flowing through the tissues, where it is exposed to an increased CO$_2$ pressure (PCO$_2$), and low PO$_2$; hemoglobin rapidly becomes deoxygenated and thus less acid, binding to CO2 in the red cell. CO2 pressure is lowered, and CO2 rapidly diffuses into the red cell, where its hydration to carbonic acid is catalyzed by carbonic anhydrase. Carbonic acid is unstable, and splits into bicarbonate and hydrogen ions; the process is described by the reaction—

$$CO_2 + H_2O \rightarrow H_2CO_3 \rightarrow H^+ + HCO_3^-$$

The hydrogen ions combine with the amino acid histidine on the (less strongly acidic) reduced hemoglobin—

$$(Hb)\text{-}N + H^+ \rightarrow (Hb)\text{-}NH^+$$

thus allowing the bicarbonate concentration [HCO$_3^-$] to increase. At the same time CO$_2$ combines with amino acid groups on hemoglobin to form a "carbamino" compound—

7   There is no doubt of CG Douglas's generosity, however, in the case of an important paper on lactic acid production in exercise when he removed himself from authorship, so that his New Zealand pupil J. Harding Owles would gain first credit for the work.

$$(Hb)\text{-}NH_2 + CO_2 \rightarrow (Hb)\text{-}NHCOO^- + H^+$$

and again the hydrogen ions may be buffered by histidine. These reactions result in a potential move to the alkaline side of equilibrium and in so doing they activate a chloride (Cl^-) channel, allowing chloride to move into the red cell, and lowering the chloride concentration in plasma, in turn favoring movement of bicarbonate from the red cell. This process is known as the "chloride shift" or the "Hamburger effect" (after the Dutch physiologist Hartog Jacob Hamburger, who described the effect in 1902). The only problem with this mechanism is that it is relatively slow; its "half time" is 15 seconds, which means that during exercise it will not be complete by the time blood reaches the lungs; more critically, the reverse reaction cannot reach completion during the time blood is in the lungs (about 1 sec).

The end result of these complex, interrelated and coexisting reactions is that blood takes on CO_2 in both the red cell and plasma as it passes from the arterial to the venous side of the tissues; a small amount of the increase (about 7%) is due to dissolved CO_2 and H_2CO_3; 60% is carried as HCO_3^- in plasma, 8% as HCO_3^- in red cells, and 25% as a carbamino compound with hemoglobin. The "punch line" is that most is carried in plasma as bicarbonate, and that in the absence of red cells this amount would not exceed 10%. Teleology may be allowed to rear its head here: we have evolved a system in which the oxygen carrying protein also provides a mechanism for CO_2 carriage. The ways in which the two gases are carried by hemoglobin are quite different: oxygen binds to a specific site related to iron (ferrous Fe^{2+}) ions, whereas CO_2 is carried in relation to amino acids. The carriage of some CO_2 in association with hemoglobin in the red cell protects tissues from big swings in acidity.

When venous blood reaches the lungs, reverse reactions take place; rapid oxygen uptake converts reduced hemoglobin to its oxygenated form, and it becomes a stronger acid; carbon dioxide is released from the carbamino compound and H^+ ions are also released. Carbonic acid is formed rapidly and red cell CO_2 pressure increases to drive CO_2 out of the cell and plasma into the lung alveoli—

$$H^+ + HCO_3^- \rightarrow H_2CO_3 \rightarrow CO_2 + H_2O$$

Conceptually, the transport of CO_2 from the tissues where it is produced to the lungs where it is eliminated, is simple. The whole process is driven by pressure differences; the tissue PCO_2 is greater than the PCO_2 of arterial blood, and venous blood PCO_2 is greater than the PCO_2 in alveolar gas. However, when we come to express the process quantitatively we find two factors that complicate matters. First, as we have seen, the blood oxygen saturation influences the amount of CO_2 carried (and the PCO_2 influences the O_2 saturation). And second, the acidity (concentration of H^+ ions) influences, and is influenced by, the PCO_2.

GAS TRANSFER IN THE LUNG

In the early part of the 20th century, the leading researchers in the field of lung gas exchange, were the Danish couple, August Steenberg Krogh and his wife (a former student of his) Birthe Marie Jørgensen. Working in Christian Bohr's laboratory in Copenhagen, the Kroghs reported refinements in the measurement of oxygen pressure in blood, and showed that pressure of O_2 in arterial blood was always less than in alveolar air; the findings were published in 1910 as seven short papers that the Kroghs nicknamed "the seven small devils". In the last of these, August Krogh apologized for having "to combat the views of my teacher Prof. Bohr on certain essential points"—after all, he was putting the topic of oxygen secretion in the lung, strongly held by Christian Bohr in Copenhagen and also John Scott Haldane in Oxford, finally to rest. Krogh goes on to acknowledge "the debt of gratitude" he owed to his teacher, and everyone owed to him, for the advances in knowledge made by him in the field "due to his labours and to the refinement of methods which he has introduced"—a touching and fitting tribute, the like of which is never seen in drier present day publications. August Krogh became Denmark's foremost physiologist, and was awarded a Nobel Prize in 1920 for his work on the regulation of blood flow through capillaries. Marie Krogh also made an exceptional contribution to lung gas exchange in 1915; she used gas mixtures containing small concentrations of carbon monoxide in a method for measuring gaseous diffusion into the lungs that continues to be used to this day. Carbon monoxide is taken up by hemoglobin at least as well as oxygen, and may be easily measured. Oxygen diffusion could be derived from the known molecular differences between O_2 and CO. Marie Krogh showed that the lungs' diffusing capacity increased with exercise.

VENTILATION-PERFUSION RATIO

During the Second World War it became important to understand what happened to lung gas exchange at altitude and during sudden decompression experienced by airmen. Highly talented physiologists were recruited to specialized research laboratories, such as the Royal Air Force Research Establishment at Farnborough, England, and the U.S. Naval School of Aviation Medicine in Pensacola, Florida. These groups brought modern analytical methods and sophisticated mathematics to bear on many topics related to the lungs, addressing such questions as what happens to atmospheric

pressure as altitude increases, and what factors influence the pressure of oxygen and carbon dioxide in arterial blood.

What was already known by the 1940's? It was known that oxygen uptake and carbon dioxide output in the lungs were driven by oxygen consumption and carbon dioxide production in the tissues, and pulmonary blood flow—cardiac output—also increased in parallel with these metabolic demands. Alveolar ventilation also increased, so that an equal amount of oxygen left the alveoli as entered the capillaries, and vice versa for carbon dioxide. It was known that gases moved between these two "compartments" according to pressure differences, acting in both the smaller airways to move gases to and from the alveoli and across the alveolo-capillary barrier. And, as Dr. Willis had pointed out in the 17th century and quoted at the start of this chapter, the efficiency of gas exchange depended crucially on an even distribution of alveolar gas to capillary blood flow through the lung. Any amount of ventilation would not be of any use if there was no blood flow to the same part of the lung. Similarly, lots of blood flow in a poorly ventilated area would add blood that was relatively unchanged from its venous state to the rest of the lung blood flow. These relationships became known as ventilation-perfusion matching (or mismatching).

Dr Richard L. Riley and his colleagues, first at Bellevue Hospital in New York and later at the U.S. Naval School of Aviation Medicine in Pensacola, set about clarifying the mathematics inherent in these complex relationships, no mean task in the era before computers. In a series of papers in the *Journal of Applied Physiology* between 1945 and 1950, the theory was set out beautifully in a set of equations and graphs. Riley's elegant work represented a great advance: he was one of a number of physicians who were

54

"turned on" to respiratory medicine at the time, because he had contracted pulmonary tuberculosis as a medical student. Treatment consisted mainly of resting at home and he later observed "never was enforced confinement given more profitable psychotherapy". Riley proposed that as the lung alveoli received inspired air, expressed as alveolar ventilation (V_A), and venous blood through capillary blood flow (Q_c), and because the amount of oxygen entering the lung's capillaries had to equal that leaving alveolar gas (and *vice versa* for carbon dioxide), all combinations of O_2 and CO_2 in the alveoli and capillaries could be calculated. Further, the combinations in any part of the lung depended on the ratio of ventilation to perfusion in (V_A/Q_c). Areas with a high V_A/Q_c contained gas and

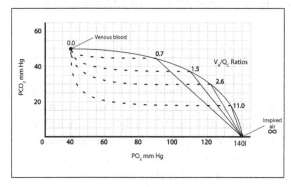

Figure 17 Riley's O2/CO2 diagram, showing the alveolar gas pressures in areas of the lungs having differing ventilation - perfusion (V_A/Q_c) ratios.

blood with low PCO_2 and high PO_2; and areas with a low V_A/Q_c had a high PCO_2 and low PO_2. The relationships were elegantly presented in a graph, the "O_2/CO_2 Diagram", in which all possible V_A/Q_c ratios fell on a curve that extended from the venous blood composition (v) to inspired air (I). These two extremes represented the effect of areas with a V_A/Q_c of zero (areas receiving no ventilation but still perfused with blood) and infinity (areas being ventilated but with no blood flow) respectively,

and the intervening values on the curve (in Figure 17 - V_A/Q_c ratios of 0.7, 1.5, 2.0 and 11.0 are shown) demonstrate the different effects that V_A/Q_c ratios have on the oxygen (PO_2) and carbon dioxide (PCO_2) pressures. The approach was published in 1949, in two papers, one by Hermann Rahn in Buffalo and the other by Dick Riley and André Cournand of New York, and represented a huge advance in our understanding of the effects of variations in V_A/Q_c on the efficiency of gas exchange, the effects of disease on function, the effects of altitude and exercise and other aspects of lung function. To those who, like myself, were struggling to understand the apparent complexities of lung function, there came a sense of revelation together with awe at the intellectual power of the analysis.

Riley went on to develop the "three compartment lung model", a simplified analysis that allowed the efficiency of lung gas exchange to be applied to clinical medicine. The analysis used measurements of lung exchange of O_2 and CO_2 and of the arterial pressures of the two gases, to describe the lung <u>as if</u> it were composed of three compartments—an "ideal" compartment in which <u>all</u> gas exchange took place, and two other compartments in which <u>no</u> gas exchange occurred—a "dead space" compartment, ventilated but not perfused with blood (V_A/Q_c of infinity) and a "venous admixture" compartment that was perfused but not ventilated (V_A/Q_c of zero).

The key measurement needed for the three compartment analysis was the arterial partial pressure of CO_2. Long before, in 1889, Christian Bohr had suggested that <u>arterial</u> PCO_2 represented the average alveolar PCO_2 because CO_2 was relatively unaffected by mismatching

55

SYMBOLS

Scientists have evolved a system of symbols, a sort of shorthand that they use particularly to identify measurements. This chapter contains several, so it may be a good place to demystify them.

The symbols are used in a set order—

First comes the *function* being measured—V, volume or ventilation; P, pressure; Q, blood flow; S, saturation..

Second comes *where*—this is added as a subscript, Such as V_A, alveolar ventilation; P_a, arterial pressure; Q_c capillary blood flow. Often omitted, if it's obvious or stated in full (eg "arterial PO_2".)

Third comes *what* is measured, such as O_2 or CO_2. Thus P_ACO_2 refers to alveolar carbon dioxide pressure.

Finally comes the measurement and unit; thus an arterial oxygen pressure of 100 millimetres of mercury is expressed as P_aO_2 100 mmHg.

of ventilation to perfusion.[8] Knowing the alveolar PCO_2 means that the "ideal" alveolar PO_2 may be calculated and compared to the measured arterial PO_2; if the lung behaved perfectly, or "ideally", the two would be the same (an "alveolo-arterial PO_2 difference" of zero); the extent to which arterial PO_2 is lower than the alveolar value reflects the "venous admixture" compartment.

8   The reason for this is not intuitively apparent, but is due to the CO2 dissociation curve, which compared to oxygen is steep (a large change in content for a given pressure change); in spite of the fact that the change in content is roughly the same, PCO2 in venous blood is 46 mmHg, and in arterial blood 40 mmHg, but for oxygen the corresponding figures are 40 and 100. This means that if venous blood bypasses gas exchanging alveoli the result will be a much lower PO2 with little change in PCO2.

The three compartment lung analysis satisfied everyone in the 1950s, but with the advent of computers more elegant analysis was possible. A leader in this field was John Burnard West, who began extensive work on ventilation-perfusion (or V_A/Q_c) relationships at the Royal Postgraduate Medical School at the Hammersmith Hospital in London, and later at the University of California in San Diego, with his Australian compatriot Peter D. Wagner. John was already working in the Respiratory group at "the Hammersmith" with Philip Hugh-Jones when I became a clinical registrar (senior resident) there in 1961. We were all housed in a wooden "outhouse" attached to the Hospital—the "lower medical corridor"; a ramshackle edifice that doubtless would be banned as a site of clinical investigation nowadays, but then housed the most up-to-date investigational equipment. John and Philip might both be classed as "Renaissance Men"—John was preparing for a Himalayan expedition (The "Silver Hut" expedition of 1961 on the Mingbo glacier, 12 miles from Everest), and Philip was shortly off on a dangerous expedition into the Bolivian jungle. They used the newly developed respiratory mass spectrometer to study variations in gas exchange, and later employed radioactive oxygen and carbon dioxide to expand their findings. The exposure to brilliant and innovative research was an extraordinary experience that would influence the rest of my career.

Most disorders of lung function, due to pneumonia or asthma for example, lead to changes in the V_A/Q_c ratio in different parts of the lungs, whose effect may be quantified with the "three compartment" analysis. However, it may come as a surprise that regional differences in V_A/Q_c also occur in the normal lung; surely the way the lung is constructed will lead to uniform ventilation and blood flow? Well, no; the lung is the only internal organ that is exposed directly to the atmosphere, and more importantly, to atmospheric pressure. This means that the lung and its blood are directly exposed to gravity. The weight of the lung leads to alveoli at the top (or apex) of the lung to be more expanded than those at the bottom (or base), as described in the first (1858) edition of Henry Gray's *Anatomy*. We used to teach this concept with the use of a "slinky", the coiled steel toy that performs tricks like descending a flight of stairs in an almost purposeful way. Hold one end of a slinky and raise it a foot or two and the coils become widely separated at the top, and successively less towards the bottom; the weight acting on the upper coils is greater than on the lower, leading them to be stretched farther apart. The effect in the lung is that—perhaps counter-intuitively—during breathing the alveoli at the base expanded relatively more than those at the apex, which are already partly expanded even before the

breath commences. Similarly, blood in the lung circulation will only rise to a level equal to the pressure in the pulmonary artery; at rest in the upright position this means that the apical alveoli may not have any blood flowing in their capillaries, and the basal alveoli have more blood than they can handle. Such factors mean that the distribution of V_A/Q_c ratios can vary all the way from zero (perfusion but no ventilation) to infinity (ventilation but no perfusion), even in normal healthy lungs.

Of course, it comes as no surprise that disorders of lung function are associated with profound mismatching between V_A and Q_c, either on a localized or generalized basis. Pneumonia in one lobe of the lung leads to poor or absent ventilation with the affected lobe still being perfused; a blood clot in one of the arteries (a pulmonary embolus) will lead to zero perfusion of the affected segment, but it may still be ventilated. The situation is even more complex because there are localized reflexes that combat these effects; an unventilated area becomes short of oxygen, leading to constriction of small blood vessels and reduction in its blood flow; unperfused alveoli lead to constriction of small airways to limit the ventilation of the affected area. Finally, there are responses that involve the whole respiratory system rather than localized effects in the lung. If there are areas in the lung that are underperfused (high V_A/Q_c) this will lead to a reflex increase in breathing in order to maintain normal blood gases; similarly, the presence of low V_A/Q_c areas in the lung will lead to a reflex increase in total blood flow in an attempt to maintain oxygen delivery to tissues.

In spite of the effects of gravity on the lungs, the distribution of air and blood to them is remarkably even, especially during exercise when breathing and blood flow both increase. However, efficient gas exchange (with minimal "dead space" and "venous admixture") depends on normal airway caliber and alveolar structure and adequate lung blood flow and pressure. Because the lungs are the only vital organs to be in contact with the environment, and because all the body's blood flow passes through them, they are especially prone to damage. The airways and alveoli may be damaged by particles and chemicals in the air, and blood flow and pressure in the lungs are compromised by disorders of the heart and circulation; both alveoli and capillaries may become involved in inflammation secondary to infection and immune reactions.

ALVEOLAR VENTILATION

The upshot of all the factors we have been considering in this chapter, is that the pressures of carbon dioxide (PCO_2) and oxygen (PO_2) are regulated to within quite small ranges in the arterial blood supplying the tissues of healthy (young) subjects both at rest and during exertion. Expressed conventionally in millimeters of mercury (mm Hg), arterial PCO_2 lies between 35 and 45 mm Hg, and arterial PO_2 between 85 and 105 mm Hg—high enough to occupy at least 95% of the oxygen binding sites in the blood's hemoglobin, an oxygen saturation (SaO_2) of 95% or more. Deviations outside these ranges are basically due to three factors—changes in inspired air (such as at altitude), changes in alveolar ventilation, and mismatching between alveolar ventilation and capillary blood flow (V_A/Q_c). A fourth factor related to incomplete gas diffusion between alveoli and capillary blood has been debated for decades, but for simplicity is usually "lumped" with V_A/Q_c mismatch, because its effect is mainly to influence blood oxygen. The effects of altitude may be left for the moment, but we should briefly consider the other two factors, even

if it is at the risk of repeating the previous discussion.

Changes in alveolar ventilation are quantitatively reflected in the arterial PCO_2—a doubling of ventilation reduces PCO_2 by half (i.e. from 40 to 20 mm Hg); this is hyperventilation, brought about by the respiratory control mechanisms (as a response to low oxygen pressure, or as a panic effect, for example). Similarly reductions in ventilation are associated with increases in PCO_2—halve ventilation and you will double PCO_2 (to 80 mm Hg); this is termed hypoventilation, although "underbreathing" might be safer, to avoid confusion with its same-sounding but opposite "hyperventilation". So long as the lungs are normal, the changes in PCO_2 are accompanied by changes in PO_2 that are quantitatively similar but opposite in direction—a 20 mmHg fall in PCO_2 from 40 to 20 mmHg is accompanied by a 20 mmHg rise in PO_2 from 100 to 120 mmHg, and vice versa.

Our knowledge of the gas exchange process in the lungs began with the necessarily crude anatomical observations of Marcello Malpighi and the intuitive ideas of Thomas Willis and proceeded through increasingly precise anatomical observations and mathematical treatment of the variation in ventilation of the alveoli and their perfusion with blood, to our present day understanding of ventilation/perfusion relationships. Even the normal lung does not behave in an "ideal" way, because the effects of gravity lead to a wide range in the relation between ventilation and perfusion. In the normal lung these effects have little impact on the efficiency with which the lungs take up oxygen from, and release carbon dioxide into the alveoli. Disorders of lung function impair this efficiency, leading to reductions in the oxygen saturation of arterial blood and to a need for greater ventilation to clear carbon dioxide. Furthermore, during increased oxygen demands, for example during exercise, the normal lung becomes more efficient, whereas in the diseased lung the situation worsens, leading to falls in blood oxygen saturation and increases in breathing.

CHAPTER 5

HOW BREATHING HELPS TO CONTROL OUR "INTERNAL ENVIRONMENT"

"The stability of the milieu intérieur is the primary condition for freedom and independence of existence..."

Claude Bernard, 1859.

"The principle enunciated by Claude Bernard, if dressed up in modern language, seems to me to be just a little grotesque...The accuracy of the first clause contrasts almost comically with the vagueness of the second."

Sir Joseph Barcroft, Features in the Architecture of Physiological Function, 1934.

"Two chemical individuals stand alone in importance for the great biological cycle upon the earth. The one is water, the other carbon dioxide."

Lawrence Joseph Henderson, The Fitness of the Environment, 1913.

The principle of the constancy of the internal environment is one of the major tenets of modern physiology, just as Claude Bernard is acknowledged as its Father. Almost a century later, Bernard is being taken to task by Barcroft, who as Professor of Physiology at Cambridge fathered major research into hemoglobin structure and function. The point is, what do we take as the internal environment, and how constant does it have to be? The arterial blood plasma gets close to all body cells, so we'll take that to represent the *milieu intérieur*. Blood is the medium used to transport oxygen and carbon dioxide, in sufficient quantity to maintain our metabolism for all our activities. But importantly, our breathing plays a major role in maintaining plasma acidity within acceptable limits. L.J. Henderson was Professor of Physiology at Harvard, was a prolific and innovative researcher and thinker, who laid the foundation for the quantitative description of the systems that control the acid-base balance in blood. In his book *The Fitness of the Environment* he provided an unparalleled description of what we might call "the big picture" in this topic. He understood the links between our internal and external (the ocean and atmosphere) environments, even identifying the main factors contributing to global warming many decades before it became a fashionable *cause célèbre*.

Claude Bernard, France's most celebrated physiologist and the father of clinical physiology, wrote his major work—*An Introduction to the study of Experimental Medicine* in 1865. He pointed out that animals live in two environments, the external—which varies greatly even over short periods of time, and the internal (the *milieu intérieur*)—whose composition must be kept constant within narrow limits, whatever the changes that occur in the external environment. This is the concept of homeostasis. It is worth reflecting that the only external environment that remains relatively constant is in the ocean, and that the composition of sea-water is similar to that of the fluids that make up the internal environment. In evolution, the sea was the only environment that could provide the constant chemical state needed to allow primitive organisms to survive, even though they had not yet developed mechanisms to combat environmental changes. Comparison of the relative proportions of major constituents of sea-water and the body fluids of widely different organisms, shows a remarkable agreement—not really surprising when we consider that life originated in the primeval soup of oceans. In terms of constancy, what is important is the ionic composition. Humphry Davy's pupil Michael Faraday introduced the term "ion" in 1834, after their experiments in which electric currents were passed through solutions of salts, to designate the particles that migrated to the positive and negative terminals of Alessandro Volta's battery. The electrode to which different particles migrated (either + or -) not only identified their charge, but also their designation as acids or bases according to their ability to generate hydrogen ions (H^+)—acids—or hydroxyl ions (OH^-)—bases. Water contains both of these ions, but is present in the body almost completely in its combined form (H_2O), making it the most important chemical player that determines the ionic state of the internal environment.

The physico-chemical implications of ionic dissociation were first advanced by a trio of geniuses who were all awarded Nobel prizes in the early years of the 20th century—Svante August Arrhenius, Wilhelm Ostwald and Jakobus Hendricus van't Hoff. Van't Hoff was a distinguished Dutch chemist who made an intuitive leap by concluding that Boyle's Law relating pressure and volume of gases might be applied to ions in solution, where the osmotic pressure is proportional to concentration. He thought of this effect as being exerted through dissolved molecules and their attraction to water, with water moving across semi-permeable membranes. These ideas were transmitted to the Swedish Academy of Medicine in 1885. Previously, in 1883 and at the age of 24,

Arrhenius had presented his thesis at the University of Uppsala on the conduction of electricity by electrolytes in solution. Shortly after he visited van't Hoff and Ostwald, and learning of their work, proposed a theory of electrolyte dissociation which was published in 1887. Arrhenius made many contributions to both chemistry and physics, and was the first to predict that the widespread combustion of fossil fuels would inevitably lead to an increase in CO_2 in the earth's atmosphere with climatic effects, the prime concern of present-day environmentalists. Ostwald, born of German parents who later emigrated to Russia, studied chemistry at the technical college in Riga. He wrote his doctoral his thesis on the chemical reactions between acids and bases and this earned him a chair of chemistry there. A few years later he was appointed professor in Leipzig, where he developed a remarkable department that garnered several Nobel prizes. The work of these three scientists led to a theory of ionic dissociation, whereby electrolytes split when dissolved in water into their component electrically charged ions. The extent to which they split, or dissociate, may lead to increases in hydrogen (H^+) or hydroxyl ion (OH^-) concentrations depending on whether they act as acids or bases, respectively. Strong acids and bases are completely dissociated; for example hydrochloric acid (HCl) in solution exists only as H^+ and Cl^-; and sodium hydroxide similarly exists only as Na^+ and OH^-. Salts that are combinations of strong acids and bases (such as sodium chloride, NaCl) will in solution exist as their component strong ions (Na^+ and Cl^- in this example), rather than in the combined form. Weak acids and bases (such as the amino acids that form proteins), on the other hand, exist in the partly dissociated state in aqueous solution; as explained below, because they are only partly dissociated they are able to combine with H^+

or OH⁻, and thus act as "buffers" to minimize changes in acidity.

Ionic reactions obey three basic physico-chemical laws—of Conservation of Mass (discovered by Lavoisier, and enabling chemical reactions to be measured in balance-sheet form), Electrical Neutrality (in water, the sum of the positive charges always equal the negative charges), and the Law of Mass Action (which governs the ratios between reactants).

The key to understanding the reactions, and the importance of water to living systems, is to consider its dissociation.

WATER, AND ITS DISSOCIATION CONSTANT

Water (H_2O) exists mainly in its tightly bound form, but it provides a huge reservoir of H^+ and OH^- ions, as expressed by the chemical reaction—

$$H_2O \rightarrow H^+ + OH^-$$

In pure water, as no other ions are present, the concentrations $[H^+]$ and $[OH^-]$ are equal, maintaining neutrality, and are very small. At room temperature, only 1 gram of each exists in 10,000,000 litres of water; their concentration is 1/10,000,000; there are 7 zeros here—in mathematical notation 10^{-7}. The "dissociation constant" of water (Kw) is small, as defined by the Law of Mass Action—

$$[H^+] \times [OH^-] = 1 \times 10^{-14}$$

This expression means that in an aqueous solution $[H^+] \times [OH^-]$ always has to equal 10^{-14}, and that in pure water $[H^+]$ (and OH^-]) is 10^{-7} equivalents (Eq) or ions, per litre (l); both these facts are helpful in understanding and calculating the effects of different ions that enter the solution.[1] For example, if we add 100 Eq (10^2) of a strong base, such as caustic soda (NaOH) to a litre of water, then

$$[H^+] + [Na^+] = [OH^-]$$

as $[Na^+]$ is 10^2 Eq/l, and because

$$[H^+] \times [OH^-] = 10^{-14}$$

$[H^+]$ will fall to 10^{-9} and $[OH^-]$ will increase to 10^{-5} ; the solution is alkaline because $[OH^-]$ exceeds $[H^+]$.

Dealing with large numbers of decimal places is difficult, so two conventions were adopted. The first introduced units to deal with the numbers, such as centi- for 10^{-2} (as in centimeter, cm), and 10^{-6} is "milli" (m); 10^{-9} was denoted "nano". Thus 1 x 10^{-9} equals 1 nanoequivalent (nEq), and 1 x 10^{-7} equals 100 mEq. In pure water the "neutral" concentration of hydrogen ions is 100 nEq/l. The second convention was introduced by the Danish scientist Søren Peter Lauritz Sørensen, who after training as a physician, followed a career in biochemistry, becoming the head of the prestigious Carlsberg laboratory in Copenhagen. He became a foremost authority on enzyme activity (so important in brewing Carlsberg beer), which is greatly influenced by changes in hydrogen ion concentration. To simplify handling the small concentrations, Sørensen introduced the concept of the "hydrogen ion exponent" expressed as "pH", where "p" denotes the negative power of $[H^+]$. Thus an $[H^+]$ of 10^{-7} is denoted as a pH of 7. This is all well and good, but in some ways many people find it difficult to understand

---

1   This value applies at a temperature of 22 Celsius, and changes predictably with changes in temperature and some other physical properties.

the implications that changes in pH, say from 7.4 to 8.0, have for changes in [H$^+$]. This was brought home to me many years ago when Moran Campbell, with whom I was working at the Royal Postgraduate Medical School, set what he termed a simple problem, for attendees at the weekly "Grand Rounds". He asked "What will the final pH be, if the hydrogen ion concentration doubles from its normal value at a pH of 7.4?" From the couple of hundred at the meeting, representing the cream of academic trainees and their mentors, only seven correct answers were obtained.[2] However, the pH notation is firmly fixed in many sciences, and is used as a measure of hydrogen ion activity to a far greater extent than [H$^+$] in medical science; that said, I will use both values where necessary.

"STRONG" ACIDS AND BASES

Turning now to strong acids and bases, which exist in solution only as their constituent ions, if we add the same number of molecules of each, no change in pH will occur; for example, if we add equimolecular amounts of hydrochloric acid and caustic soda we will end up with

$$NaOH + HCl = Na^+ + Cl^- + H^+ + OH^-$$

Although a mixture of two deadly liquids, the end product is an innocuous drink having a pH of 7, because [H$^+$] = [OH$^-$]. If, on the other hand, unequal amounts of NaOH and HCl are mixed, there will be a change in pH. In blood plasma [Na$^+$] is 140 mEq/l, and [Cl$^-$] 100 mEq/l; if these ions existed alone in the solution, the difference would be made up with OH$^-$, in a

concentration of 40 mEq/l. Of course, there are other ions in plasma, so [OH$^-$] is not normally in that concentration. Other strong ions in plasma are in much lower concentration than sodium and chloride—the positively charged calcium (Ca^{2+}), magnesium (Mg^{2+}) and potassium (K$^+$); and negatively charged sulphate (SO$_4^{2-}$), carbonate (CO$_3^{2-}$) and lactate (La$^-$); these ions do not change their concentrations much in health, although lactate may increase to as much as 25 mEq/l during severe exercise.

"WEAK" ACIDS AND BASES

Weak acids and bases are only partly dissociated, to an extent expressed in their dissociation constants. For example, the extent to which a weak acid, which we will conventionally designate HA, dissociates into H$^+$ and A$^-$ is expressed in the following way—

$$K_A [HA] = [H^+] \times [A^-]$$

This equation may be rearranged to show that K$_A$ is the [H$^+$] at which [HA] equals [A$^-$]—ie. half the HA has dissociated. This value is usually expressed as pH to obtain "pK".

Because they are only partly dissociated, weak acids have the power to absorb hydrogen ions to increase the concentration of HA; in this way they act as "buffers"—the term indicating the analogy to train buffers absorbing impact.

There are three groups of weak acids that are important in blood—the amino acids that constitute plasma proteins (PPr), the protein molecule of the two forms of hemoglobin, and to a lesser extent phosphates. In normal plasma the proteins have the potential of providing up to about 20 mEq/l of A$^-$. Amino acids can act as acids or bases, depending on their composition and the hydrogen ion concentration of their

63

2　This is not a difficult problem if the pH notation is understood and the logarithm of 2 is known (0.3). We wish to know what 2 x [H+] will be if we start from a pH of 7.4. Start with log 1/[H+] =7.4; then log 1/2[H+] will be 7.4 – log 2, or 7.1.

environment. This property is due to presence of both amino and carboxyl groups; amino groups can take up hydrogen ions when their concentration increases—

$$R\text{-}NH_2 + H^+ \rightarrow R\text{-}NH_3^+$$

and the carboxylic acid groups can release hydrogen ions when their concentration falls—

$$R\text{-}COOH \rightarrow R\text{-}COO^- + H^+$$

The final system to be considered is carbon dioxide, which exists in several forms in blood, of which the largest is the bicarbonate ion (HCO_3^-); smaller amounts are present in simple solution and in combination with amino acids in proteins and hemoglobin (carbamino compounds).

CARBON DIOXIDE, AND THE INFLUENCE OF BREATHING ON HYDROGEN ION CONCENTRATION

So, at last, we come to CO_2, which Lawrence Henderson considered second only to water in importance for the control of both the internal and external environments.

Diabetes has been a serious problem since the earliest times, and became the subject of intense research in the latter half of the 19th century. The clinical picture was recognized to include a comatose state associated with acidic plasma and urine, and deep breathing (termed Kussmaul's breathing after the eminent German physician who described it in 1874). In what was probably the first experimental demonstration of the effectiveness of breathing in the regulation of the body's hydrogen ion concentration ([H^+]), Friedrich Walter gave rabbits dilute hydrochloric acid, and noted that their breathing increased greatly. Walter's studies, conducted in 1877 at the University of Strasbourg, were followed by

many other animal experiments on the effects of various acids and alkalis, and provided a clue as to why breathing is stimulated in patients with severe diabetes.

In 1907, Lawrence Henderson was the first to place the role of CO_2 on a firm theoretical basis, when he modified the "concentration law" (Law of Mass Action), and applied it to the CO_2 system

$$CO_2 + H_2O \rightarrow H_2CO_3 \rightarrow H^+ + HCO_3^-$$

to obtain

$$[H^+] = k \ \times [H_2CO_3] / [HCO_3^-]$$

then, knowing that the content of carbonic acid ([H_2CO_3]) is dependent on the pressure of CO_2 (PCO_2), he derived

$$[H^+] = k \ \times \alpha PCO_2 / [HCO_3^-]$$

since known as Henderson's equation, later simplified to

$$[H^+] = \ 24 \, PCO_2 / [HCO_3^-]$$

where the variables are in their usual units—nEq/l, mm Hg and mmol/l, respectively.[3]

If we use usual numbers for arterial blood plasma

$$40 = 24 \ \times \ 40/24$$

Useful mathematically, because if two variables are measured the third may be derived, the

---

3   In 1917 Karl Albert Hasselbalch rewrote Henderson's equation, using SPL Sørensen's pH notation to derive pH = pK + log [HCO3-]/ [CO2]—known ever since as the Henderson-Hasselbalch equation.

expression is even more valuable conceptually, because it shows the extent to which [H⁺] is changed by a change in PCO_2 or [HCO_3^-]. For example, if PCO_2 is halved (by a doubling of ventilation), [H⁺] will also be halved, unless [HCO_3^-] is lowered.

One of the difficulties in understanding these relationships is that the reactions

$$CO_2 + H_2O \rightarrow H_2CO_3 \rightarrow H^+ + HCO_3^-$$

can be approached from both ends. From the left, a change in PCO_2 through a primary change in breathing, tends to change [H⁺] ; and from the right, a change in [HCO_3^-] will be accompanied by a change in [H⁺].

The ideas in this chapter, and the one that preceded it, have been quite complex, partly because they are all interrelated. Arterial blood has to carry sufficient O_2 to tissues to maintain metabolism, and similarly venous blood has to remove CO_2. It's no surprise that the content of O_2 affects the amount of CO_2 carried in blood, and *vice versa*, and that the effects aid O_2 uptake and CO_2 unloading in the lungs (also *vice versa* in the tissues). Furthermore, the control of acidity ([H⁺], pH) is similarly linked to O_2 and CO_2; a primary change in [H⁺] influences both, and changes in O_2 and CO_2 contents lead to changes in [H⁺]. The great American physiologist Walter Bradfield Cannon coined the phrase "homeostasis" , and popularized the concept in his book *The Wisdom of the Body* in 1932. Whilst we may question our body's wisdom from time to time, the properties of blood that we have been considering seem to be very wise.

CLINICAL DISORDERS OF ACID-BASE HOMEOSTASIS

In routine clinical practice homeostasis in the body is assessed by measuring components of the scheme described above, found in arterial blood plasma. We have identified the three major systems involved in this control—

1. Strong ions, of which the most important in blood plasma are Na⁺ and Cl⁻, in concentrations (approximately 140 and 100 mEq/l, respectively) that normally leave a "strong ion difference" ([SID]) of 40 mEq/l, that has to be filled with other negatively charged ions to obey the law of electrical neutrality.

2. The total concentration of weak acids in 20 mEq/l plasma proteins provides about 16 mEq/l of anion equivalents ([A⁻]).

3. Carbon dioxide, whose pressure (PCO_2) is controlled by breathing and which exists in several forms, of which bicarbonate (HCO_3) is in the highest concentration (about 24 mEq/l, to complete the balance sheet).

Nowadays, these three independent variables are easily measured, together with plasma pH. Normally the plasma reaction is slightly alkaline, with a pH of 7.40 ([H⁺] of 40 nEq/l), with a range (95% confidence) of 7.35-7.45.

Traditionally, a surprising degree of confusion surrounded the terms *acidosis* and *alkalosis*. It would seem easy to define these terms on the basis of a measured plasma pH that is outside the normal limits—acidosis where pH is less than 7.35, and alkalosis where the value is above 7.45. Two main subtypes were recognized- the change being termed *respiratory* when due to a primary change in PCO_2, and *metabolic* or *non-respiratory* when due to

65

changes in [SID], and, less commonly, plasma protein concentration. However, matters are made less straightforward by the adaptive responses that follow an initial perturbation. Thus, acidosis due to an increase in PCO_2, a respiratory acidosis, is countered by an increase in [SID] due to excretion of chloride in urine, and an accompanying increase in $[HCO_3^-]$, which could be termed a metabolic alkalosis. Of course, the adaptive response, or "compensation" is usually incomplete, so that pH ends up slightly reduced. A metabolic acidosis, due to reduction in [SID] (due to accumulation of acid, or increase in $[Cl^-]$ relative to $[Na^+]$) is usually accompanied by increases in ventilation and consequent lowering of PCO_2, a compensating respiratory alkalosis, and so on. Many serious illnesses, especially with multiple organ failure, are accompanied by changes in several of the independent variables, each of which has to be treated on its own merits.

Only the CO_2 system is able to change rapidly through control of its pressure, via changes in breathing. This is why breathing plays such a large part in the rapid control of Claude Bernard's *milieu intérieur*, and how breathing can affect all the functions of the body. The concentration of the strong ions can only be controlled slowly, mainly through their excretion of Na^+ or Cl^- by the kidneys; of course, other strong ions can accumulate in plasma, such as lactate in exercise and ketones in diabetes, but we are talking control here rather than perturbations. Finally, plasma protein concentration also can only be controlled slowly, mainly through changes in water content. Similarly, treatment of acid-base disorders involves appropriate reversal of abnormal strong ion concentrations, water and protein deficits, and measures to improve breathing.

Because all the systems contributing to acid-base homeostasis influence each other, the relationships are complex, especially in clinical medicine. Thus, although the physico-chemical relationships were well established in the first few decades of the 20th century, several short cuts were adopted, and the basic facts to some extent forgotten. However, in the 1980s, Peter Stewart, a Canadian physiologist at Brown University, Rhode Island, pointed out that modern computers were able to handle the mathematics with ease. He advocated a return to the classical physico-chemical relationships. His seminal book *How to understand acid-base* was published in 1981. In it, the relationships were described together with the computer algorithms that made it possible for anyone to solve the six simultaneous equations that quantify the roles of each of the three independent variables—the strong ion difference, the total weak acid concentration and the PCO_2. Stewart's approach has clarified the factors contributing to acid-base disturbances, and has proved especially helpful when applied to tissues, such as the red blood cells and muscle.

CHAPTER 6

THE ACT OF BREATHING

"The matter of this communication is founded upon a vast number of facts—immutable truths, which are infinitely beyond my comprehension. The deductions, however, which I have ventured to draw therefrom, I wish to advance with modesty, because time, with its mutations, may so unfold science as to crush these deductions, and demonstrate them as unsound. Nevertheless, the facts themselves can never alter, nor deviate in their bearing on respiration—one of the most important functions in the animal economy."

John Hutchinson, On the Capacity of the Lungs, and the Respiratory Functions, 1846.

"the mechanics of breathing is a problem requiring on one hand the detailed knowledge of a classical anatomist and on the other hand the analytic understanding of an engineer"

Wallace O. Fenn, Mechanics of Respiration, 1951.

Most of the time we breathe without giving it much thought, and we all "know" how to breathe; given these two facts, it's strange how often experts tell us that we are not breathing "correctly", or, for example, that we should "breathe more with the diaphragm". Different strategies are often proposed for breath control in such activities as singing and competitive sports, or to achieve relaxation, as in yoga. Whilst not denying some aspects of the effects of breathing in different ways, we

need to understand how we breathe in order to judge the validity of the advice. In this chapter we will consider breathing in terms of depth (or volume of each breath, usually expressed in liters), rate (how frequently we breathe, breaths per minute) and air flow (the velocity with which we breathe in and out, liters per minute or second). These parameters determine the way in which we achieve the total amount of breathing (litres of ventilation per minute) to supply oxygen and remove carbon dioxide. The work involved in breathing is carried out by the respiratory muscles acting against forces that impede lung expansion and air flow; the forces are related to the change in volume and stiffness of the chest cage and lung, and to the resistance to flow in the airways. The processes involved are sufficiently complex for there to have been several books on the topic; we need to consider the structure of the thorax, lung and airways and the actions of the respiratory muscles.

EARLY CONCEPTS OF THE THORAX AND MUSCLES OF BREATHING

The Greek word "thorax" began life as a surrounding protective wall for a city, boat or body, and later more specifically for protective armour that surrounded the trunk—the soldiers in Homer's *Iliad* wore a copper and leather thorax to protect the chest and its vital organs. The present-day Greek respirologist Charis Roussos traces its change in meaning—to the chest cavity—at least as far back as Plato, who viewed the "cavity of the thorax" to be in two parts, an upper containing the heart and lungs and the lower containing the liver and intestines, the two being separated by the diaphragm. Galen provided a definition which could stand to this day—"that cavity bounded by the ribs on both sides, extending to the sternum and diaphragm in front and curving down to the spine in the rear". Galen's many animal vivisections and observation of injured gladiators, showed that breathing was accomplished by the intercostal muscles and diaphragm. As with many other features of human anatomy, the structures of breathing were revealed by Andreas Vesalius' meticulous dissections in the 16th century.

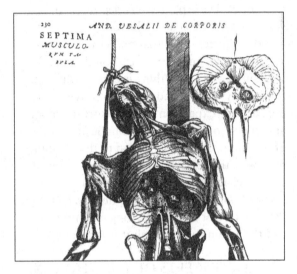

Figure 18 The thorax with the diaphragm dissected out, in Veasalius' Fabrica.

The bony thorax is composed of 12 ribs, attached to the spine by joints that allow them to swing out and up like the handles of buckets; at the front they are attached to a flat bone, the sternum, by flexible cartilage. The upper ribs are attached to muscles in the neck, and lower ribs to the powerful abdominal muscles; there are also muscles running diagonally between adjacent ribs, the intercostals, acting to narrow the space between them; there are two layers—the internal contracting during expiration, and the external aiding inspiration. Being attached to the spine, the ribs are expanded by straightening

the spine, and crowded by bending the spine. Importantly, the thorax contributes a stable base for muscles acting on the upper arms; because the abdominal and back muscles are recruited for changes in posture and movement, all activity has implications for the muscles of breathing.

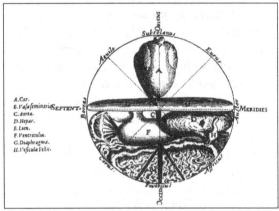

Figure 19 Robert Fludd's (1628) perception of the diaphragm separating the thorax (containing air and heart) from the abdomen (containing stomach, intestines and liver).

Historically, the muscles involved in breathing were recognized early, beginning with Galen, who described the diaphragm and its main nerve supply by the long phrenic nerve that courses down from the neck alongside the spine. The Greek derivation of "diaphragm" indicates that it was first considered mainly as a partition, between organs to do with breath and spirit and the less lofty digestive systems. Leonardo drew the first anatomically correct diaphragm and correctly inferred its function; under the drawing he penned in his mirror writing—"The functions of the diaphragm are four. First, it should be the origin of dilatation of the lung by which the air is attracted. Second, that it should press on the stomach covered by it and drive out of it digested food into the intestines. Third, that together with the abdominal wall it should squeeze and help compress the intestines to help drive out the superfluities. Fourth, that it should separate the spiritual from the natural organs". An example, perhaps, of the danger in saying more than is strictly necessary; his fourth function harks back to Aristotle and Plato.

John Mayow has often been described as the first pulmonary physiologist; his experiments on pulmonary gas exchange have already been described, but also he made the first study of respiratory muscle function. An illustration in his *Tractatus Duo: De Respiratione* shows the attachments of the two sets of intercostal muscles, internal and external, but also a small

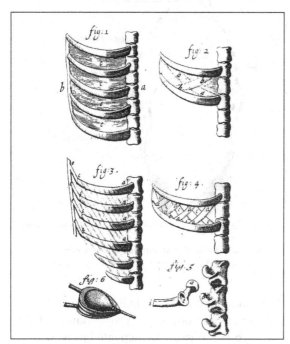

Figure 20 Mayow's illustration of the action of intercostal muscles; note the bellows "model", lower left.

cartoon showing a balloon inside a bellows— the "mechanical model" adopted by nearly all teachers ever since. In his 1669 treatise, he shows his understanding of the physical principles previously put forward by Torricelli

and Boyle—"With respect, then, to the entrance of air into the lungs, I think it is to be maintained that it is caused in the following manner by the pressure of the atmosphere. For as the air, on account of the weight of the superincumbent atmosphere, not only rushes in to all empty places, but also presses forcibly on whatever is next it (as Boyle's experiments have proved beyond doubt), it follows that the air, passed through the nostrils and the trachea, up to the bronchi or gates of the lungs, presses against the lungs from within and seeks an entrance into them. Hence it is that when the inner sides of the thorax (which by compressing the lungs from without were resisting the pressure of this air) are drawn outwards by muscles whose function it is to dilate the chest, and the space in the thorax is enlarged, the air which is nearest the bronchial inlets, now that every obstacle is removed, rushes under the full pressure of the atmosphere into the cavities of the lungs, and by inflating them occupies and fills the space of the expanded chest." Nearly 200 years were to pass before Mayow's analysis was improved by the addition of the concept of the elastic recoil of the lungs and thorax in aiding respiration; in 1820 the Scots physician James Carson suggested that the "elasticity or resilience of the lungs" aided both respiration and the motion of the blood through the lungs. This set the scene for the modern views on lung mechanics of the 20th century.

69

THE MUSCLES OF BREATHING

Respiratory muscles are usually classed as inspiratory or expiratory, but we need to appreciate that because nearly all the work of breathing occurs during inspiration, the main inspiratory muscle, the diaphragm, carries the brunt of this load; all the other muscles play supporting roles by stabilizing the ribs, anchoring the chest cage or providing space for the diaphragm to move. Expiration is achieved mainly by recoil of the expanded lung and thorax, but the expiratory muscles allow the lung to be deflated to below its resting volume. As Vesalius first showed, the diaphragm is a wide but thin muscle attached around the inner border of the lower rib cage and sitting like a dome over the liver and stomach; a large proportion of its area is occupied by a flat central tendon; because of this the muscle fibres run almost vertically between the tendon and ribs. Although we always think of the diaphragm as a single muscle, and normally it acts that way, there are really two parts to it; the rear portion, attached to the spine gains its nerve supply from nerves coming locally from the spinal column, whereas most of the diaphragm is supplied by the phrenic nerve, which travels down the thorax from the third and fourth spinal nerves in the neck. During inspiration, the muscle fibres of the diaphragm contract, and because they run almost vertically their shortening can have two possible outcomes; if the abdominal muscles are fully relaxed, the abdominal wall protrudes, and the liver and abdominal contents descend—this is often termed abdominal or diaphragmatic breathing. If the abdominal muscles are contracted, or some other impediment prevents descent of the diaphragm, the ribs are pulled up and rotated to expand the chest—so-called intercostal breathing. As you can find out by yourself, by contracting the abdominal muscles consciously, we can limit the movement to the chest, with little downward movement of the diaphragm, and conversely by relaxing abdominal muscles we can breathe without much chest movement; normally both occur without our thinking about it. Deep inspiration is aided by contraction of the external intercostal muscles and muscles of the neck, both favoring upward movement of the ribs. In expiration the diaphragm and thorax revert back to their resting position;

70

further expiration, to below "functional residual capacity", is achieved by contraction of abdominal muscles, forcing the diaphragm upwards, and by contraction of the internal intercostal muscles. Although the action of both intercostal muscles is similar, causing narrowing of the ribs, during expiration the lower ribs are pulled down by the abdominal muscles; in consequence all the ribs are pulled down, contributing to expiration. The opposite is the case during inspiration, because then the upper ribs are anchored, by the neck muscles.

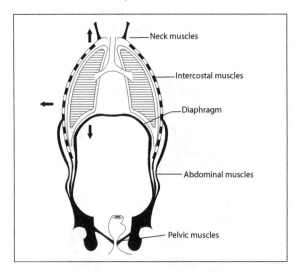

Figure 21 Diagram of the thorax and abdomen, showing the dome of the diaphragm which acts to lift the ribs

Breathing movements are highly integrated and complex; in addition to the prime movers of the thorax, other muscles are activated to reduce resistance to flow during inspiration; these include the muscles of the nose and throat, the larynx and larger airways.

STRENGTH OF RESPIRATORY MUSCLES

The muscles of breathing are subject to similar constraints as any skeletal muscle; as they shorten they become weaker, and they also fatigue during repeated contractions. Surprisingly perhaps, for a set of muscles so essential to life, in the population there is as large a variation in their strength, as there is for skeletal muscles; some of us are the Charles Atlases of breathing and others resemble the puny guy who gets the sand kicked in his face. In healthy subjects studied in our laboratory at McMaster, the maximum inspiratory pressure was found by Kieran Killian to vary between 40 and 200 cms H_2O—a five-fold variation, comparable to the variation in skeletal muscle strength. In the same way that people with weaker muscles find that a given activity takes more effort than someone with stronger muscles, those who achieve lower inspiratory pressures experience more effort in breathing—they are more "breathless"—than subjects capable of higher pressures. It might seem a good idea to train the respiratory muscles, but unfortunately, it is not as easy to train these muscles as those of the arms or legs.

THE VOLUME OF THE LUNGS

The first systematic measurements of the size of the lungs and the capacity to breathe were carried out using methods that have hardly improved to this day. In 1846 John Hutchinson read his paper "On the capacity of the lungs, and of the respiratory functions" to the London Society of Physicians and Surgeons.[1] It must have been a marathon meeting, because when published the paper ran to 125 pages. Based on measurements made on 1775 healthy subjects he established the effects of stature on lung volume, and proposed that the measurement of vital

---

1 His subjects included "Members of the Fire Brigade, Metropolitan Police, Thames Police, Paupers, Mixed Class (artisans), Grenadier Guards, Royal Horse Guards, Chatham Recruits, Woolwich Marines, Pugilists and Wrestlers, Giants and Dwarfs, Printers, Draymen, Girls, Gentlemen and Diseased Cases".

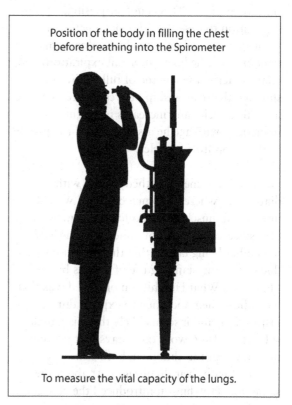

Position of the body in filling the chest before breathing into the Spirometer

To measure the vital capacity of the lungs.

Figure 22 Silhouette of Hutchinson demonstrating the use of his spirometer

capacity would allow early diagnosis "of the disease which ultimately caused death, and that before the usual means availed" (the disease referred to is tuberculosis). Here, as in several other instances of major advances in understanding lung function, innovative ideas had to wait for decades before they were applied in patient care. Early in my training in the 1950s we had no readily available spirometer measurements in my London teaching hospital. In the 1960s the picture changed, but even then the clinical spirometer was almost identical to the one devised by Hutchinson 100 years before. In presenting his data, Hutchinson observed "The matter of this communication is founded upon a vast number of facts—innumerable truths, which are infinitely beyond my comprehension". This is not surprising, because in addition to describing his spirometer and its proper use, defining residual volume (that remaining in the lungs after full expiration) and vital capacity (the volume of full expiration), showing the relationship between increases in vital capacity and increases in height and reductions with age he also measured the power of the respiratory muscles.[2]

He noted that men breathed mainly with the diaphragm whereas women breathed with the intercostal muscles; this notion has remained ever since, almost without question, and I can remember being taught that this behaviour was due to the longstanding use of corsets by the "fair sex". What Hutchinson observed was that men allow their abdomen to expand during inspiration, and it seems likely that his female subjects in 1846 wore tight stays that prevented movement of the abdomen; both sexes breathed with their diaphragm. At about the same time Hutchinson introduced the concept of pulmonary elastance (or its reciprocal, compliance), by measuring the pressure required to inflate excised lungs to increasing volume. Ever since, the "pressure-volume curve" of the respiratory system, analogous to the stress-strain diagram of the engineers, has remained the standard way in which respiratory mechanics, and the related topic of the work of breathing, has been analyzed. In Canada, Hutchinson's landmark paper continues to be celebrated; the black silhouetted figure of the author, showing the use of his spirometer, is the logo used by the Meakins-Christie Institute at McGill University,

Canada's foremost centre for research in respiratory physiology.

THE PRESSURE REQUIRED TO EXPAND THE SYSTEM

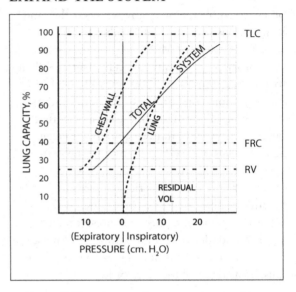

Figure 23 The pressure-volume curve, showing the pressure required to expand the lungs and chest wall, separately and together.

As with other aspects of respiratory function, research into the mechanical characteristics of the respiratory system received a considerable boost during World War Two, and the seminal papers were published by groups at the University of Rochester, Harvard and the Johns Hopkins University. "The pressure-volume diagram of the thorax and lungs" was published in 1945 by the famous triumvirate of Wallace O. Fenn, Arthur B. Otis and Hermann Rahn in Rochester, New York; it presented an elegant graphical analysis of the pressures needed to expand the lung and thorax, both contributing to the forces required to move the total respiratory system (the solid line in figure 25). At full inspiration the inspiratory muscles generate their maximum force against the sum of both thoracic and lung recoil; this recoil

2   In fact the only factor he apparently did not assess, of those presently used to predict lung volume, was that of gender—for given age and height, vital capacity in females is about 80% of the male value, in common with other organ dimensions such as the heart and muscles.

provides most of the energy for expiration, and at the end of a relaxed breath the inward recoil of the lung is exactly balanced by the outward recoil of the thorax. If expiration is continued, the expiratory muscles work against the outward recoil of the thorax to compress the lung to its residual volume; this provides energy for the beginning of the next inspiration. It must have come as a shock to Fenn, Rahn and Otis to find, as they describe in their paper, that "since completing this work we have discovered similar diagrams from papers by Rohrer (1916) …as well as a partially similar effort by Jacquet (1908) and Bernouilli (1911)". All three of these earlier authors came from Switzerland, Rohrer from Bern and the others from Basel, emphasizing the extraordinary contributions, albeit largely forgotten for decades, of Swiss physiologists and physicians of the time.

Fritz Rohrer, called "the Mozart of respiratory mechanics" by the foremost expert of the 1960s, Jere Mead, appears to have been a driving force in Swiss respiratory physiology, having made exhaustive studies of bronchial branching and dimensions, with a theoretical analysis of the forces impeding flow in airways, and later going on to calculate the forces needed to overcome elastic recoil of the lung and thorax, before dying at the early age of 37. Presumably also, the Rochester group was unaware of the work of Rohrer's pupil Karl Wirz and his colleague Kurt von Neergaard in the late 1920's, which with hindsight was a great pity, for two reasons. First, Wirz and von Neergaard realized that the important pressure was the intrapleural pressure—in the potential fluid lined space between the lung and thorax. They took advantage of the need to induce a pneumothorax in a tuberculosis patient (a procedure in which air is allowed into the pleural space through a needle, in those days a common treatment used to collapse TB cavities in the lung). They measured

the pressure through the needle, simultaneously with breath volume, and so calculated lung elasticity during normal breathing; this serendipitous study provided the rationale for several methods for measuring intrapleural pressure, but many years later. Second, von Neergaard ,who was a chest physician as well as physiologist, had a brilliant intuition—he hypothesized that the lung might not behave in the same way during expiration as during inspiration, which was when the measurements conventionally were made. He found that the pressure required to maintain a volume during expiration was less than that needed to inflate the lung to the same volume; the respiratory system exhibited *hysteresis*—in which the stress-strain relationship was not the same during imposition of stress as on its withdrawal. This meant that there was a factor tending to maintain volume during expiration, and von Neergaard proposed that the force was due to the presence of an air-liquid interface in the alveoli; a force that reduced the surface tension tending to collapse the alveoli. He predicted that if the interface was eliminated experimentally by filling the lung with fluid, the effect would be lost and hysteresis abolished.[3] Neergaard tested this hypothesis in animal lungs by measuring pressure-volume curves in air filled and water filled lungs, and the results clearly showed that the major elastic force resisting expansion was due to surface activity, which also lessened recoil during expiration. The effect was consistent with the physics of soap bubble formation.

SURFACE-ACTIVE FORCES IN THE LUNG

Von Neergard's experiments were published in 1929; they showed conclusively that surface

---

3   Among its many unique qualities, water has the highest surface tension of any liquid except mercury; its molecules have a large tendency to stick together.

tension is a more important retractive force than tissue retraction, but also that in air filled lungs the surface tension effect was reduced in deflation compared to inflation; the liquid filled lungs did not show hysteresis. Von Neergaard's paper includes an elegant theoretical application of the relationship between volume and pressure in spheres established by Lavoisier's mathematician friend Laplace, and concludes with the prophetic statement—"the consequences [of the findings] in terms of pulmonary elasticity in neonates… [in whom]… surface tension in the alveoli is of vital importance". It would be many years before von Neergaard's concepts would be applied in the investigation of neonatal respiratory distress syndrome; indeed, his paper was forgotten for almost 20 years.

The discovery of a surface active material in the lung fluid of rabbits exposed to phosgene was made by Richard Pattle, whilst working at the Chemical Defence Experimental Establishment of the British Ministry of Supply at Porton Down, in 1955. Pattle observed that bubbles formed in the lung fluid were extremely stable, suggesting a very low surface tension (he thought zero); he appeared ignorant of von Neergaard's work of almost 30 years before. The same cannot be said of John A. Clements who, working at the US counterpart of Porton Down—The Chemical Warfare Laboratories in Maryland—measured the relation between the area and tension of a film of lung fluid, and confirming a very marked hysteresis between expansion and compression of the film. John Clements was to devote the rest of his long and distinguished career to the study of the surface active film in the lung alveoli, and the clinical condition of neonatal respiratory distress (a topic to which we will return in a later chapter).

Part of Clements' work was to uncover the composition of the fluid that he proposed lined the alveolar surface. Von Neergaard felt the fluid was probably a type of mucus secreted by the lung. In 1954 the Canadian histologist Charles Clifford Macklin, on the basis of careful microscopical studies, agreed and proposed that the film was secreted by a cell found around the alveoli, that he termed a granular pneumocyte. The application of the electron microscope would eventually show that the surface film consisted of a one-molecule thick fatty acid compound (dipalmitoyl lecithin), secreted by what became called the type II alveolar cell (Macklin's granular pneumocyte). Thus, the ancient advice to "pour oil on troubled waters" and the observation by whalers that whale lung fluid stilled the water around their boats finally gained physiological and medical importance. Eventually, new-born infants whose lungs would not expand normally due to the lungs' immaturity would be treated by administration of synthetic dipalmitoyl lecithin, thus providing them with a film that lessened surface tension.

The tissue elasticity observed by von Neergaard is related to the structure of the bony thorax which after expansion tends to revert to its relaxed position, and the structure of the lung. Charles Macklin showed that the major bronchi provided much of the lung's tissue elasticity; they expanded and lengthened in inspiration and recoiled on expiration; the fine tissue between airways and alveoli also contributes to this recoil. Although physiologists like teaching about lung elasticity as if the alveoli are a collection of little balloons that expand and contract, the reality is that in full inspiration alveoli are polyhedrons and composed of more-or-less straight wall segments; as their volume decreases in expiration the corners of the polyhedrons fold to reduce volume. It is the alveolar surfactant that maintains a more spherical shape, as it does not enter the folded angles. This behaviour leads to a relatively large decrease in alveolar surface area relative to the change in volume, and allows surfactant to exert a large surface active effect that resists alveolar collapse; were it not to lower surface tension, a large proportion of the alveoli would become airless, especially at the lung bases where gravity has a large effect.

At the end of a normal breath, the outward recoil of the chest cage balances the inward lung elastic recoil; the "transpulmonary pressure" is zero, and the lung is still about 40% expanded. We begin to breathe in, exposing the alveoli to a pressure that is slightly negative with respect to the atmosphere and doing work mainly against lung recoil; at about 70% of lung expansion we have to work against the recoil of both the lung and chest wall, so that at full inspiration—at total lung capacity the respiratory muscles are generating a tension of about 30 cms of water.[4] As we can generate a maximum inspiratory pressure of well over 100 cms H_2O, you'd think we have more than enough strength to do this, but inspiration is accomplished by a shortening of the respiratory muscles, and like all muscles they get weaker as their length shortens; it appears that the volume of the lung is perfectly matched to the muscles, such that 30 cms H_2O

is their maximum tension at the total lung capacity. At this point the elastic recoil of the lung and chest wall equals the maximum tension developed by the muscles. During expiration we can relax and the elasticity of the lung and thorax bring volume back to where we started; at this point, functional residual capacity (FRC), there is a small lung recoil pressure that equals the outward recoil of the thorax. Then if we need to recruit extra volume below the resting 40%, for example during exercise, we have to contract the expiratory muscles against the outward recoil of the thorax, finally reaching a residual volume of 20% of capacity. This gives us a potential usable volume (vital capacity) that amounts to 80% of the available volume in the lungs—ie. total lung capacity. Of course, it is hard to use this potential, because it would require a great deal of effort if we tried to maintain it for more than a few breaths. Usually only about 2/3 of the vital capacity is used as a tidal volume during exercise. The elasticity of the lungs is gradually lost in old age, so that even though the total lung capacity remains the same as we age, the reduced elastic recoil means that the volume of air left in the lungs at the end of expiration (residual volume) is increased.

---

4   Units of pressure can be very confusing; Torricelli measured pressure with a closed tube containing mercury, thus pressure is often measured in millimeters of mercury (mmHg), as commonly used for blood pressure); sometimes this unit is called a Torr. At sea level, atmospheric pressure is about 760 mmHg—this can be known as 1 atmosphere, or even as 100 kilo Pascals, after the French physicist Blaise Pascal. When pressure measuring devices came into widespread use, it was impossible to read fractions of a millimeter and water filled manometers were used instead, thus the unit cmH2O, which is close to 1.3 mmHg.

A neat example of the connectivity between the heart and lungs is that the relatively negative pressure in the chest during active inspiration aids the return of blood into the chest and heart. The negative pressure surrounding the heart also helps the output of the right ventricle as it sends blood into the lungs. It might be thought that this effect might be cancelled during the subsequent expiration; however, because expiration is mainly passive, there is little impediment to blood flow. For its part, the heart helps gas exchange through pulses of blood flow and pressure in the lung that occur with each beat, helping to mix gases in the deeper areas of lung, where mass flow due to ventilation has stopped.

At this point we will not consider disorders associated with reductions in the lung volume, lumped together into the terms atelectasis (airless lung as in pneumonia) and fibrosis (scarring of the lung), except to say that much more pressure than normal is required to expand the lung, and thus much more tension has to be developed by inspiratory muscles.

RESISTANCE TO AIRFLOW IN THE AIRWAYS

We now turn from the forces needed to achieve a volume of breath to consider the rate of flow through the airways, which is also driven by pressure differences between the alveoli and the atmosphere. Airway resistance is the term that describes the impedance to flow, just as elastance describes impedance to volume change; the units of resistance are litres/sec/cmH$_2$O (i.e. flow divided by pressure). The French physician Jean-Leonard-Marie Poiseuille made measurements of flow and pressure in glass tubes of varying length and caliber with a new manometer in 1828. Purely on the results of the measurements he derived an equation that showed that flow in a tube is directly related to the driving pressure and the fourth power of the radius, and inversely to the length of the tube and viscosity of the fluid, thus establishing the overriding importance of the tube's caliber. He was also the first to show that arterial blood pressure varied with the phase of breathing. The importance of the equation was not recognized until Fritz Rohrer applied the equation (now known as Poiseuille's Law) some 80 years later to all the measurements he had made on the length and radius of the airways in a single human lung. This was an astonishing achievement, made as it was well before the era of computers, in 1915, and it allowed Rohrer to show that most of the resistance to air flow is in the upper airways, from the nose to the larynx. Flow depends on the gradient of pressure between the alveoli and the atmosphere, and because of this the lung elastic recoil assumes a dominant role, although not an obvious one. During inspiration the alveolar pressure is determined by the forces generated by the respiratory muscles minus the elastic recoil; inspiratory muscle forces tend to open the airways. During expiration, lung elastic recoil provides virtually all the force needed for adequate flow; indeed sometimes this flow is actively "braked" by the action of inspiratory muscles. Excess forces developed by expiratory muscles tend to reduce flow by subjecting the airways to pressure surrounding them, thus tending to narrow them. These facts explain why in patients with emphysema, who have lost elastic recoil due to the destruction of alveolar walls, inspiration is easy, but expiration very hard. Inspiratory flow is often normal, with the negative intrathoracic pressure tending to hold airways open, whereas expiratory flow is drastically reduced. To recruit elastic recoil, patients inspire to a larger and larger lung volume, requiring greater inspiratory effort.

MODERN SPIROMETRY

Rohrer's followers, Wirz and von Neergaard, took advantage of new technology to measure flow and alveolar pressure in human subjects to clarify the relationships between alveolar pressure and flow; their work was expanded by Fenn, Rahn and Otis and their contemporaries in the 1940's. The new understanding took time to be incorporated into clinical practice; the French physician Robert Tiffeneau helped the process in 1945 by suggesting that airflow could be assessed by timed measurements of expired volume, later standardized to the volume expired in the first second of a forced expiration; in the late 1950's the "FEV$_1$", together with the total expired volume—or vital capacity (VC)—became the internationally accepted measurement to quantify breathing capacity, assess impairment of ventilatory function, and to follow progress in patients with asthma, chronic obstructive pulmonary disorders, and other generalized pulmonary diseases. The FEV_1 is expressed in units (litres per second) appropriate to flow, and as it is measured after taking a deep breath, it represents maximum expiratory flow capacity. In healthy people it is influenced by the same parameters as those identified by John Hutchinson as influencing VC—height, age and gender—and is usually about 80% of VC; ie. most healthy people can breathe out 80% of their VC in one second, and a reduction in this proportion represents airflow slowing, due to airway narrowing or inability to achieve peak alveolar pressure.

As a measure of the capacity to breathe, the FEV_1 has a major drawback—it measures maximum flow achieved in underline only; breathing capacity depends as much, if not more, on the ability to inspire. In recent years, it has become easy to measure the "flow/volume loop"; flow is measured during both inspiration and expiration and represented on a graph as a function of volume; this shows both components of breathing together, and represents the "envelope" available to achieve breathing, for example during exercise. Athletes typically have a large envelope and are able to use most of it if required; at the other end of the spectrum, patients with emphysema may show very poor expiratory flow, but still have an adequate envelope, due to well maintained inspiratory flow.

Although we know a lot about the forces involved in breathing, we remain quite ignorant about how the individual muscles are coordinated in order to achieve the required ventilation with the greatest efficiency. In a way, it's lucky that we don't have to think about it;

the brain takes care of the cooperation between the diaphragm and intercostals and the muscles in the larynx and upper airways, completely automatically. We tend to think of this automatic control in terms of reflexes, such as the Hering-Breuer reflex, which acts to inhibit inspiration at the end of a breath. However, it seems more likely that the "pattern" of breathing—the amount of each breath, and the time spent inspiring vs. expiring—is at least in part "chosen" to minimize the effort in breathing; in other words to make breathing as comfortable as possible. Thus, the total amount of breathing is regulated in response to blood carbon dioxide and oxygen pressures; the way this is achieved is through a pattern of breathing that depends on nerve messages from the inspiratory muscles to the brain, which in turn dictates the pattern of breathing. This is not a real reflex response because it can be appreciated consciously. The sense of effort in breathing increases with the rapidity and extent to which the respiratory muscles contract, as well as how frequently. There are many combinations of depth of each breath, how deep the inspiration, how far we breathe out, and how long we spend breathing in versus breathing out, but for any required breathing load the brain is able to coordinate the respiratory muscles in such a way as to make life comfortable. That said, we have to admit that sometimes we come across individuals who breathe at very low frequencies, such as 3 breaths per minute, that most of us would find uncomfortable.

CHAPTER 7

THE CONTROL OF BREATHING

"...the adjustment of the ventilation is like the adjustment of an electric blanket. When you feel cold you turn the heat up a little and leave it there until you feel too hot, then you turn it down. If you guess right the first time no abnormal signals are received and no adjustments are necessary...This is the kind of behavior that we could reasonably expect from a respiratory center in our highly efficient and talented brains."

Wallace O. Fenn, 1964, introducing a symposium on breathing control at the New York Academy of Sciences.

We have already noted that breathing incorporates a number of unique features; although not normally consciously regulated, its control can be overridden at will or by subconscious events; changes in breathing potentially affect function in a variety of body systems; and conversely, impaired function in these systems can themselves influence breathing. No wonder then that our understanding about how breathing is controlled has a long and complex history, and many features of respiratory control remain controversial. Perhaps it may help if I begin by giving the short message, before going on with a more complete story.

In 1994, Elliot Phillipson and his colleagues at the University of Toronto presented the results of studies made in adult sheep and dogs. They attached an artificial membrane lung, similar to that used in open heart surgery, to the main vein returning blood to the heart, and removed

carbon dioxide progressively. As the amount of CO_2 removed increased, the animal's breathing fell until eventually breathing ceased completely; thus, the short message is that breathing control is geared to the amount of CO_2 returning to the lung. Phillipson's results also call into question whether there sits in the brain a centre that sends out a central nervous message to breathe, the respiratory rhythm generating centre.

Whilst Galen, and others that followed him, had some theories on breathing control, its scientific study could not begin until Lavoisier and Séguin showed that breathing was related to the uptake of oxygen and output of carbon dioxide that accompanied metabolic combustion. It was much later that the two gases were considered important in regulating breathing. Early studies were stimulated by the observation that it was impossible to hold one's breath for longer than a minute or two. At the "breakpoint", when blood oxygen was low and carbon dioxide high, the intense "drive" to breathe that develops during the breath-hold was ascribed to the effects of increased CO_2 and low O_2 on the brain.

THE CENTRAL (BRAIN) CONTROL OF BREATHING

Galen described his observations on the effects of neck injuries in gladiators and carried out complex vivisection experiments on several animal species to show that high spinal cord lesions led to cessation of breathing. His studies were the start of animal experimentation in the search for the site of nervous control of breathing, but further understanding had to wait until the purpose of breathing and the function of the lungs had been established.

In 1811 Julien-Jean-César Legallois showed in rabbits that removal of a small area in the lowest part of the brain (the medulla) stopped breathing. Legallois was a Breton who as a young man took part in the French Revolution, and after was forced into hiding for several years; he did not obtain his medical degree until the age of 31, and then began his career as an experimental physiologist. As one of the first modern experimenters his technical skills were outstanding, but he gained a reputation for conducting crude and brutal experiments; it was rumored that his interest in the role played by the brain and spinal cord in breathing was stimulated by the gasping movements observed briefly in heads severed by the guillotine. In his studies of the role of the brain in regulating the heart and respiration, he usually began by opening the skull of a young rabbit and progressively removing more and more of the brain until he obtained a response; he found that he could remove the whole of the brain cortex, the cerebellum, and upper part of the medulla without stopping breathing, but once he cut the medulla at the level of the eighth cranial nerve, "it instantly ceases". Nowadays we might question both the approach and its ability to answer specific hypotheses of physiological control, but there is no doubt that the experiments won him a place in the history of respiratory physiology. His work indicated the presence of a "respiratory centre", and provided hypotheses that later physiologists tested with methods of increasing complexity, eventually using microelectrodes to stimulate different parts of the medulla, and applying solutions of varying composition to its surface.

PERIPHERAL (OUTSIDE THE BRAIN) MECHANISMS

Many physiologists applied themselves to finding the stimulus to which the control system responded, whether CO_2, O_2, hydrogen ion concentration, or some other "signal". In the last decade of the 19th century, Leon Fredericq, a colleague of Nathan Zuntz in Bonn, carried out a series of experiments on dogs that reflected his extraordinary imagination and technical expertise. The technique is now known as a "cross-circulation" experiment, and it has been used to test a variety of reflexes that depend on changing the flow or composition of blood supplying the brain. The arteries and veins supplying the head of one dog are connected to the head of another, and the effects of some experimental perturbation on breathing or some other function in the two dogs is observed. Fredericq blocked the trachea of one dog, so that blood with a high CO_2 and low O_2 passed to the other dog's brain; that dog increased its breathing, and in so doing delivered blood with low CO_2 and high O_2 back to the other, whose breathing thereby diminished. In another experiment he artificially increased breathing in the first dog, producing breathing cessation (apnea) in the second. Together with many other observations made in subsequent studies Fredericq concluded that breathing was controlled by changes in the amount of CO_2 going to the head. Soon after, John Scott Haldane and John Gillies Priestley, at the University of Oxford, investigated the effects of changes in O_2 and CO_2 content in the air breathed by human subjects. In one of many experiments they found that an increase of only 1 or 2 mmHg in inspired CO_2 pressure could lead to a doubling of ventilation, whereas it needed a reduction of 50 mmHg in O_2 pressure to effect a change. Because increases in blood CO_2 usually make blood more acid, there was some debate at the time as to whether the increase in ventilation produced by changes in CO_2 were actually due to changes in hydrogen ion concentration. However, Haldane and Priestley showed that the effect of CO_2

was much greater that an acid injection of comparable strength; this experiment did not rule out an effect of hydrogen ion concentration locally, in the chemically sensitive cells of the respiratory centre. Subsequent work on where and how CO_2 has its central effect uncovered several sites in the region identified by Legallois in the medulla, that respond to changes in hydrogen ion concentration. In reviewing research in this topic one is struck by the extent and quality of the work done in an area scarcely larger than a dime, less than 1 ml in volume. Also one is left wondering why so much effort has been expended on questions whose answer can at best be only a small part of a very complex control system. At least in part, this is because other "chemosensitive" tissues have long been known to influence breathing.

"CHEMORECEPTORS"

The carotid body is a tiny organ in the right side of the neck; it is situated in the fork where the common carotid artery divides into its internal and external branches—it is close to the heart and in an ideal position to respond to changes in the blood coming from the lungs. It has the dubious distinction of having been "discovered" half a dozen times—that is, several people described it without referring to others who had already done so. Although pride of place is generally accorded Hartwig Wilhelm Ludwig Taube, who presented his doctoral dissertation in 1743, even he found it hard to get proper credit for the work—his supervisor was the famous and influential professor of physiology at the University of Göttingen, Albrecht von Haller, whose name appears on the front page of the thesis in much larger letters than his student. In spite of its rediscovery on several occasions through the next century and a half, it was not well recognized during this period—it does not feature in Gray's *Anatomy* of 1858;

its structure and function were not identified until the 20th century. In 1926, Fernando De Castro y Rodriguez, a histologist working at the Cajal Institute in Madrid provided the first microscopic description of fine nerve endings in the capillaries of the very vascular structure. De Castro inferred that the carotid body "sensed" chemical changes occurring in the aortic blood, and was the first to realize its function differed from other nearby structures that responded to changes in aortic pressure. The early physiological studies had not differentiated between these functions.

The father and son team of J F and Corneille Heymans worked at the University of Ghent, where Heymans *père* was professor of physiology, being later succeeded by his son. In 1924 they began experiments that used Leon Fredericq's cross-circulation technique to isolate the circulation to the head of one dog, whilst retaining its nerve supply. When the aortic blood pressure was changed, breathing was affected; these physiological changes were due to nervous impulses traveling to the brain, rather than any direct effect of blood pressure on the brain, because the brain's circulation was supported by the second dog. Low aortic pressure stimulated breathing, and elevated pressure inhibited the respiratory centre, sometimes to the point of stopping breathing completely. The studies provided the first evidence of reflex regulation of breathing, and the Heymans went on to study the reflex effects of changes in the composition of aortic blood on breathing; using the same animal preparation, they found that increases in CO_2 and hydrogen ion concentration, and reductions in O_2 content, led to a reflex stimulation of breathing. When the nervous connections from the aortic and carotid region to the lower part of the brain were cut, low O_2 content actually depressed breathing, suggesting that the respiratory centre in the brain, in contrast to the carotid body, is depressed rather than stimulated by low O_2 in its local blood flow; this was not the case with elevated CO_2 which acted in the same way, whether stimulated directly or reflexly. Corneille Heymans was awarded the Nobel Prize for Medicine in 1938, and gave his acceptance speech in 1945; in this, he refers to the "glomus caroticum" rather than the more usual "carotid body", perhaps to emphasize his own contributions to the mechanisms which "by regulating the activity of respiratory centre through the vascular presso- and chemo-sensitive reflexes establishes, thus, an even closer functional correlation between the blood circulation, the metabolism, and the pulmonary respiratory exchanges". His work, together with the microscopical descriptions of de Castro, remains the bedrock of subsequent investigations on the nervous control of breathing, that have tried to establish the cellular mechanisms or signals that set in train the relevant nervous impulses. Heymans strongly espoused the idea that the effect of chemical changes in blood on breathing are mediated entirely through reflexes that originate in the chemosensitive carotid body. This view is not accepted today, as it was shown by Julius Comroe in 1938 that removal of the nerves supplying the carotid body does not abolish the effect of CO_2 on breathing. The links between respiratory centres in the mid-brain and higher levels in the brain, and the role of a possible respiratory "pacemaker" remain topics of debate. These links, or neuronal networks, are needed to explain such observations as the effects of emotion and mental activity, and personality, on the responses to chemical stimuli, and changes in the pattern (rate and depth) of breathing that minimize the sense of effort that is consciously appreciated when breathing increases.

INTEGRATION BETWEEN FACTORS CONTROLLING BREATHING

Where does this leave us in understanding how our breathing is regulated? First, the production of CO_2 from metabolic processes in the body exerts the dominant effect on breathing, through changes in blood CO_2 pressure, acting on both chemo-sensitive areas, central (medullary) and peripheral (carotid body). Second, low O_2 pressure, either in inspired air (eg. at altitude) or arterial blood (eg. due to problems in the lung) stimulates breathing at the level of the carotid body, but usually not until arterial PO_2 has fallen from its normal value at about 100 mmHg to below 60 mmHg. Third, changes in blood pressure may affect breathing due to aortic receptors). Finally, the activity of the central rhythm generator in the brain stem is influenced by nervous input from the chemosensitive tissues. It all adds up to a complex interaction that can be seen as working to maintain Claude Bernard's *mileu intérieur,* by controlling the blood level of CO_2 within narrow limits and to prevent serious reductions in the level of O_2. We will need to return to breathing control at several points in the book, as we explore what happens to breathing when you climb mountains, or exercise, or battle with chronic respiratory disease. Although the general responses to such situations are more or less understood, we still struggle to understand differences in the responses between individuals, which vary widely.

ALVEOLAR PCO_2, INDICATOR OF ADEQUACY OF BREATHING

In 1915 Haldane and Priestley described a non-invasive method to measure alveolar CO_2 pressure; the subject breathed out into a long tube, and a sample of the gas nearest the mouth was taken at the end of expiration. The gas sample was analyzed in Haldane's chemical analyzer; in healthy subjects this end-expired or "alveolar" PCO_2 is a close approximation to the arterial blood value. They found that PCO_2 was quite constant from over time in a given individual, but varied widely between individuals; nowadays this PCO_2 is referred to as the "set point" of PCO_2, and averages 40 mmHg. The Haldane-Priestly method could not be used during exercise, because the PCO_2 in alveoli is always changing and an average cannot be calculated easily. For similar reasons, the method could not be used lung disorders. However, in 1889 Christian Bohr had reasoned that the PCO_2 of mixed blood from all alveoli, as in arterial blood, would represent average or "effective" alveolar PCO_2. As we saw in Chapter 4, this concept was adopted universally, once Riley and his colleagues had established the theoretical foundations of ventilation/perfusion relationships. Their work showed how PCO_2 could be used to calculate the effective alveolar oxygen pressure. The "normal" range of the arterial PCO_2 is between 34 and 46 mmHg. Although this may seem a narrow range, implying little variability, it is easy to calculate the implications that this variation has for ventilation (breathing volume per minute).[5] If we assume an average resting output of CO_2 to be 200 ml/min, a PCO_2 of 46 implies an alveolar ventilation of 3.2 litres/min, which translates into a total ventilation of 4.4 litres/min. In contrast, a PCO_2 of 34 implies an alveolar ventilation of 5.1 and total ventilation of 7.0 litres/min. The difference seems small, but were we to make a similar calculation for exercise the

difference becomes very large, putting someone whose set point is 34 at a distinct disadvantage compared to someone with a set point of 46, because their breathing is at least 35% (46/34 = 1.35) greater. Such differences imply differences in individual "responsiveness" to CO_2.

MEASURING "CO_2 RESPONSIVENESS"

Haldane and Priestley found large increases in ventilation as they increased the inspired CO_2 concentration, associated with only a small increase in the alveolar PCO_2. This was because the large increase in ventilation minimized the increase in PCO_2. Control engineers term this a feed-back control system in "closed loop" conditions. In the 1960s, Moran Campbell thought that a better idea would be to study "open loop" conditions, in which increases in breathing would not reduce the extent to which PCO_2 rose. These conditions apply to a rebreathing system.

In the early 1960s it was difficult to obtain a measurement of blood PCO_2 yet this was crucial to the management of many patients with lung problems, and the methods available were time-consuming. Moran Campbell decided to modify a method first proposed by Clarence Collier of the University of California, which depended on the much simpler gas, as opposed to blood, measurement. The principle was to rebreathe from a small rubber bag (normally found on anaesthetic machines) so as to equilibrate the gas in the bag with that of blood flowing through into the lungs (the "mixed venous" PCO_2), and then to analyze the gas in the bag for CO_2. As the rebreathing took only 2 minutes and the analysis less than 10, one had one's answer very rapidly, and we could perform the method without even leaving the patient's bedside. We studied the method intensively, and it became the bedrock of a new approach to patient management.

---

5   Alveolar ventilation (VA) is calculated from the ratio of CO2 output (VCO2) to alveolar CO2 pressure PACO2, as in the equation— VA = 0.863VCO2/PACO2; to obtain the total expired ventilation (VE), the contribution form "dead space" in airways, of approximately 150 ml per breath, is added on.

Rebreathing from the rubber bag was accompanied by a progressive rise in breathing rate and volume, both easy measurements to make. As PCO_2 in the lung and bag increased so breathing increased linearly, allowing an index of breathing control to be expressed in terms of litres of ventilation for each mmHg increase in PCO_2. The measurement took about 5 minutes and had a great advantage over the previous methods—the system was studied under "open loop" conditions; the extent of breathing had no effect on the stimulus (PCO_2) because CO_2 was retained in the bag. In 1965, David Read came to the Hammersmith from Sydney, Australia, and undertook a series of studies that established the "Read method" as the preferred method for measuring CO_2 responsiveness world-wide. David continued this work on his return to Sydney, but tragically succumbed to cancer a few years later.

A surprising but important early finding was that CO_2 responsiveness was much more variable than previously recognized; even studies with relatively few subjects showed that responsiveness ranged from 1 liter of ventilation for every 1 mmHg increase in PCO_2, to more than 10 liters. The variability accounted for variability in the resting ventilation, and the variation in arterial PCO_2 between 34 and 46 mmHg, and for differences in ventilation during exercise. In all cases, ventilation was higher in those having a greater response to CO_2. Some of the variation was shown to be due to genetic influences; for example, in 1976 Nick Saunders and his colleagues in Sydney, Australia, studied elite swimmers and their non-swimming siblings, and found that responsiveness to CO_2 did have a familial link; one of the swimmers showed a very low response to PCO_2 (only 0.42 litre per 1mm Hg rise in CO_2); her sister similarly had a low response (0.5 l/mm Hg); two years later she had broken world records for both 800

and 1500 meters freestyle. It seems likely that a reduced demand for breathing contributed to her success.

It may seem odd that up to now there has been little mention of oxygen, or the lack of it, providing a stimulus for breathing, but there are a number of reasons. First, breathing "tracks" metabolic CO_2 production more closely than O_2 consumption. Second, we cannot use arterial PO_2 as an index of breathing control, as we do with PCO_2 because PO_2 is affected by ventilation/perfusion distribution to a greater extent than PCO_2. Finally, although reductions in arterial PO_2 do stimulate breathing, the effect is non-linear. Whereas an increase in arterial PCO_2 of only a few mmHg will normally lead to a prompt ventilatory response, PO_2 has to fall from its normal range of 80-100 mmHg to below 60 mmHg before there is much effect.

Modulating the overall control of breathing, with its emphasis on maintaining arterial PCO_2 and hydrogen ion concentration within narrow limits, are a variety of factors related to the act of breathing itself. Nervous impulses travel to the brain from receptors in the muscles of breathing, providing information on the depth of each breath and the effort expended by the muscles; these give rise to a consciously appreciated sense of breathing effort, but also may act to automatically govern the pattern (depth and rate) of breathing. There are also impulses that arise in small nerve endings in the lung, which were discovered a surprisingly long time ago and reported in two remarkable scientific papers.

REFLEX CONTROL OF BREATH VOLUME

In 1868, Dr Joseph Breuer and Professor Ewald Hering, of the lowly Josephs-Akademie in Vienna, published their only full paper and Breuer presented a communication at a local meeting. Breuer was born in Vienna and qualified in medicine in 1867; the two papers were published in April and November of the following year which, considering the number and complexity of the experiments he described, is little short of miraculous. It is clear that Breuer was the driving force for the work; his rank is described as Clinical Assistant; Hering was the departmental head and sponsor for the papers. Both papers have the same title—*Self-steering of respiration through the vagus nerves*. "Self-steering" is the usual translation of the term *Selbststeurung* then used in engineering to denote feedback control through mechanical regulators in devices such as large pumps, but it seems to be the first time it was used in a physiological context to denote negative feedback control through nerve reflexes. For this reason, the work was extremely important, although in common with other innovative concepts it took many decades for this fact to be realized. In their own words, their studies in dogs revealed that "I. The lung, when it becomes more expanded by inspiration, or by inflation, exerts an inhibitory effect on inspiration and promotes expiration, and this effect is the greater the stronger the expansion. Every inspiration, therefore, in that it distends the lung, brings about its own demise by means of this distension, and thus initiates expiration". "II. Reduction of the size of the lung affects the movements of respiration in the opposite sense". Breuer and Hering showed that the nerve impulses arose in the lung itself, rather than the chest wall or diaphragm, and that the reflexes were abolished by section of the vagus nerve. They suggested that the vagus contained two separate sets of nerve fibers, one activated by lung expansion and the other by deflation. Finally they described an odd finding that they felt would have to be mediated by a third receptor; occasionally when inspiration was

terminated by occluding the trachea, the animal responded by making a forceful <u>inspiratory</u> effort. Nowadays, this reflex is ascribed to the activation of fine irritant "C" fibres in small airways. The so called "Hering-Breuer inflation and deflation reflexes" (the master taking precedence over the student who did the work!), has been a major tenet of respiratory physiology, as the mechanisms that reflexly determine the rate and depth of breathing. Many sophisticated techniques, including recordings of single nerve fiber impulses, have been used to study and validate the mechanisms involved, although what part it plays in humans is still debated. Some sceptical wags used to say that the reflex could only be demonstrated in medical students, and then only in those that had read the textbook!

Another remarkable fact about Breuer and Hering's paradigm-changing work, is that neither of them carried out any other respiratory research; Hering gained a reputation as a leading expert in vision research and became Carl Ludwig's successor as professor in Leipzig; Breuer went into private practice and later achieved considerable fame as one of the founders of psychoanalysis, coauthoring with Sigmund Freud *Studies on Hysteria* in 1895.

Much of the recent research on the Hering-Breuer reflex suggests that it is just one of the mechanisms that influence the breathing pattern, together with other stimuli that arise in the muscles of breathing, as they contract, and in the pulmonary circulation, responding to increases in pressure. Such reflexes probably account for changes in the pattern of breathing seen in disorders of the lung, airways and circulation. More intriguing is the importance of the vagus nerve in mediating the responses.

THE ROLE OF THE VAGUS NERVE, AND SYMPATHETIC NERVOUS SYSTEM

The vagus nerve is the tenth cranial nerve, but its distribution and influence are far greater than any other cranial nerve. Also, unlike some cranial nerves, it carries messages both to (afferent) and from (efferent) the medulla of the brain stem. This small area contains clusters of nerves that act as coordinating "centres" for many functions that are unconsciously controlled by what is known as the autonomic nervous system. In addition to inspiratory and expiratory centres, it contains a vasomotor centre that mediates control of blood vessel constriction and thus blood pressure through the sympathetic nerves, and a cardiovascular centre regulating heart rate and force production. Although termed centres, the nerve groupings behave as relay points in a variety of reflexes, and also receive input from other "higher" areas in the cortex of the brain, and sensory nerves that supply the head and neck. Afferent nerve fibers travel in the vagus from the heart and major blood vessels, lungs and airways, and efferent fibers from the medulla travel in the vagus to the airways (causing them to narrow and produce mucus) heart (causing a slow heart rate and decrease in blood pressure), stomach (causing increased activity and acid secretion), glands (increased secretion of sweat and digestive enzymes) and many other organs. Efferent nerves from the medulla also contribute to the sympathetic nervous system, a chain of nerves that travels parallel to the spinal column to mediate functional reflexes throughout the body. Sympathetic nerve impulses activate two types of receptors (α and β), providing a great range of responses; they are usually classed as "fright and flight" responses, and include increase in heart rate and force of contraction, increase in blood pressure, relaxation of airway muscle, release of glucose from the liver,

and so on. As we will see in a later chapter, these autonomic reflex activities explain the physiological links between breathing and the function of the heart and other organs, which underlie many daily experiences both in health and disease.

DISORDERS OF BREATHING CONTROL

To come back to breathing control and the punch line that began this chapter, none of the central controls work adequately in the absence of the normal response to carbon dioxide, so called chemosensitivity. There are individuals in whom CO_2 responsiveness is severely blunted, either congenitally or because of injury to the brain stem.

In 1976, Dr Stanley Epstein, a Toronto colleague who had trained with me at the Hammersmith Hospital, phoned to ask if we might investigate a teenaged patient who had presented with heart failure: her heart was large but there was no sign of any cause and the diagnosis was initially that of primary heart muscle disease (cardiomyopathy). However, Dr Charles Bryan, at the Toronto Sick Children's Hospital had picked up that she became blue at night and that her blood bicarbonate was very elevated, suggesting that perhaps she was retaining CO_2. Blood gas analysis confirmed his suspicion, showing an elevated PCO_2, and reduced PO_2. Our studies at McMaster confirmed the blood gas changes, which became much worse at night, when the PCO_2 rose to 90 mmHg, more than twice what it should have been. Her lung function was normal, but she showed no response to CO_2 increases during rebreathing or to falls in O_2; she could hold her breath almost indefinitely—she had to be asked to stop holding her breath, or she might have passed out due to lack of oxygen. During exercise her breathing increased, but not enough to prevent large increases in PCO_2 and falls in PO_2. She was clearly suffering from "Ondine's Curse".

The term "Ondine's curse" refers to a number of fairy tales that feature an ondine (mermaid) who falls in love with a mortal, and after marrying him is jilted; all this after being warned by the King of the Ondines that this outcome will lead to an unpleasant end. It's the King who imposed the curse, but the curse itself has been subject to considerable editorial license—from the mermaid returning to the sea as foam, through to dire effects on the unfaithful mortal. In the latter category is one version of the story in which he (the mortal Hans) loses all the body's automatic functions, one of which is breathing. The unfortunate Hans bemoans his fate—"If I relax my vigilance for one moment, I may forget to hear or to breathe. He died, they'll say, because he could no longer bother to breathe". Julius Comroe, renowned director of the Cardiovascular Research Institute in San Francisco, in one of his lighter publications, chronicles but also criticizes the use of the term "Ondine's Curse" on both literary and scientific grounds—it was not Ondine that cursed, and lack of automatic breathing was only one of the problems facing Hans. However, once a picturesque eponym has been invented it's hard to replace it, in this case with "congenital central hypoventilation syndrome". Our patient showed the widespread effects of not maintaining the *milieu intérieur* when breathing fails to respond normally to the body's needs. The resulting increase in PCO_2 maintained over a long period of time caused changes in the heart muscle cells (contracting poorly), in the blood vessels of the lung (narrowing to increase pressure) and in the kidneys (retaining water and sodium), leading her to death's door. Fortunately, improvements in breathing with a rocking bed and later electronic pacemaker for the phrenic nerve led to an excellent outcome.

The control of breathing is yet another example of the complexity of interactions between the external and internal environment, and involving, directly or indirectly, as well as the lungs, many other systems of the body— including the heart and circulation; the brain and nervous system; all tissues capable of large changes in metabolism, such as muscle; and blood. This complexity has made it impossible to explain how the system works in different situations merely by using analogies to engineering control systems. The changes in breathing that occur during sleep and exercise, at altitude or during diving, and as a response to stress or its opposite (such as yoga), all have aspects that are unique to each, probably because each system adapts differently. However, the overriding importance of controlling the blood gas and hydrogen ion concentration of circulating blood is clear, and this provides us with a starting point for thinking about what happens to breathing in these various situations.

CHANGES IN BREATHING CONTROL IN LUNG DISORDERS

Anything which makes it hard for you to breathe, leads to extreme discomfort; just try breathing through a drinking straw to experience this feeling. Whatever it costs in terms of the effort required to keep PCO_2 from increasing is accepted as the only way to stay alive. Patients who have a severe asthma attack become very distressed but manage to maintain normal blood PCO_2; doctors who find an elevated PCO_2 in this situation become as anxious as the patient, because it is a sign that he or she is at death's door. However, in patients with chronic obstruction to bronchial air flow, there is often an adaptive response which tends to ease the distress; the blood PCO_2 gradually increases, and the kidneys have time to respond, minimizing any increase

86

in the blood's acidity. In patients with chronic obstructive pulmonary disease (COPD) this underbreathing tends to occur more often in patients with chronic bronchitis than in those with emphysema. Interestingly, this is not the only difference between these two groups of COPD patients; the chronic bronchitics are overweight whereas emphysema patients are frequently very skinny. When they exercise, the bronchitics tend to improve their blood oxygen, whereas emphysema patients usually show large reductions in PO_2. Also, their personalities differ; the patients that underbreathe tend to be placid and less extraverted than those who fight to maintain their blood gases normal. Unfortunately, chronic underbreathing leads to a lowered blood oxygen, and to retention of fluid in the body, leading to these patients being called the "blue bloaters", as opposed to the "pink puffers" with emphysema. Although these differences were first described more than 50 years ago, the mechanisms that underlie them remain a matter of debate. The complex interactions, apparently involving personality and nutritional state, as well as the damage to the bronchi and lung alveoli, make it hard to separate the main causes from the effects of the problems these individuals face.

It would be easy to conclude that breathing is controlled so as to maintain oxygenation of arterial blood, removal of carbon dioxide, and alkalinity of body fluids. However, these three objectives are often not tightly linked, leading to a debate as to which takes precedent. Furthermore, the ways in which the objectives are met vary between species, with each employing a strategy that maintains life and activity of the organism. For each organism, breathing control involves coordination between systems that respond in very different ways to the challenges presented by changes in activity, the environment, and the structure of the body.

The coordination is so complex that we cannot hope to describe it completely. The simple explanation has to be viewed with scepticism, if not suspicion.

CHAPTER 8

ALL CREATURES GREAT AND SMALL…BREATHE

"First forms minute, unseen by spheric glass
Move on the mud, or pierce the watery mass;
These as successive generations bloom,
New Powers acquire and larger limbs assume;
Whence countless groups of vegetation spring
And breathing realms of fin, and feet, and wing."

Erasmus Darwin (1731-1802), The
Temple of Nature

"…while this planet has gone cycling on
according to the fixed law of gravity, from
so simple a beginning endless forms so
beautiful and most wonderful have been,
and are being evolved."

Charles Darwin, 1859, The Origin of Species

Erasmus Darwin was more poetic and less scientific than his grandson, but seems to have had an innate understanding of the evolutionary process. Some 50 years after his death, in the last few words of the most influential and most widely read scientific work of all time, *The Origin of Species*, Charles Darwin expressed the wonder and fascination everyone feels when they consider the development of the myriad life forms on our planet. The extension of the book's title is seldom mentioned—"by means of natural selection or the preservation of favoured races in the struggle for life"; it expresses the notion of "survival of the fittest". The expression, first used by Darwin's colleague Herbert Spencer, may be overused, but as we now define fitness in terms of maximal oxygen consumption, survival is clearly dependent on the capacity to breathe.

Among the myriad fields of scientific inquiry, that of comparative physiology is one of the most fascinating. Its scope ranges from changes during evolution, through differences between species, and mechanisms that allow adaptation to different environments, to the implications of size differences both between different species and within a given species. Thus, the present chapter will explore not how different creatures breathe to exchange oxygen and CO_2 with their environment but also why it matters whether they are large or small.

DIFFERENT STRATEGIES TO SUPPORT METABOLISM

All animals, large and small, use metabolic chemical reactions to generate energy. The processes in animal tissues link chemical energy to oxygen, with production of CO_2 and water. Oxygen is supplied to tissues and CO_2 is removed; this "respiratory exchange" takes place with the environment, whether it's water or air. The metabolic production of water is handled by evaporation and the kidneys. For these reasons it will come as no surprise that the mechanisms that accomplish oxygen intake, CO_2 output and water loss are closely linked. What may come as a surprise is the variety of strategies that different species employ to achieve these essential functions. The differences between different evolutionary "branches" (phyla), or classes, are so marked that they have become part of their defining characteristics. In this chapter we will briefly explore the gas exchanging organs of single celled organisms, worms, fishes, amphibians, reptiles, birds and mammals. Before delving into complex differences between species, we can boil them down into two major objectives that all animals have to achieve; the first is the extraction of oxygen from the environment and the second is its delivery to tissues. The efficiency with which these two objectives are met, determines the fitness of the organism. Removal of CO_2 naturally goes along with the two objectives, being removed from tissues, transported to the gas exchanger, and transferred to the environment. The transfers are always down a <u>pressure</u> gradient, but metabolism involves <u>amounts</u> of O_2 and CO_2. The relationships between pressures and volumes of the gases, both in the environment and the organism, show considerable variation, leading to a wide variety of strategies being employed to achieve gas exchange.

The main source of oxygen is the atmosphere, receiving the benefits of plant photosynthesis; in water, most of the oxygen has diffused from air until its pressure at the surface equals that in the atmosphere; only a small amount comes from submerged plants. Unfortunately, oxygen is not very soluble in water—the amount of oxygen in a litre of water is about 30 times less than in a litre of air, and the speed with which it moves through water is thousands of times less. For these reasons much more water has to be supplied in order to deliver the same amount of oxygen when delivered by air. Once the oxygen has diffused into the animal, various strategies are used to deliver it to the tissues. Getting rid of CO_2 poses fewer problems, because the pressure of CO_2 is always greater than in the environment, and because CO_2 is more soluble in water than oxygen.

PRIMITIVE SYSTEMS

Very small organisms obtain oxygen directly from the environment; in some, diffusion is aided by very fine hairs (cilia) that move the surrounding water. In more complex animals respiration is closely linked to digestion, water or air being taken in at the mouth and absorption of oxygen occurring directly from the digestive tract or in specialized organs that developed as offshoots from it. Most use some sort of blood, containing an oxygen carrying pigment, and circulated to tissues where oxygen is off-loaded. A simple system exists in worms, where air is taken in at the mouth and forced down the gut by circular muscles; oxygen is taken up in the gut, and circulation is effected by small blood vessels that contract rhythmically. CO_2 diffuses out of blood and through the skin. The arrangement is sufficient to support the worm's metabolism (they are sluggish!); however, the skin has to be kept moist or too much water will be lost and the worm dries from inside out.

GAS EXCHANGE IN FISH

Blood circulates in fish in a simple, single circulation. The heart pumps blood through the gills, on into the tissues and back to the heart. Fish take in water through the mouth and it

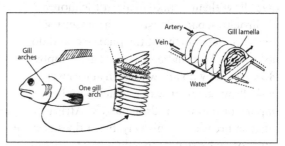

Figure 24 Gas exchange system in the fish

passes through the gills, containing delicate membranes supplied with blood. When the fish is motionless, the water is forced through the gills by muscles in the mouth and pharynx, and muscles in the gills also control the flow. Large increases in metabolism are mainly associated with movement and thus accompanied by large increases in water flow through the gills; fish with larger gills are capable of greater activity. Two other factors help oxygen absorption in fish. First, blood flow in the gills is in the opposite direction to the water (a counter-current). Because the blood exiting the gills is meeting the highest PO_2, this helps to maintain a high pressure difference between water and blood. And second, the blood contains hemoglobin, which carries oxygen as a function of its pressure. As the pressure of oxygen in water is the same as in the air (or higher, at depth) the amount of oxygen being supplied to tissues is similar to that of air-breathing animals. However, because of the large amount of water flowing through the gills, CO_2 is washed out of blood and exists at a pressure that is only one-tenth of that found in air breathers. Consequently blood bicarbonate is also low, which reduces fishes' ability to adapt to acidic environments. This is one factor contributing to the lifeless lakes affected by acid rain, but that's another story.

Some fishes have developed primitive lungs that allow them to take in air at the mouth or through separate nostrils. The primitive lungs are outgrowths of the pharynx, and do not sustain large increases in oxygen supply. However, they do allow some fish to survive in shallow, stagnant water, which may be important in times of drought. The African lungfish breathes in this way, but it doesn't have much of an existence, spending most of its life dozing. The lungfish has always been considered a link between fish and amphibians, as animals evolved from water to air breathers.

AMPHIBIANS—DWELLERS IN AIR AND WATER

Amphibians, such as frogs, have lungs that are ventilated by the muscles of the mouth, but also exchange oxygen and CO_2 through the skin. Early in their development, as tadpoles, amphibians possess external gills; water circulates through the gills when the tadpole swims. As adults they have a parallel two-part circulation and a three chambered heart having two atria and one ventricle. Oxygenated blood from the skin mixes with venous blood from the rest of the body in the right atrium, and the left receives blood from the lungs; the single ventricle delivers blood to the lungs and general circulation. This may appear inefficient, but the two streams remain almost separate through the action of a spiral valve, with most of the blood that passes through the right atrium going to the lungs. A final implication of the three chambered heart is the fact that blood is delivered at high pressure equally in the lungs and general circulation. This is in contrast to mammals, where a four-chambered heart allows the lungs to be supplied with blood at a fraction of the pressure needed to deliver blood to the rest of the body.

REPTILES, THE FIRST TERRESTRIAL VERTEBRATES

The lungs of reptiles are more developed than amphibians, being of larger relative volume and providing greater surface area for diffusion. The air passages (bronchi) end in air sacs (alveoli); the lungs are enclosed in a fairly rigid cage (thorax) and air is moved by the abdominal muscles; there is no diaphragm. Most reptiles spend their days resting in the shade or half-submerged in water and they do not need to maintain high levels of oxygen consumption for long periods of time. In common with amphibians most reptiles have a three chambered heart, but there is even less mixing of oxygenated and deoxygenated blood than in amphibians; indeed, crocodiles have four completely separate chambers, similar to mammals.

90

INSECTS—A RADICALLY DIFFERENT APPROACH

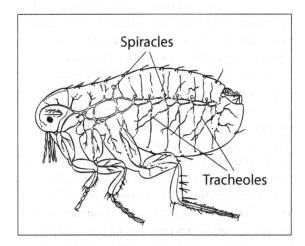

Figure 25 In the flea—(total length 2mm) fine tubes distribute air directly to the tissues

Insects are interesting because they supply air directly to muscles through fine air passages (spiracles) which reach right down to the cells; the action of the muscles moves air to help with the diffusion of oxygen in the spiracles. Also the spiracles can be closed, allowing CO_2 release to be regulated and avoiding excessive water loss. Most insects are tiny; the system would not work well for large animals because of the distances over which the oxygen would have to travel. Some insects have air sacs connected to the spiracles, which are filled through the action of the abdominal muscles. Insects that live in water take their air down with them in bubbles.

BIRDS, FLYING AND BREATHING

Birds draw in air through quite rigid tubes into large air sacs in the abdomen. These sacs are filled periodically and act as bellows, sending a continuous stream of air forward through fine tubes arranged in parallel. These have thin walls containing tiny blood vessels, acting as lungs. The outflowing air is collected in large anterior air sacs, which can be vented back into the main airway (trachea). Although measurements in flying birds are difficult, this intriguing arrangement may allow birds to extract oxygen from the air more efficiently than other animals. Birds such as the bar-head goose are capable of flying at altitudes that are higher than those where pilots require oxygen masks. It seems likely also that water loss is minimized during breathing—another problem that birds seem to have solved more effectively than mammals. In common with mammals, they have two separate circulations, for the lungs and rest of the body.

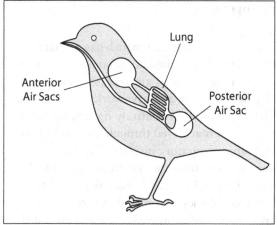

Figure 26 In birds, the lung is supplemented by storage air sacs

DO EGGS REALLY BREATHE?

Before leaving birds, we should mention their eggs. There is a constant requirement for oxygen, to sustain the metabolic demands of the developing chick. Air diffuses into the egg through minute pores in the shell—the average egg has 10,000 of them, and they afford an example of evolution following the precept of "not too little, not too much, but just enough". Too many pores would weaken the shell and also lead to the contents drying out through excessive loss of water; too few, would limit oxygen delivery and removal of CO_2. The mathematics involved in these relationships has intrigued comparative physiologists, like Knut Schmidt-Nielsen. In his book *Scaling: why is animal size so important?* he considers the differences between the egg of a hen, weighing 60 grams, and that of the South American ostrich-like Rhea, which weighs ten times as much. It turns out that the pores in the larger, thicker shelled egg have an average area that exactly compensates for their greater metabolic requirements and greater pore length.

MAMMALS, FROM MICE TO ELEPHANTS

The structures that accomplish gas exchange in mammals, described in chapter 4, consist of a branching system of air passages ending in alveoli containing a fine network of capillaries. The lungs occupy a relatively rigid thorax and ventilation is achieved through the diaphragm and other respiratory muscles. The major improvement from the system in reptiles is the muscular diaphragm, which achieves greater inspired volumes, and may therefore allow greater specific metabolism. In using the word "specific" I mean the metabolic demands in relation to the mass, or volume, of the animal.

Which brings me to the second major endeavour of comparative physiologists—crudely put, what are the differences between the lungs of elephants as compared to mice? Further, what are the structural and functional implications of the huge differences between animals of differing size; an elephant weighs 100,000 times as much as a mouse?

"SCALING" THE ORGANS OF BREATHING

The first person to apply scientific method to the structural implications of animal size, seems to have been Galileo, possibly taking note of Leonardo's geometrical studies of the human body. Galileo started out with the principles of Pythagoras, to reach the conclusion "the Book of Nature is written in characters of geometry". Observations of the dimensions of bones in different animals showed that the bones of large animals were proportionally thicker than their smaller relatives. Galileo concluded "… nor can Nature construct an animal beyond a certain size, whilst retaining the proportions and employing the materials which suffice in the case of a smaller structure". This seminal idea was developed further in a book that Sir Peter Medawar described as "beyond comparison the finest work of literature in all the annals of science that have been recorded in the English language". The book *On Growth and Form* was written by D'Arcy Wentworth Thompson and published in 1917. Thompson held many appointments as a naturalist, classicist and mathematician, all three disciplines being well represented in the book. He was skeptical of Darwin evolutionary theory and probably his analysis of animal structure could be used nowadays to support "intelligent design". The Laws of Nature exhibit a form of mathematical beauty, with relationships between structure and function and between different species showing consistent geometric similarities. Comparative zoologists are driven by the notion that studies of relative dimensions in different species will reveal universal principles linking structural design to optimal function.

IMPLICATIONS OF BODY SIZE TO METABOLISM AND THE LUNGS

The geometric similarities have a very simple basis. Starting with a line of length L, the area of a square having sides of that length is given by L^2 (L x L), and the volume of a similar cube by L^3 (L x L x L). It may seem odd that animals of different shapes can be compared in terms of lines, squares and cubes, but similar relationships exist for other shapes. In a sphere of radius r, surface area is a function of r^2 (4 πr^2) and volume a function of r^3 (4/3 πr^3). In using the concept of geometric similarity, we are proposing, for example that someone who is 10% taller than, say, the average height (ie. L is 1.1 times the average), will have a surface area that is 21% larger ($1.1^2 = 1.21$), and a mass or volume that is 33% larger ($1.1^3 = 1.33$). We may then choose some measurable attribute, such as the volume of the lungs and test whether it scales as a function of body length, area or volume, or somewhere in between. The justification for this is to judge whether some structure, for example lung size, is a limiting factor for the metabolic requirements of the whole animal. The concept was termed "symmorphosis" by Ewald Weibel and Charles Taylor, who carried out the most comprehensive study in this field, to be described below. Behind it, also, is the hypothesis (or belief) that "animals—and man—are built reasonably. Thus there should be no waste, or as little waste as possible… There should be just enough, but no more, alveolar surface in the lung; just enough, but no more, mitochondrial mass to support the largest energy needs of the body".

The respiratory function that has been most extensively studied in a wide variety of animals is oxygen uptake, VO_2. This is a measure of metabolic rate, and to begin with it was felt that metabolism was a function of mass; in other words, specific VO_2 (VO_2/kg) would be the same for large and small. Indeed, when it came to expressing fitness in terms of maximum exercise VO_2 (VO_2max), VO_2max/kg became the measure of choice, and it remains so—surprisingly, as we shall see.

As long ago as 1838, a professor of mathematics at Strasbourg University, Frédéric Sarrus had argued that metabolism in animals was related to heat production, and that heat loss—which has to equal production—was a function of body surface area. Applying the strategy of geometric similarities, he argued that because area is equivalent to length^2 and volume$^{2/3}$, VO_2 should vary as mass$^{2/3}$ ($M^{0.66}$). The relationship seemed to fit changes in size associated with growth, and later Max Rubner obtained data on resting metabolic rate in animals varying in size from a mouse (18 grams) to swine (128 kilos), to confirm that metabolic rate expressed per unit surface area was the same. This became known as Rubner's surface area rule. Basal metabolic rate (BMR) became a standard measurement in the early 20th century, used mainly in the diagnosis of thyroid disorders; normal standards were established and an equation was used that expressed BMR as a function of height^2. The relationship was also used to define lean body mass (LBM), or desirable weight, as a function of height^2; ie. LBM = k / H^2. This relationship was used to describe average body weight in a population, and known as the Quetelet index. Alphonse Quetelet (1796-1874) was one of the first to apply statistics to the population, so-called vital statistics, and was a forerunner to modern biometricians.

Many years after Rubner, in the 1920s and 30s, many more data were obtained in animals, by Max Kleiber at the University of California, Davis, and Samuel Brody at the University of Missouri. They found that resting VO_2 increased as a function of mass raised to ¾ power ($M^{0.75}$); this exponent lies between the 2/3 ($M^{0.66}$) suggested by the surface rule, and 1 (M), which would express BMR as a function of mass.[1] Although the difference may seem rather

1   The equation for the relationship was VO2 = 0.19 x M0.75 (Taylor et al, 1980)

esoteric, it becomes important when the factors affecting BMR were being debated—whether related to heat loss or to the mass of tissue contributing to metabolism. Using the mouse-to-elephant analogy, the mouse's resting VO_2, expressed per kg weight, is 30 times that of the elephant's. Relative to its weight, the mouse has to eat 30 times more than the elephant to sustain life. Expressed as a function of $M^{0.75}$, metabolic rate in the two animals is the same. It is a remarkable fact that the relationship holds for all classes of the animal kingdom.

SUPPORTING MAXIMAL EXERTION

Of course, when we consider "Survival of the Fittest", the VO_2 achieved during exertion (maximal VO_2, VO_2max) seems more relevant than resting VO_2 (BMR). In one of the most remarkable studies in comparative physiology C. Richard Taylor, of Harvard University, in the 1980s, measured VO_2max in over 20 species of mammal, from mice to elephants. All the animals were successfully exercised, on suitable treadmills, at the East African Veterinary Research Organization at Muguga in Kenya. The relationship was proportionally similar to that found for resting VO_2; VO_2max increased in proportion to the 0.8 power of body mass. Not surprisingly there were some differences between wild and domesticated animals, and between "active" and "inactive" species. For example, dogs and horses have VO_2max values that are about 3 times those found in cattle and sheep. In humans, also, VO_2max is 2-3 times larger in trained athletes that untrained people. After reviewing previous studies, Weibel and Taylor proposed that VO_2 max increased in proportion to $M^{0.75}$, and was about 10 times the resting metabolic rate in all the species they studied.[2] The results were very close to those obtained by Kleiber and Brodie, and they felt that the relationship between VO_2 max and mass$^{3/4}$ "best reflects the optimization of design of respiratory structures as demands for oxygen change with size". We may ask the question, what are the implications in relation to humans?

The standard measure of fitness for many decades has been maximum exercise VO_2, measured on a treadmill or cycle, expressed per kilo weight (VO_2max/kg). No doubt it is used as one measure to choose athletes for representative teams, and one might argue that in some running events in which one has to shift one's weight, the athlete with the higher VO_2max/kg is expected to perform better. However, weight often is not so relevant to performance. What then might be a better index of performance when comparing athletes of different heights and weights?

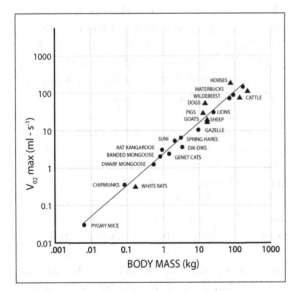

Figure 27 The relationship found by CR Taylor, between maximal oxygen consumption and body weight (logarithmic scales) in a wide range of animals

2 The equation for the relationship was VO2 = 1.94 x M0.75 (Taylor et al, 1980)

MAXIMAL OXYGEN CONSUMPTION IN HUMANS

Without doubt the doyen of the modern world's exercise physiologists is Per-Olof Åstrand. As the Director of the Gymnastik - och Idrottshogskolan in Stockholm in the second half of the 20th century, he spearheaded the successful drive to improve fitness in Scandinavia. Also, he popularized and simplified exercise testing techniques so that they became a mainstay in assessing cardiac and pulmonary disorders. Finally, he was the principal investigator in many oft-quoted studies, during which he mentored several of the world's premier exercise physiologists. In 1962, as a fledgling exercise physiologist, I had the great good fortune to visit him in Stockholm. He picked me up at the airport in his battered Volkswagen, transported me to his department, and soon after I was pedalling hard on the cycle ergometer, with one of the technicians waving a Union Jack to provide suitable encouragement. After it was over Per-Olof informed me that I was much fitter than the average US Marine, but not quite up to the average Swedish housewife. Another lesson learnt—that however eminent one becomes, it's important not to take life too seriously!

Even before the study of Taylor and Weibel, Åstrand realized the implications of dimensional analysis; it meant that VO_2max, expressed per kilogram of body weight, was not a valid index to compare fitness in different individuals. He took data obtained in a group of elite athletes, members of Norwegian national teams in whom VO_2max had been measured. He assumed they must all be of similar fitness, but that VO_2 would not be the same across different statures. Sure enough, VO_2max expressed per kg yielded higher values for the smaller athletes than the larger, to an extent expected from Rubner's $M^{2/3}$ rule. For example an elite athlete weighing 60 kg had a VO_2max of 4.3 litres/min (expressed per kg, 72ml/min/kg); the comparable value for an athlete weighing 100 kg was 6.3 litres/min (63 ml/min/kg). Assessed by VO_2max/kg, the smaller athlete appears fitter by almost 20%; however, expressed in relation to mass$^{2/3}$, the values were comparable. Incidentally, if mass$^{3/4}$ is used, the agreement is even closer.

Of course, when it comes to assessing fitness in a general population, one cannot use weight to predict maximum exercise capacity, because it would imply that obese individuals achieve higher performance that lean subjects. For this purpose, a power function of height (H)

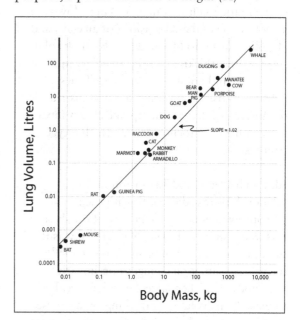

Figure 28 The "mouse to elephant" graph for lung volume.

makes better sense. In the Exercise Laboratory at McMaster, we eventually had a large enough population to establish an appropriate prediction; as we expected, the power function was between H^2, expected from the surface area rule, and H^3, expected from ideal (fat-free) body mass. It is , of course, much more difficult to demonstrate the validity of a particular scaling factor in a population with a 2-3-fold variation in mass, as compared to the animal studies of Weibel and Taylor, where the variation was as much as 20-30-fold.

In pursuing their objective of defining structural "optimization" to achieve the needed oxygen consumption, Taylor and Weibel systematically analyzed the structures involved in the oxygen flow pathway, in their mammals—representing a huge size range. Structures that scaled similarly to VO_2max would potentially be limiting to oxygen transfer. The conceptual model was that of sequential processes that linked inspired air to the mitochondria in muscle. Thus, flow to the alveoli involves the dimensions of airways and alveoli; transfer to blood, depends on alveolar surface area, thickness of the alveolar-capillary "barrier", and number of lung capillaries; delivery to tissues, on heart size and distribution of muscle capillaries; and uptake of oxygen, on the volume of mitochondria in which oxygen combustion takes place.[3]

Although Weibel and Taylor found some relationships that did not fit with their preconceived notions, the beauty of the data was unquestioned. To start with, there was the tight fit between VO_2max and body mass$^{0.75}$; oxygen consumption changes non-linearly with body size. Then, alveolar volume scaled to mass$^{1.0}$; the volume of the lungs in a mouse was proportionally smaller than in an elephant; in both, lungs were approximately 7% of body mass, where volume in litres is equivalent to

mass in kilograms. Alveolar surface area also scaled to mass$^{1.0}$. The capacity to diffuse oxygen across the alveolar-capillary barrier scaled to mass$^{1.0}$, rather than VO_2max. Heart size also scaled to mass$^{1.0}$, being approximately 6% of body mass across species. Finally, muscle mitochondrial volume was closely related to VO_2max, independent of mass. Some years earlier, in 1973, Thomas McMahon, a colleague of Richard Taylor, had made a complex engineering analysis of the structures that contributed to running speed. Larger mammals, with longer legs and larger muscles, ran faster and incurred larger metabolic costs. The oxygen demands scaled with $M^{3/4}$, lending support to the dominance of muscle in determining VO_2max.

Most of Weibel and Taylor's findings make intuitive sense, but they had not expected to find a discordance between VO_2max and the lung's capacity for oxygen diffusion. They pointed out that lung oxygen transfer in the mouse was 10 times less than in a cow, for a comparable mass-specific oxygen flow; there was far less reserve available in lungs of smaller animals. This did not fit with the notion that a structure that was rate limiting for oxygen intake, would scale across species to the maximal oxygen requirements. This follows from "the hypothesis that the respiratory system of mammals scales optimally at each step in the system, from the oxygen store in environmental air to the oxygen sink in the mitochondria". Two questions followed; first, is the analysis valid; and second, are there factors that help smaller animals to adapt to the relatively lower lung transfer capacity? In answering the first question, help came from an unlikely source; for the second, a more integrative view of respiratory gas transport would be needed.

---

3   Mitochondria are unique cellular bodies (because they have their own DNA) in which the oxidative metabolic processes take place (such as the Krebs Cycle). They have been termed the body's "power house"; their inner membrane is greatly folded, giving a huge surface in relation to their volume.

A NEW APPROACH—FRACTAL ANALYSIS

Up to this point in the attempts to define the structures that limited oxygen supply in animals used relationships based on classical (Euclidean) geometry. That is, circumferences and areas were assumed to behave similarly to a perfect circle or square, and volumes as if they behaved as perfect spheres, cubes or cylinders. But structures in the body are not regular and their sizes are not describable by simple equations. As already discussed to relation the sizing of airways, a new way of analysing structure was pioneered by the Polish mathematician and physicist Benoit Mandelbrot. His book *The Fractal Geometry of Nature*, published in 1982, has had a profound impact on science and art in general, and dimensional analysis in particular. Mandelbrot argued that, in thinking of complex structures that are capable of being viewed all the way from a total body down to a minute cell, "fractal dimensions" were more revealing than the classical three dimensions. The branching of airways and blood vessels exhibit fractal behaviour to a marked degree; this fact has great functional implications. If one examines part of the bronchial tree, one cannot tell whether it is at, say, the level of a fourth branching or a tenth; they are (self) similar. At every branch the diameter is reduced by about 0.8, and each branch shortens by 0.6. The branching in a true fractal would go on to infinity; in airways and blood vessels it continues until a functional minimal diameter is reached; airways have to feed alveoli, and capillaries have to allow blood cells to reach tissues.

Mandelbrot's reasoning and Weibel's measurements of airways and blood vessels were used by Geoffrey West and his colleagues to construct a model of the respiratory and cardiovascular systems. The model had three defining features: airways and blood vessels branched fractal-like to fill the entire volume of the organism; the final branch in the system was always the same size; and the energy required to supply air and blood was at a minimum. Almost uncannily, the model predicted all the relationships found by the researchers that had preceded them. Tellingly, the close relation between metabolic rate and mass$^{3/4}$ was predicted, as was oxygen diffusing capacity and mass$^{1.0}$. West's paper was published in the journal *Science* in 1997; the journal's editor asked Ewald Weibel for his comment on the work. "I'm not sure their model is the final one, but it has good predictive power, and study of the deviations from it is going to be very interesting".

We are left with the conclusion that the supply of oxygen for maximal activity is that expected from the branching airways and blood vessels that are perfectly distributed for the size of the lungs and the body's muscles. It does, however, serve to emphasize the fact that many processes have to integrate to maximize delivery of fuels and oxygen, and maximize the removal of CO_2 and the associated acid-base homeostasis. How else can we explain the fact that a dwarf mongoose studied by Weibel and Taylor, sustains a specific maximal oxygen consumption (VO_2max/kg body weight) that is about 3 times that of a wildebeest, in spite of having similar weight-specific airways, lungs, heart and circulation?

97

Although the capillaries and the blood corpuscles they contain are the same size in small compared to large animals, there are more capillaries in a given volume of muscle in the smaller than the larger. The total amount of hemoglobin is relatively larger in smaller mammals. Furthermore, the oxygen carrying characteristics of hemoglobin (the relation between oxygen pressure and content, expressed in the O_2 dissociation curve) favours the unloading of oxygen in the tissues of smaller animals. The red cells of smaller animals also have a higher concentration of the enzyme carbonic anhydrase, which speeds the unloading of CO_2 in the lungs, and also indirectly speeds the uptake of oxygen. The frequency of breathing and heart beat are systematically higher in smaller animals. It is likely that the maximum rate that muscle can use oxygen plays a role in the differences, through differences in mitochondrial enzymes.

Also not explained by in studies of metabolic rate related to body size are the large differences between active and inactive individuals in the same species, who are identical in size and have similar lungs, hearts and blood vessels. The differences between athletes and untrained humans, and trained and untrained horses, for example, can be as much as 3-5 fold. Trained athletes have as much as 8 times the number of mitochondria in their muscles, together with a greater number of capillaries and more efficient distribution of blood flow to go with them. They are also able to supply fuels for muscle contraction at a greater rate.

So closely connected are the processes and systems involved in maximum exercise, that it becomes impossible to identify which play limiting roles to explain differences in performance between different species. Even within a species, predicting performance from measurements of height and weight, lung capacity and heart size, is a chancy business at best. There is too much room for adaptation at various points in the transport lines between the lungs and tissues, for the major structures to become limiting. We may echo the feelings of Giovanni Alfonso Borelli, who was professor of mathematics at Pisa University in the mid-17th century—"But so great a machinery of vessels and organs of the lung must have been instituted for some grand purpose, and that we shall try to expound if possible, though we shall stammer as we go along".

One last point in the discussion regarding VO_2max is worth making. It may not deserve its almost mythical reputation as the index of performance, which when reached, leads to muscle failure. Instead, it may merely be the metabolic rate at which the human, or animal, finds the effort is too great to be tolerated. This intolerable effort may be due to high muscle acidity, or to fuel shortage. Both these factors can be prevented and thereby allow exercise to be continued. There are situations in which fuel delivery and homeostasis take precedence over oxygen delivery, and where CO_2 removal becomes the more pressing need.

CHAPTER 9

THE AIR *GAIA* BREATHES

"Pure country air, freed from moisture, contains 20.93 per cent by volume of oxygen, 0.03 per cent of carbon dioxide, and 79.04 per cent, of a residue usually designated as "nitrogen", although of this 79.04 per cent about 0.94 per cent consists of argon. Careful analyses have indicated that over all the earth's surface, including the tops of high mountains, the proportions are the same, though they may be expected to vary appreciably in the stratosphere. Very minute traces are also present of hydrogen and various rare gases. Ordinary atmospheric air, contains, however, aqueous vapour in varying proportions: about 1 per cent is an average content present in a climate such as that of Great Britain, with more being present in summer than winter. In summer weather the percentage of CO_2 near the ground may be as low as 0.025 during the day, and as high as 0.035 during the night, owing to the influence of vegetation, etc.; and doubtless the oxygen percentage rises or falls correspondingly, though this has not been shown directly."

John Scott Haldane and his long-time colleague John Gillies Priestley, in their book *Respiration*, were able to write this paragraph about air in 1935. It is remarkable, in view of all the technological advances of the last 70 years, that this quantitative description cannot be improved upon. Only those respiratory physiologists who lived in an era when the chemical analysis of gases constituted the only sure way to measure the composition of respired gases, will be able to appreciate the amount of work and skill that this paragraph represents. Technological advances have lessened the required work and skill, but have not improved the quality of the observations. Perhaps what we need to ask first, is how the concentration of oxygen in the atmosphere came to increase to a level that sustains life as we know it, because it was not always so.

THE EVOLUTION OF ATMOSPHERIC OXYGEN AND CO_2

From an evolutionary point of view, we know from analysis of ancient rocks that atmospheric oxygen has risen from being virtually zero to constitute a fifth of the earth's atmosphere, and conversely that carbon dioxide was initially high but fell to a low concentration. One hundred million years ago, in the time of the dinosaurs, atmospheric carbon dioxide was some five times greater than it is today. More recently, in the past few million years or so, the composition of the atmosphere appears to have remained virtually constant. However, during the past few decades carbon dioxide has increased steadily, making it a major culprit of global warming. There is general anxiety that air quality is gradually deteriorating because of the accumulation of potentially toxic particles and chemicals. Because the lung is the only major internal organ to be in constant and intimate contact with the atmospheric environment, it is constantly at risk from changes in the composition of air. The need to understand the changes and their effects is underlined by the broadcasting of "smog alerts" with their advice that people with lung diseases should stay indoors and the general population should not exercise. The present chapter and that which follows will attempt to provide some perspectives on these topics, if only briefly.

The evidence for what happened "in the beginning" is buried in the earth's crust and the province of palaeontologists and physical chemists. However, the topic has engaged the minds and imagination of a much larger audience, which for centuries was dominated by the upholders of religious dogma. What we now know is that life on earth became possible once the temperature of its crust had fallen sufficiently for there to be an atmosphere and for water to exist in its fluid form. The oldest rocks date from at least 4,000 million years ago, and even those must have been the result of countless physico-chemical reactions in which new elements and compounds were forming. They would have formed a "sink" for any oxygen that was around, for oxygen is a highly reactive element; most rocks consist of oxides, and the abundance of carbon in meteorites must indicate that carbon dioxide would have been abundant in the atmosphere. There must then have been a long wait for the earth to cool, and for steam to form water, before conditions were right for chemical reactions to occur between water, carbon, nitrogen and the sun's energy, to create the early forms of life. Charles Darwin conceived of a "small, warm pond with all sorts of ammonia and phosphate salts" where the first protein might have been formed.

In 1953, Stanley L. Miller, a graduate student working under the supervision of Harold Clayton Urey[1] at the University of Chicago, experimentally tested Darwin's concept, by connecting two flasks, a small one containing water (H_2O) and the other a large flask in which vapour could be subjected to electrical

sparks delivered by tungsten electrodes. The water was boiled and a mixture of ammonia (NH_3), methane (CH_4) and hydrogen (H_2) was introduced into the system; the sparks flew to simulate lightning. A few days later the water was murky and contained a variety of organic compounds, including the "building blocks of life"—amino acids (the simplest of which is glycine, $NH_2.CH_2.COOH$). The gas mixture in the flasks did not contain oxygen, but even so critics felt that it was more complex than one might have expected. However, Miller and Urey later obtained the same results with nitrogen, hydrogen, carbon dioxide and carbon monoxide. Whatever the postulated initial mixture, all seem to be agreed that there was very little oxygen in the atmosphere, and that its concentration took billions of years to increase. The early organisms were anaerobes, requiring no oxygen to flourish; indeed, oxygen would have prevented them flourishing as well as they did. Then came photosynthesis in plants, a turning point in the development of life on our planet.

PHOTOSYNTHESIS

Photosynthesis uses the sun's energy radiation to make carbohydrates (sugars) from CO_2 in the air and water, thereby releasing molecular oxygen into the atmosphere—the basic chemical reaction is written—

$$6CO_2 + 6H_2O \rightarrow C_6H_{12}O_6 + 6O_2.$$

Gradually the oxygen concentration in the atmosphere climbed, and CO_2 fell; animal cells evolved the machinery to reverse the process, burning sugars with oxygen and producing CO_2, with the liberation of metabolically essential energy. The two linked processes of photosynthesis and oxidation form the *Oxygen Cycle* or *Carbon Cycle*; they constitute the symbiotic relationship between plants and

100

---

1 Urey had already won the Nobel Prize for Chemistry in 1934, for his discovery of heavy hydrogen (deuterium)..

animals. If that was all there was to life, a balance between them would be associated with constant oxygen and CO_2 contents in the atmosphere. However, the balance can be disturbed by many other factors, such as the burning of carbon-containing fuels, or a reduction in the plant population. A recently recognized fact is that photosynthesis is greatest in young plants; the effectiveness of forests in removing CO_2 diminishes as the trees age.

Anaerobic bacteria still flourish in oxygen-poor situations, like the infamous *Clostridium* in our intestines, or the Komuka bacterial and fungus combination that makes a refreshing carbonated drink from a sugar solution. However, the first anaerobic bacteria could have been those that are able to exist in the very high temperatures found in the sulphurous volcanic vents or "smoke-holes" deep in the oceans. One theory is that these hyperthermophylic ("lovers of very high temperature") bacteria liberated energy by splitting off hydrogen from hydrogen sulphide to form iron pyrites (FeS_2) in combination with iron contained in the rock lining the vents. The energy could then be used for other reactions such as the splitting of carbon dioxide, thus making carbon available for organic chemical synthesis.

The next step in the ladder towards our present day atmosphere seems to have been taken by a bacterium that used the green dye chlorophyll to harness the sun's energy to build its sugars from the carbon liberated from CO_2 and thereby release oxygen into the atmosphere. The process made oxygen "the most precious waste in the firmament" to quote Richard Fortey. In his delightful book *Life*, the senior paleontologist at London's Natural History Museum describes how these first (blue-green) *cyanobacteria* rapidly reproduced, providing food for other organisms but more importantly "for every generation a thousand billion tiny

balloons of oxygen (were) released". From this beginning some 3,000 million years ago, in an atmosphere without oxygen but plentiful CO_2, the conditions began to change; there followed a thousand million years of dominant plant growth during which oxygen production exceeded its usage and its concentration rose. At its peak, the atmospheric oxygen is estimated (from the amount of rust found in ancient strata of rock) to have reached 35% some 500 million years ago. With increasing oxygen came the formation of ozone (O_3) in the upper atmosphere to absorb some of the sun's ultraviolet radiation, and a fall in CO_2, both contributing to global cooling, and a more sustaining environment for animal life. The peak concentration of oxygen is thought to have coincided with the peak of dinosaur development; perhaps it contributed to the massive size that these creatures achieved. From this peak there was a gradual fall during the succeeding 100 million years, to reach levels close to those present now, at around 21%.

GAIA: THE EARTH AS A SELF-REGULATING SYSTEM

It is a truism to say that the apparent constancy of atmospheric oxygen and CO_2 means that the processes of production and consumption of the two gases must be equal. However, how our atmosphere, dominated by nitrogen and oxygen and with very little CO_2, is maintained constant has proved remarkably difficult to establish mathematically, if only because the amounts are so large. So large are they that a new unit was proposed, the *Erda*, signifying the magnitude 10^{18}. I mention this, not because I propose to use it, but because it resonates with *Gaia*; both words, the first Teutonic and the second Greek in origin, signify Mother Earth. In the Gaia Hypothesis proposed in 1979 by the British independent scientist James Lovelock, the Earth is viewed as a vast self-regulating, living organism. On this scale the global system is seen to be composed of the "lithosphere" (rocks), "hydrosphere" (water), "biosphere" (living organisms) and "atmosphere" (air), all in a constant state of flux, with exchange of gases and other elements between them, but achieving a "steady state" in the contents of their constituents. Thus, the biosphere generates (via plants) and absorbs (via animals) oxygen, with reverse effects on CO_2; water, mainly the oceans, takes up and gives off both gases according to changes in their surface gas pressures; and rocks contain huge stores of oxygen in oxides and of CO_2 in carbonates and bicarbonates, subject to physicochemical processes. This model shows that the amounts of oxygen and CO_2 in rocks and water exceed their amounts in the atmosphere by at least four orders of magnitude (ie a thousand times greater); interestingly, it also shows that most of the nitrogen, in contrast, is in the atmosphere. The bottom line is that the lithosphere and hydrosphere act as "buffers" that effectively resist any long-term change in atmospheric oxygen and CO_2. Long-term and globally that is, because short-term changes may occur in localities where some catastrophic event occurs, or where industrial production of CO_2 by the burning of fossil fuels, is greatly elevated. Carbon dioxide, being heavier than other atmospheric gases, may accumulate at ground level if winds do not clear it, for example in a valley. One potential source of catastrophic amounts of local CO_2 is volcanic activity; the massive combustion of carbon that occurs generates large amounts of CO_2 that can lead to large increases in its concentration close to the ground; in 1969 the inhabitants of a village situated deep in a valley in Tanzania were wiped out by volcanic CO_2. Such happenings might lead one to be scared that all increases in CO_2 could be potentially lethal; however, the ambient CO_2

has to rise several hundred-fold, to above 15% from its usual 0.035%, before death is likely.

One of the intriguing attributes of James Lovelock's Gaia is that she "breathes". Just as Haldane and Priestley were able to measure small fluctuations in atmospheric CO_2 during a day, Charles David Keeling was able to show similar fluctuations of about 0.005% in atmospheric CO_2 during the year. In his book *The Discovery of Global Warming* Spencer Weart describes the meticulous way in which

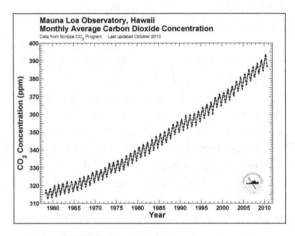

Figure 29 The Keeling Curve

Keeling, then a young geochemist working at the Scripps Institute of Oceanography, went about the task of measuring CO_2 with the greatest accuracy and precision in the late 1950s. He sampled air at a site remote from any source of pollution, at the summit of the 4170m high Mount Mauna Loa in Hawaii over four decades—one of the most sustained pieces of research ever accomplished. Keeling found that each spring there was a fall in CO_2 that he ascribed to its absorption by new leaves in the forests of the Northern Hemisphere; then, at the end of each summer there was a swing back up as vegetation decomposed, to release CO_2 into the atmosphere. As interesting as these observations of our planet breathing are, their importance is dwarfed by another of Keeling's findings—an inexorable steady trend upwards in CO_2 concentration, from a yearly peak of 0.032% in 1960 to 0.037% in 2000. Thus, during the past 40 years, CO_2 production has exceeded its uptake to rise by 15%. This trend can be extended back two centuries to a time when the burning of fossil fuels, the manufacture of cement, and the large scale cutting of trees all took off in earnest. Then, in around 1800, the average atmospheric CO_2 was probably around 0.025%. More recently, radiocarbon studies have revealed that of the total amount of CO_2 emitted into the atmosphere between 1800 and 2000, almost a third occurred during the last two decades of the 20th century. In view of the fact that we are so dependent on oxygen, it's intriguing that we know less about the downward trend in atmospheric O_2 during this time, than we do about the upward trend in CO_2. At least in part this is due to difficulties in analysing O_2 with comparable precision; whereas the observations imply changes in % that are to the third decimal place per decade, O_2 is assumed to be stable at 20.93%, and no one seems to know if anything has happened to its third decimal.

The increase in CO_2 concentration over the past two centuries seems very small in absolute terms, especially when compared with the relative abundance of other gases—for example the concentration of oxygen is about one thousand times as large as CO_2—so why worry? The reason for worry is that carbon dioxide has as one of its most potent properties the capacity to selectively absorb energy wave lengths in the infra-red range;[2] this warms the molecules to slightly raise the temperature of air. Although CO_2 concentration is small, the depth of the atmosphere through which the infra red rays pass is large, amounting to huge numbers of CO_2 molecules. Furthermore, any increase in air temperature leads to an increase in water vapour content; as water concentration is about one hundred times that of CO_2, the effect is much larger. Water absorbs infrared energy to the same extent as CO_2, thus leading to a potential vicious cycle, which is to some extent damped by cloud formation—clouds reduce the amount of the sun's energy reaching the earth's surface. The global warming effect associated with increases in CO_2 concentration was first recognized by the great Swedish physicist Svante August Arrhenius at the turn of the 19th-20th century. Arrhenius won the Nobel Prize for Chemistry and Physics in 1903, not for this intuitive leap that was to become such a concern a century later, but for his mathematical descriptions of the dissociation of acids and bases.

THE INFLUENCE OF THE EARTH'S OCEANS

The atmosphere, because of its huge volume, can take up large amounts of CO_2 without much change in its concentration; however this great capacity of the atmosphere is exceeded by that of the oceans, which absorb almost 50% of the planet's emissions of CO_2. Just as we can measure fluctuations in atmospheric CO_2, it has proved possible to measure the storage of CO_2 in the planet's water. The ocean's handling of CO_2 is almost as complex as the body's. The effects of gas exchange on the air we breathe are simpler than its effects on body fluids; similarly, changes in atmospheric CO_2 are easier to understand than changes in ocean stores of

103

2   The commonest physical analyzer used to measure CO2 concentration uses this property; the introduction of the infra-red analyzer into clinical use in the 1950s, made a huge impact in monitoring expired CO2, for it allowed

precise adjustment of ventilation during surgery and intensive care situations.

CO_2. The differences in complexity are due to three main reasons. First, CO_2 in solution exists in several forms—in simple solution, as bicarbonate and carbonate. Second, just as in the body, CO_2 moves between different sites—in the body from tissue water to plasma to the red cell, and in the ocean from surface water to the depths of the sea, from ocean to ocean, and into the rocks below. Finally, the capacity of seawater to contain CO_2 in its various forms depends on the concentration of ions—charged particles that act as acids or bases.

Carbon dioxide, in common with other soluble gases, moves from the atmosphere into water, and *vice versa*, according to pressure differences—which are always tiny, bearing in mind that the CO_2 pressure in the atmosphere is seldom higher than 0.3 mmHg (remember that in the body its pressure is normally around 40 mmHg). The CO_2 that enters water becomes converted into four molecular forms, which are all linked chemically. It dissolves in water and a very small amount exists merely as CO_2 in solution; it forms carbonic acid ($CO_2 + H_2O \rightarrow H_2CO_3$), most of which splits (dissociates) into hydrogen and bicarbonate ions ($H_2CO_3 \rightarrow H^+ + HCO_3^-$). Bicarbonate ions can dissociate further to carbonate ions

$$(HCO_3^- \rightarrow H^+ + CO_3^{2-}).$$

The dissociation reactions proceed in one direction or the other according to an equilibrium constant that governs the concentrations of the ions in the individual reactions; for this reason the acidity (concentration of H^+ ions) is especially important, as we shall see. Temperature and pressure—important parameters in the sea—also affect the reactions. The extent to which the progressive dissociation outlined above occurs, depends both on the pressure of CO_2,

and on the balance between all the positively charged ions (cations) and negatively charged acid anions. In sea water the main cations are sodium (Na^+), calcium (Ca^{2+}) and magnesium (Mg^{2+}), and their total ion concentration usually exceeds the sum of the anions, mainly chloride (Cl^-) and sulphate (SO_4^{2-}), but by only a small amount. Electrical neutrality, where the sum of positive charges equals the sum of negative charges, is always observed, and the bicarbonate (HCO_3^-) and carbonate (CO_3^{2-}) ions make up the difference. The result is that seawater is slightly alkaline; the pH is around 8, neutral (neither acid nor alkaline) pH being 7. In any situation where the negatively charged anions exceed the sum of the cations, the water will be acidic, with a pH below 7; all the reactions in the previous paragraph would shift back to the left, there would then be no bicarbonate or carbonate ions present, and the amount of carbon dioxide would be minute, consisting only of dissolved CO_2. This situation may occur in some lakes, where sodium concentration is relatively low but sulphates— from acid rain—are in high concentration; such lakes contain no CO_2 in any form, and in consequence sustain no life. There are many lakes in Ontario that are superficially beautiful—crystal clear because of the lack of small plant life, but disappointingly free of fish also.

Normally the balance of the ionic charges is amazingly stable in seawater; the difference between the cations and anions is only a few milliequivalents per litre (mEq/l) in a total of around 600 of each; bicarbonate ions are in a concentration of only 2-4 mEq/l and carbonate ions exist in a concentration that is one-hundredth of this. Although CO_2, existing mainly as bicarbonate ions, is in a low concentration compared to the other ions in seawater (constituting about 1%), it is still much higher than in the atmosphere, where it constitutes only 0.035%.

There are some serious misconceptions regarding CO_2 in the sea. One is the belief that it mainly exists as carbonate, whereas bicarbonate is the predominant form. Another is that increasing CO_2 concentration will cause oceans to become more acidic; the fact is that increasing acidity reduces the capacity of seawater to contain CO_2. The concentration of CO_2 can only increase so long as the sum of strong cations ($Na^+ + Ca^{2+} + Mg^{2+}$ etc) exceeds the sum of strong anions (mainly $Cl^- + SO_4^{2-}$). Can we identify a dangerous adversary here? The sulphate ion concentration has only to increase by 1 or 2% to completely prevent seawater taking up CO_2; this is because the concentration of sulphate is about 25 times that of all the CO_2-derived molecules. Sulphur dioxide (SO_2) is one of the most important and prevalent pollutants liberated into the atmosphere when fossil fuels are burnt;[3] volcanic eruptions are another potent, if localized source of the gas. In the atmosphere, SO_2 combines with water vapour to form very fine particles (aerosols) of sulphuric acid, and being very soluble in water it also is avidly taken up by water in lakes, rivers and the oceans. The aerosols are incorporated into clouds, where they reflect the sun's rays back into space, and eventually fall back to earth in "acid rain". We will encounter SO_2 again when considering health aspects of air pollution, but should note in the context of global warming that it actually contributes to global cooling, through reflection of the sun's rays, and to the acidity of the oceans, thus tending to limit their capacity for uptake of CO_2. It's ironic that one of the more successful measures taken to limit

air pollution, the use of SO_2 absorbers in the smokestacks of coal fired industries, will also contribute to global warming.

Oceanic surveys have shown the highest contents of carbon compounds in the surface waters of the North Sea, which take up large amounts of CO_2, especially in the summer months. The CO_2 is transported mainly as bicarbonate into the Atlantic, where it slowly distributes to greater depths, and lower temperatures; because the equilibrium constant governing ionic reactions is affected by temperature, sea water becomes more alkaline at depth, and thus able to absorb more CO_2, and form more carbonate ions. The ultimate sink for CO_2 is the combination of carbonate with calcium to form chalk and limestone, and calcify coral. A monumental study was carried out in the 1990s by an international group coordinated by the US National Oceanic and Atmospheric Administration; water was sampled at different depths at almost 10,000 oceanic sites, and the dissolved carbon subjected to tracer analysis so as to identify the man-made (anthropogenic) CO_2 from 1800 to the present day. The results were published in 2004, and showed that 50% of the carbon load during these two centuries remained at depths that were less than 400 m. Bearing in mind that the average depth of the planet's oceans is 4,000 m, the findings indicated that vertical mixing of bicarbonate and carbonate is very slow, and that only a fraction of the oceans' long term capacity to absorb CO_2 have so far been used. The authors of the report predicted that over a time scale measured in thousands of years, some 90% of anthropogenic CO_2 "will end up in the ocean".

GLOBAL WARMING

Thinking about how Gaia breathes has led us into the topic of global warming, now a clear

105

---

3   We should remember two facts related to global industry—first, in spite of all the potential sources of energy, 85% of the global energy production is from the combustion of fossil fuel; and second, that the production of sulphuric acid exceeds all other industrial chemical processes. .

and present danger facing humankind in the present century. The topic is confusing, not least because a few decades ago experts were warning that we were doomed to a new ice age, but more recently the evidence has been mounting for the opposite trend. More confusing, for expert and non-expert alike, is the number of factors that have to be taken into account when anyone attempts to predict what will happen in the future. There are factors tending to influence the amount of energy reaching the earth from the sun—cloud formation, aerosols, reflection from snow and ice, and thinning of the ozone layer. To these must be added factors that impede the outward radiation of heat energy, of which the most important appears to be the gradual accumulation of CO_2 in the atmosphere. The initial brilliant calculations of Arrhenius were followed almost a century later by computer models of increasing sophistication. As recounted by Tim Flannery in his acclaimed book *The Weather Makers*, the largest study was carried out in 2005 by a group at Oxford University who linked 90,000 personal computers during their downtime in order to calculate the effect of a doubling in atmospheric CO_2. The results indicated an average rise in the earth's temperature by 3.4°C; as this was what Arrhenius had calculated in his head, this was rather underwhelming; however, it was the possible range of warming that might occur that impressed Flannery. This Australian professor of biology noted that the low end of the range of global warming was an increase of 1.9°C, which he considered inevitable and probably unavoidable. The upper end of the range was 11.2°C, a possibility that would have catastrophic results, should it occur.

ATMOSPHERIC WATER

A variable constituent of clean air is water, a thoroughly unique substance, existing in many forms that obey a myriad of physical laws and essential to life as we know it. Furthermore, because there is nearly always more water in our expired breath than in the air we breathe in, loss of water from the lungs can lead to problems.

In his ground-breaking book *The Fitness of the Environment* Lawrence J Henderson in 1913 emphasized the importance of water's high latent heat of evaporation. As liquid water is turned into vapour, energy is lost and the water cools. The property acts to stabilize the temperature of both the Earth's atmosphere and its animal inhabitants. Increasing temperature increases evaporation, which in turn exerts its cooling effect.

In common with all liquids, water exists in equilibrium with its vapour, whose pressure depends on the ambient temperature. At the interface between a liquid and the surrounding gas, molecules exchange between the two phases (liquid and gaseous) according to the pressure in each, until at equilibrium the number of molecules entering the liquid equal the number leaving. The gaseous pressure at equilibrium is termed the vapour pressure. An increase in the temperature of the liquid increases its pressure thereby causing molecules to enter the gaseous phase and increasing the vapour pressure. At a normal body temperature of 37°C, water vapour pressure is 47 mmHg, or about 6% of the sea level pressure (760 mmHg). The amount of water in the air we breathe depends on atmospheric conditions that determine the humidity as well as temperature; in Death Valley it is usually zero in spite of temperatures in excess of 100°C, because there simply is no water to be found there. At the Poles it is similarly dry in spite of plenty of water, because the temperature is well below zero; the water is present as ice. The factors of temperature and humidity become of great importance during activity in very cold environments, when the amount of air going in and out of the lungs is greatly increased, and when the air is cold and dry. The cold incoming air meets the warm moist lining of the airways and water moves out until water vapour pressure is equalized in the two sites. This process is rapid, and in quiet breathing is complete by the time air reaches the trachea; during exercise the process may not be complete until well down in the small airways. This movement of water has two main effects—first, there is the loss of water from the body, and second, the airways are dried.

People with asthma commonly experience symptoms if they exercise in cold weather and most of us experience an irritating cough when we go out in very cold and dry conditions. The cough is due to the drying of airways which stimulates sensitive nerve endings in large airways. In susceptible asthmatic individuals there is also a cellular response, with mast cells liberating histamine and other chemical mediators, leading to constriction of smaller airways. The situation is termed "exercise induced asthma", and may be life-threatening.

The loss of water from the respiratory tract is particularly severe at altitude, where the boiling point of water is lowered. In physical terms, boiling occurs when the liquid's vapour pressure exceeds the atmospheric pressure as it falls with increasing altitude. This fact lies behind the complaint of mountaineers of the impossibility of making a good cup of tea at high altitudes; the water boils at a lower temperature than that recommended by Mr Twining. It also accounts for the huge amount of water lost from the respiratory tract during Everest attempts, which for many years was an unappreciated contributor to the severe fatigue experienced by climbers. The water loss leads to a reduction in blood volume, thereby reducing blood

flow and oxygen delivery to muscles. During the preparation for the 1953 British Everest Expedition, its physiologist Dr L.G.C.E. "Griff" Pugh measured water loss from the lungs at altitude, and found that it was about four times that experienced at sea-level. On the basis of his findings, fluid intake was increased to 3-4 litres per day, and this was counted as one of the factors that contributed to the success of the expedition.

As mentioned briefly above, the increase in atmospheric water vapour that occurs as temperature rises, makes it a very important factor contributing to global warming; this is because water vapour, just like CO_2, is a potent absorber of infra-red rays. Thus, as atmospheric CO_2 increases, the associated warming increases atmospheric water vapour and leads to even more warming. The scene is set for a positive feed-back loop which serves to progressively magnify an effect, in this case temperature. There are many other feed-back loops that influence global warming, and most of them seem to have a positive, rather than negative effect. It's an interesting contrast between our own bodily physiology and the systems involved in the control of the global environment. Most of our physiological systems—with breathing being an outstanding example—involve negative feedback loops to achieve homeostasis. An increase in breathing leads to a fall in arterial blood CO_2, which tends to inhibit breathing through the action of chemoreceptors. Gaia is less lucky, for increases in environmental CO_2 tend to lead to changes that further increase its concentration and its effect on warming. There is also the potential for negative feed-back; plants grown in a CO_2-enriched atmosphere tend to grow faster and take up CO_2; unfortunately this mechanism is unable to cope with the huge amounts of man-made CO_2.

OTHER GASES IN THE ATMOSPHERE

Nitrogen. The most prevalent gas in the atmosphere, at 78.04% of dry air, is nitrogen (N_2), considered an inert gas, because it does not take part in the body's chemical processes. The body does not take up nitrogen from the air to make its amino acids and proteins; it obtains most amino acids from plants, which in turn made them from nitrates in the soil; indeed the only organisms that can use atmospheric nitrogen are very primitive "nitrogen fixing" bacteria, and blue-green algae that live in soil and oceans. Nitrogen is poorly soluble in blood, and thus is not taken up or released by the lungs. Inert it may be, but nitrogen still deserves respect, from two main perspectives. First, it protects the lungs from collapse, because however much oxygen is absorbed from the alveoli, there is always nitrogen that remains to maintain their volume. During World War II, fighter pilots breathing 100% oxygen at high altitudes often developed "atelectasis" at the lung bases—airless areas caused by total absorption of the nitrogen-free alveolar gas. This effect was combined with G-forces tending to pull blood into the lower parts of the lung. Second, although the solubility of nitrogen is low, it is not negligible; as liquids take up gases in proportion to their pressure, more nitrogen is taken up by the lungs into the blood when air is breathed under pressure. Furthermore, the solubility of nitrogen varies in tissues, mainly in accordance with their fat content; gases are roughly six times more soluble in fat as in blood; for this reason, during prolonged conditions of high pressure nitrogen is gradually transferred to fatty tissues, most tellingly the brain and spinal cord. John Scott Haldane calculated that the amount of nitrogen held in the body during prolonged hyperbaric conditions was as much as 26 times the amount held in blood. Rapid decompression after air breathing under pressure leads to nitrogen coming out of solution, in the form of bubbles, which can block small vessels, and distort structures such as nerves; this is the condition known as "the bends", which we will consider again in Chapter 13.

Argon (*the inactive*) is present in air in a concentration (1%) that is about 30 times that of CO_2—which bearing in mind that we can't do without CO_2, but have no need of argon, is an extraordinary fact. It is a member of a group of gases, that includes neon, xenon and krypton, usually termed "inert" or "noble". They do not react with anything,[4] and from the standpoint of the lung, argon merely takes up a little space but otherwise may be safely forgotten. Quantitatively, it is usually lumped together with nitrogen, to increase its apparent concentration to 79% of the atmosphere.

It may strike you as odd that we are almost at the end of this chapter, without much mention of the changes that have occurred in atmospheric O_2 during the past century. Although it seems quite likely that changes have occurred that are similar in extent to those occurring in CO_2, relatively speaking these would have been so small that they would be impossible to measure. Dave Keeling's findings of an increase in atmospheric CO_2 from 0.032% in 1960 to 0.037% in 2000 are significant and accurately measurable, but a comparable change in O_2, from 20.930% to 20.925%, would have been almost undetectable.

---

4   Well, almost never; Primo Levi, in Il Sistema Periodico, observes "As late as 1962 a diligent chemist, after long and ingenious efforts succeeded in forcing The Alien (xenon) to combine fleetingly with extremely avid and lively fluorine, and the feat seemed so extraordinary that he was given a Nobel Prize."

Fortunately, Dave Keeling's monumental work has been carried on by his son Ralph, now also a Professor at the Scripps Institute at the University of California at San Diego. As well as extending the "Keeling Curve" for CO_2 to the present day (Fig. 29) Ralph Keeling has overcome many of the analytical problems for oxygen and has followed the trends in atmospheric O_2 concentration in several sites. The results are as informative as they are (at first sight) unexpected. For San Diego, between 1990 and 2010 the peak annual CO_2 concentration has increased from 0.0350% to 0.0390%, an increase of 40 parts per million (ppm), or 2 ppm/yr, with an average yearly fluctuation (the height of the waves in Fig 29) of 10 ppm. For O_2 over the past two decades Ralph Keeling has found a decrease of 90 ppm, or 4.5 ppm/yr, and an average seasonal swing of 30 ppm. Thus the changes in O_2, both in total and in the seasonal swing, are more than twice the comparable changes in CO_2, which he believes are due to at least two factors. First, there is a greater "sink" for the CO_2 taken up by ocean water due to the physicochemical reactions, and second, the O_2 consumed during the burning of fossil fuels exceeds the CO_2 evolved by a factor of about 1.4.

Unlike the changes in CO_2, the biological or physical effects of such a change in O_2 are insignificant. This is not to say that large changes in environmental O_2 are without consequence; such changes are related to the O_2 pressure. At sea level O_2 pressure is around 150 mm Hg; it has to fall below 100 mm Hg before any harmful effects occur in healthy individuals; this is the O_2 pressure at an altitude of 12,000 ft.

The human race does not need to worry that we are doomed to extinction from carbon dioxide narcosis or hypoxia. More realistic worries are global warming and the degradation of air quality due to worsening pollution.

CHAPTER 10

ATHLETIC BREATHS

"The condition of exercise is not a mere variant of the condition of rest, it is the essence of the machine."

Sir Joseph Barcroft, Features in the Architecture of Physiological Function. 1934.

"My lungs felt too small for the task"

"My effort was over and I collapsed almost unconscious, with an arm on either side of me. It was only then that the real pain overtook me. I felt like an exploded flashlight with no will to live; I just went on existing in the most passive physical state..."

Roger Bannister, First Four Minutes, 1955

THE FIRST 4-MINUTE MILE

Roger Gilbert Bannister came to St Mary's in 1953, as one of the small group of students who came yearly to complete their studies after preclinical years at Oxford. Already England's top miler, and probably better known than several international Rugby stars who were

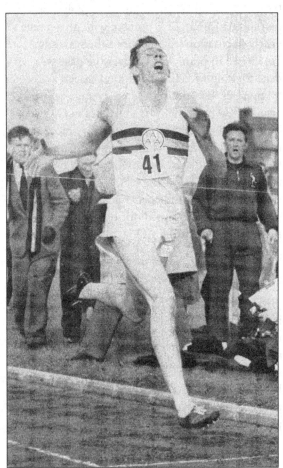

Figure 30 Roger Bannister at 3min 59.4 sec, May 6, 1954.

110

My Alma Mater is St Mary's Hospital Medical School, situated in an undistinguished triangle formed by Paddington railway station, the Grand Union Canal and Praed Street, in West Central London. At its centenary celebrations, in November 1954, the Queen placed a sealed capsule containing symbols of its history into a slab of concrete—the foundation stone for a new wing to the hospital. Only two of these symbols of achievement remain in my memory—a Petri dish containing a growth of *penicillium notatum* to commemorate the work of Sir Alexander Fleming, and a stop watch set at 3 minutes 59.4 seconds to commemorate the first 4-minute mile, by Roger Bannister, one of its students, in the previous year.

already at St Mary's, he embodied the school's recruitment credo—that achievers in sport achieve academically and in the medical profession. There is no better example of this dictum than Roger Bannister, who became Chairman of the British Sports Council during momentous years of national fitness development, a noted neurologist and Master of Pembroke College, Oxford. The emphasis on sporting achievement at St Mary's had been established by Winston Churchill's personal physician Charles Wilson, Lord Moran, a previous Dean, and always referred to—at least by the students—as "Corkscrew Charlie", referring to his Machiavellian political accomplishments during the early years of the National Health Service. No one at St Mary's at that time will forget the dreary windy day, May 6th 1954, when Roger took the train from Paddington to Oxford to be a member of the Amateur Athletics Association's team competing against the University's team; it was known that an attempt at the four-minute mile was to be made. Two more of England's premier runners—although usually at longer distances —Chris Chataway and Christopher Brasher, were there to ensure perfect pacing, which as his long-time friends they did to perfection, and the rest is history.[1] Looking at the famous photograph of Roger going through the tape it is easy to appreciate that his breathing, as well as his total effort, was at a maximum, with his head thrown back, mouth wide open, and nostrils flared, ensuring minimum resistance in the upper airway. It's the same look as another elite middle-distance runner, Emil Zatopek, who I watched as he ran away with both the 5,000 and 10,000 metres at the 1948 London Olympics, but quite different from the look of sprinters or marathoners. Breathing is not important in the 100 metres where muscle power dominates, and requires little effort in the marathon, where supplying fuel is the limiting factor. However, anyone who has run for longer than three or four minutes knows that breathing can become very hard and uncomfortable until one gets one's "second wind".

To understand these events and differences in breathing during exercise we will need to go back to Lavoisier and consider the metabolic changes in various forms of activity. It is the metabolic energy demands and the fuels that provide them that dominate the breathing demands in supplying oxygen and getting rid of carbon dioxide. In this chapter we review these complex interrelationships first from a historical point of view, then considering the chemical processes that convert chemical energy into mechanical energy, and finally contrasting different types of exercise and the implications they have for breathing.

COMBUSTION AND RESPIRATION

111

In 1789, Lavoisier and his colleague Séguin identified respiration with combustion, with consumption of oxygen and production of carbonic acid (CO_2) "in almost equal volume". The delightful sketch by Madame Lavoisier (Fig. 5) shows the experimental set-up for collecting expired gas, and Séguin performing exercise with a foot treadle. Although increases in combustion with exercise were identified by them, the accurate measurement of O_2 uptake and CO_2 output had to await improved analytical methods. It was 50 years before Heinrich Gustav Magnus, a professor of physics in Berlin, proved that the combustion occurred in the tissues, by demonstrating in 1837 that blood lost oxygen and gained CO_2

---

1   Bannister thought the pace too slow, and kept shouting "faster"; however, first Brasher and then Chataway kept their heads, to accurately pace successive laps of close to 1-minute.

as it passed from the arterial to the venous side of the circulation. Accurate measurements of respiratory gases during exercise in humans were developed by Nathan Zuntz in the last two decades of the nineteenth century. Zuntz, whom we have already met in relation to hemoglobin function, began his life as a physiologist in 1870 as an assistant to Eduard Pflüger in Bonn, and spent the next 50 years as an exceptionally productive professor of physiology in Bonn and Berlin. His gifts included a talent for devising methods for physiological studies, an intuitive understanding that physiology had to be linked to biochemistry ("die neuere Biochemie"), and a generous nature. He introduced the concept of the respiratory quotient (RQ, the ratio of CO_2out/O_2in) providing information on the fuels used for exercise—an RQ of 0.7 indicating 100% fat combusted, and of 1.0 indicating 100% carbohydrate (see below). Thus, measurement of the ratio in expired gas (now known as the Respiratory exchange ratio, RER) allowed calculation of the proportion of fat to carbohydrate used in various activities.[2]

Zuntz found that, during a 25 km walk, the RER progressively declined, indicating that as the duration of exercise increases, more and more of the energy requirements were being met by fat, less and less energy coming from carbohydrate. The higher the level of energy output, the higher the RER, indicating greater reliance on carbohydrate; indeed in very heavy exercise the RER exceeded 1.0. Zuntz interpreted this finding in the light of Claude Bernard's discovery of glycogen in muscle, and that of Berzelius, who in 1847 reported that an acid identical to that obtained from milk was present in the muscles of hunted stags. The discoveries of Bernard and Berzelius meant that lactic acid was being

produced from glycogen without the requirement for oxygen, but led to an increase in CO_2 output due to the acid accumulating in blood.[3] Thus, he presented the concept that lactic acid was produced by muscle when the demand for energy outstripped the supply of oxygen by the heart and circulation; a concept that many still hold today. Indeed, most of Zuntz's interpretations are accepted today, but took many years to be accepted then, because lactic acid production was erroneously put forward as the main biochemical event in exercise.

ANAEROBIC *VERSUS* AEROBIC PROCESSES

Walter Morley Fletcher and Frederick Gowland Hopkins improved on previous techniques, and applied them to the study of isolated fish muscle; in 1907 they showed that resting muscle deprived of oxygen produced lactic acid, and led to the evolution of CO_2. However, they apparently did not recognize glycogen as the lactate precursor; they deduced that there was an unknown store of lactic acid which could be renewed after muscle contraction stopped; also, they stated—"it is not easy to see...how the energy of a substance, oxidized after it has appeared as a product of the spalting [splitting] processes associated with contraction, can contribute to the sources of contractile activity".

Until well into the 19th century the early biochemists struggled with a philosophical problem; philosophical because it seemed impossible to study experimentally. They were unable to explain the property of living cells that allowed them to accomplish the biochemical feats associated with "Life". They

---

2   As an example, an RER of 0.85, midway between 0.7 and 1.0, indicated that the fuels consisted of 50% fat and 50% carbohydrate.

3   The acid was assumed to react with sodium, bicarbonate in blood in the reaction—
LaH + NaHCO3 → NaLa +CO2 + H2O

assumed that living organisms were endowed with a vital force that allowed them to use chemical reactions for growth, reproduction, movement and all the other life functions. The emerging field of thermodynamics, which dealt with the interconversion of mass and different forms of energy, provided ways in which the philosophical theory was replaced by experimental approaches.

Fletcher encouraged Archibald Vivian Hill ("AV") to study lactic acid production by mammalian muscle; Hill, an accomplished physiologist and athlete with a flair for applying mathematical relationships to physiological processes,[4] began by studying heat production in muscle and reported in 1912 that heat was produced during contraction, which continued after activity ceased and was associated with oxygen consumption. Later, Hill and his colleagues put forward the concept of "oxygen debt", which has been generally accepted as one of the great physiological paradigms. The concept, briefly stated, posited that at the onset of exercise there was a delay in adequate oxygen supply (oxygen deficit), due to the time it took for blood flow (heart rate, etc) to increase appropriately. The delay was associated with lactic acid formation, and an "oxygen debt" that was repaid during recovery, when oxygen consumption remained elevated, to "pay off the debt". This excess oxygen uptake of recovery was initially interpreted as being used to rebuild lactic acid into its precursor glucose. Later, when the source of lactic acid was proved to be muscle glycogen, the repaid oxygen was ascribed to the regeneration of glycogen stores. As well as "AV", the major contributors to the elaboration of the oxygen debt concept were Otto Myerhof (awarded the Nobel Prize jointly with Hill in 1922) and a celebrated trio at the Harvard Fatigue Laboratory (David B Dill, Rodolfo Margaria and Harold T Edwards). The latter group, in 1933, analyzed the oxygen debt into lactacid and alactacid components (the alactacid component was related to breakdown of creatine phosphate, below). Oxygen debt was an attractive concept, not only because the banking metaphor made it easily understood, but also because it could be used to explain why lactic acid was produced mainly at the onset of exercise, increased at altitude, and was less in well trained people, in whom heart rate increased more rapidly than untrained. The oxygen debt concept lasted untouched for decades, until the data and methods were questioned. For myself, the questioning began in 1969 after seeing a paper by the British cardiologist Peter Harris with the arresting title "The Phlogiston Debt", reflecting his view that the concept of oxygen debt should be consigned to the historical dustbin, where the concept of phlogiston—put forward in by Carl Wilhelm Scheele in 1772— already rested. However, the notion of oxygen debt lived on in the concept of the "anaerobic threshold", the level of exercise at which lactic acid appears in blood. Both concepts—oxygen debt and the anaerobic threshold—continue to spark lively debate, the controversy mainly surrounding their cause—inadequate oxygen delivery ("circulatory inertia") or insufficient oxygen uptake by muscle ("metabolic inertia"). It has proved difficult to separate the two; oxygen delivery may lag behind the demand because it takes time for blood flow to increase; and oxygen incorporation into the biochemical reactions may also take time because enzymes have to be activated before they achieve their maximum activity.

113

---

4   Amongst others, he developed equations to describe the oxy-hemoglobin dissociation curve, the fatigue process in muscle contraction and the improvement in world athletic performance.

THE BIOCHEMISTRY OF MUSCLE CONTRACTION: "HIGH ENERGY" PHOSPHATES

In the 1930s a major problem in understanding the physiology of exercise was the absence of any clue as to how glycogen breakdown and oxygen consumption were linked to the mechanical event of muscle contraction. Understanding those links had to await the discovery of high energy phosphates, metabolic cycles and their control by enzymes, and the sliding filament theory of muscle contraction. High energy phosphates, or phosphagens, were found in muscle in the late 1920s, and soon shown to be important cofactors in metabolic processes and muscle contraction. Adenosine triphosphate (ATP) was isolated in muscle in 1929, and in 1939, the enzyme myosin ATPase was discovered. When ATP was placed among myosin threads they contracted, and one phosphate molecule was split off to form adenosine diphosphate (ADP). However it was not until 1962 that it was proved that this reaction provided the energy for contraction. Creatine phosphate (CP) was discovered in 1927 by Philip and Grace Eggleton, working in the physiology department at the University of Edinburgh. During muscle contraction CP was broken down to creatine and phosphate, with liberation of energy. Grace Eggleton published her book *Muscular Exercise* in 1936, in which she puts forward the two sources of energy as the conversion of glycogen to lactate, and of CP to creatine; the reactions occur in the absence of oxygen, and then "when the muscle is subsequently allowed oxygen, the reverse happens, and some food is burnt at the same time". Thus her understanding follows that of AV Hill, with whom she later worked; the energy required for muscle contraction came from ATP conversion to ADP, and breakdown of CP and glycogen provided energy to reform ATP.

114

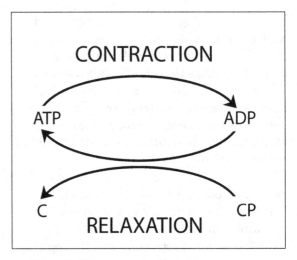

Figure 31 "High energy phosphates" in muscle contraction

Einar Lundsgard showed in 1932 that muscle could still contract when glycogen breakdown was prevented, and the CP content fell. The Harvard Fatigue Laboratory group proposed that CP breakdown to creatine and phosphate formed the "alactacid" portion of the oxygen debt. Later, CP breakdown was shown to provide an immediate source of phosphate for the regeneration of ATP from ADP. It was realized that muscle CP stores were small and would soon be depleted.[5] The energy for longer work came from the combustion of glycogen and fat in the muscle mitochondria, allowing a phosphate group to be replaced in ADP to form ATP.

GLYCOLYSIS AND LIPOLYSIS COMPARED

Glucose is stored in liver and muscle as glycogen, in the form of insoluble particles. Similarly, fatty acids are stored as triglycerides,

---

5   During the last decade, CP has become the darling of researchers, not only those who see benefits for athletic performance, but also those concerned with neuromuscular disorders, such as Parkinson's Disease and multiple sclerosis.

in adipose tissue, liver and muscle in the form of droplets of oily triglycerides. Thus, for both of our sources of energy, the first step is to liberate the active fuels from their storage form. Glucose is split off from glycogen in the first stage of glycolysis, and the glucose then transported in the blood-stream from the liver, or broken down directly in muscle. The first stage of lipolysis in adipose tissue consists of splitting off the fatty acids from their combination with glycerol and they are transported in the blood in combination with the plasma protein, albumin. Although fatty acids are also composed of carbon, oxygen and hydrogen, they are much larger molecules than glucose ($C_6H_{12}O_6$) and may contain as many as 20 C atoms, and the H and O_2 atoms are not in the same proportion as in glucose (for example, palmitic acid is represented by $C_{16}H_{34}O_4$). The first stage in fatty acid oxidation produces acetyl-CoA, and in the second stage acetyl-CoA enters the citric acid cycle and is "burnt" in the same way as the acetyl-CoA derived from glucose/glycogen. Also, the proportions of O_2 used to CO_2 produced differ from those of glucose; the ratio (RQ) is only 0.7. Thus, there are two huge advantages to the use of fatty acids as fuel in exercise; first, glucose and glycogen are spared; and second, much less CO_2 is produced, easing the load on breathing. Indeed, I believe that the next advance in performance enhancing agents (and, perhaps, weight loss) will be drugs that stimulate the release, transport and oxidation of fatty acids. Incidentally, caffeine is one such agent, but it comes with some unwanted side effects.

Before we leave this comparison of fats and glycogen as fuel sources, it is worth considering their size and efficiency. Glycogen in muscle and liver totals about 0.5 kg; if this were the only fuel, it would last for about an hour's marathon-paced running, and a few minutes at a sprint-pace. On the other hand, even an elite runner

with only 10-15% body fat, has 8-10 kg of fat, enough to keep going for 100 hours. How frustrating to have all this fuel but not to be able to use it fast enough! A well trained marathoner will employ about 50% fat and 50% glycogen; at the end of 2 hours there will be little glycogen left, and the marathoner has to guard against responding to the crowd's cheering as she arrives in the stadium; an increase in pace may bring disaster, because the brain is only able to use glucose. Run out of glucose and you'll loose consciousness, in the same way that a diabetic patient who has been given too much insulin becomes hypoglycemic .

With regard to efficiency, there is first a question of weight; because glycogen is bound to water it is relatively less efficient than fat, which contains very little; this makes fat almost twice as efficient as glycogen on an energy/weight basis. Next, the yield of ATP regenerated per molecule of oxygen used differs between the different energy sources—another aspect of different efficiencies.

The glucose molecule from glycogen that is broken down anaerobically to 2 molecules of lactate regenerates 2 molecules of ATP from 2 of ADP and 2 of Pi; no O_2 is used but CO_2 is produced by the reaction of H^+ ions with bicarbonate, mentioned above. In chemical notation the process of anaerobic glycolysis is written as follows—

$$C_6H_{12}O_6 + 2ADP + 2Pi \rightarrow 2CH_3CHOHCOOH + 2ATP + 2H_2O$$

In contrast with its anaerobic breakdown, aerobic hydrolysis of one molecule of glucose, involving the Krebs cycle, yields 36 ATP molecules from ADP and Pi—

$$C_6H_{12}O_6 + 36ADP + 36Pi + 6O_2 \rightarrow 36ATP + 6CO_2 + 42H_2O$$

From a metabolic point of view the aerobic process 18 times as efficient (36/2).

Fatty acids from triglycerides are large molecules, and their size varies, making comparison with glycogen and glucose difficult. The representative fatty acid palmitate contains 16 carbon atoms compared to the 6 of glucose; its oxidation regenerates 129 ATP molecules and requires 23 molecules of O_2—

$$C_{16}H\ COOH + 129ADP + 129ADP + 23O_2 \rightarrow 129ATP + 16CO_2 + 145H_2O$$

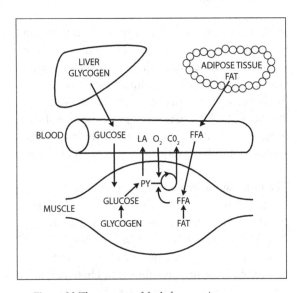

Figure 32 The sources of fuels for exercise

A way of comparing the efficiency of metabolic fuels is to calculate how many ATP molecules are regenerated for every molecule of O_2 used. For glucose this ratio is 6.0 (36/6), and for palmitate it is 5.6 (129/23)—glucose wins out in this comparison. However, if we are thinking of the load placed on breathing, perhaps the ratio of ATP gained for every molecule of CO_2 produced is more appropriate; this ratio shows palmitate to win out over glucose, with 8.1 molecules of ATP per molecule of CO_2 (129/16),

compared to 6.0 (36/6). Some runners experience a second, or third, wind, a feeling of less demand on breathing, at around 30 minutes into the marathon that is accounted for by a maximum use of fat and consequent reduction in CO_2 production.

Adipose tissue triglycerides form by far the largest fuel store, and they are never completely used, for example in a marathon run. This is because turning the oily droplets into soluble free fatty acids (FFA) that can be supplied to muscle is a coordinated process involving several hormones that control the reactions and also the blood flow to adipose tissue—not an easy task in exercise when most of the body's blood flow is being distributed to muscle. Even when FFA are mobilized at a maximum rate they are only able to provide about 30% of the energy needs during exercise; adding the FFA stored as fat in muscle raises this figure to about 50%. The corollary to this fact is that the onus is placed on glycogen to provide at least 50% of the energy required in a marathon; this means that glycogen stores in muscle and liver become progressively depleted. This is a recipe for disaster, and is one place where an experienced runner will win over an inexperienced opponent. The disaster stems from two factors—first, the muscle fatigue that occurs late in the race when you run out of muscle glycogen and you hit "the wall", after which it is impossible to run, and you have to walk; and second, the collapse into unconsciousness that occurs when liver glycogen is depleted and glucose cannot be supplied to the brain. The experienced runner is able to prevent these two potential disasters by running at a perfectly judged pace, by adjusting his diet to ensure high concentrations of glycogen in muscle and liver, and if necessary by using glucose drinks. In the history of the Olympic Games there have been many examples of runners leading late in the marathon, only to be passed as they stagger into the stadium. There are other examples of athletes performing well in heats, only to fail in the final race, often because their diet has not been adjusted to replenish their glycogen stores. A high intake of easily absorbed carbohydrate is needed for this.

Muscle glycogen is a flexible energy store, because two metabolic pathways are available for its use—one fast but inefficient and the other slower but less liable to use up glycogen rapidly. The former is usually termed "anaerobic" because oxygen is not required and the latter "aerobic"; these terms imply that that the choice between one or the other depends on oxygen supply. For decades, many changes in exercise—such as the effects of training—have been interpreted in terms of changes in oxygen delivery mechanisms. Increases in maximum oxygen uptake and reductions in lactate production were ascribed to improved oxygen supply to muscles—greater cardiac output, larger number of capillaries in muscle and so on. However, recently debate in sports sciences circles has become heated for and against this concept, versus the alternative—that changes occur that allow a greater consumption within muscle, with oxygen supply increasing in parallel. As with many famous debates, there is evidence on both sides, and probably both sides are right, with the many changes being linked.

The point at which the two pathways for glycogen breakdown diverge is at pyruvate; pyruvate is either converted to lactate "anaerobically" or enters the Krebs Cycle to be broken down "aerobically" to CO_2 and water. At this point the key regulatory enzyme complex (pyruvate dehydrogenase, PDH), increases the rate of pyruvate conversion to acetyl-CoA, the molecule that enters into the Krebs Cycle. Thus, if pyruvate appears at a higher rate than the enzyme's activity, the excess gets shunted off to lactate. Because in the resting state PDH is only 25% active, and may take several minutes to reach its full activity, during intense activity and at the start of exercise, lactate is produced—however much oxygen is supplied to the muscle. During exercise that is less intense than an all out sprint, and lasts for 2-3 minutes or longer, PDH becomes fully active and most or all of the pyruvate is metabolized aerobically. Many factors contribute to the completeness and rate at which PDHc is activated, but in the context of exercise, training is very important. Here then, is a source of controversy: trained athletes probably accumulate less lactate because they switch on PDH faster than untrained individuals, rather than because they deliver oxygen to muscles at a faster rate.

Pyruvate is first oxidized in the PDH reaction to a 2-C compound (acetate) that is bound to co-enzyme A (acetyl-CoA) with the production of CO_2. This is the central point in energy metabolism, because acetyl-CoA is also produced when fatty acids are broken down in the cell. Also, because acetyl-CoA is one of several metabolic products that affect the activity of PDH, it is where the availability of fat can reduce reliance on glycogen; increases in acetyl-CoA tend to shut down PDH. The 2-C acetyl-CoA condenses with a 4-C compound in the Cycle, and during a full turn of the Cycle 2 more molecules of CO_2 are produced. The Cycle is linked to what is termed the electron transport chain; protons (hydrogen atoms) are transported to combine with oxygen to produce water.

IMPLICATIONS FOR ATHLETIC PERFORMANCE

Let's first summarize the main features of severe exercise. Exercise is initiated by commands from the brain to the centres where movement is coordinated and thence to the muscles via the

117

appropriate nerves. Accompanying this "central command" are nerve impulses that activate (by "corollary discharge") the many body functions that contribute to exercise performance, such as increases in the heart's output and blood pressure, increases in breathing, together with secretion of various hormones (such as adrenaline and noradrenaline), and inhibition of others (such as insulin) that regulate fuel utilization. The electrical nerve impulses reach the motor end-plate to activate muscle contraction; the muscle shortens against a resistive force to produce mechanical energy. We think of this by using the analogy of a machine, but this is a simplistic model, because the energy is produced directly, rather than indirectly as in a machine. The muscle's energy is obtained from the energy stored in ATP; by action of the enzyme ATP-ase, ATP is split in a reaction with water (hydrolysis) to produce adenosine diphosphate (ADP) and inorganic phosphate (Pi). Energy is liberated because ADP and Pi contain less chemical energy than the unsplit ATP. The released energy changes the shape of the fine muscle filaments which allows cross bridge attachment between filaments; the filaments slide past each other to produce muscle shortening.[6] ATP then has to be reformed from ADP and Pi, because the amount of ATP in muscle is very small (enough

118

for less than 1 sec of a sprint). Also, because the amount of mechanical energy is directly related to the amount of ATP used up, it is obviously more difficult to reform ATP quickly enough during a 100 m sprint than in a longer race. ATP formation is a priority because it is needed for all the energy-requiring functions of the cell, and without it the cell dies.

The energy required for re-formation of ATP from ADP is obtained by coupling the process to the breakdown of energy-rich compounds. Some energy providing fuels are readily available in muscle: a tiny store of creatine phosphate and larger stores of glycogen and triglyceride.

Creatine phosphate (CP) in muscle is an immediately available source of phosphate and chemical energy to reconstitute ATP from ADP; however, if that's all there was, the 100m runner would collapse after 30 or 40 meters. To continue running, energy is obtained from the breakdown of other fuel stores that allow ATP to be reconstituted from ADP and Pi. The crucial problem facing the runner is to provide the fuels and switch on the reactions sufficiently rapidly, so that the concentration of ATP never falls. Because the use of different fuels are associated with different amounts of CO_2 produced during exercise, the choice of fuel mix has an important effect on increases in breathing as athletes perform on the track.

First, the 100 m sprinters obtain their energy mainly from creatine phosphate and glycogen breakdown to lactate; they exert themselves fully and end the race with muscles burning from lactate accumulation. They don't really need to breathe during the race, but then experience an extreme increase in breathing as CO_2 floods into the lungs.

6   This is known as the sliding filament theory, was established on the basis of animal muscle studies in which structural changes in living muscle were indirectly observed using the technique of X-ray diffraction; the findings were published in two back-to-back papers in the journal Nature in 1954, the first by Andrew Fielding Huxley of University College in London, and the second by Hugh Esmor Huxley from the Massachusetts Institute of Technology (MIT); the unrelated Huxleys had developed their theory simultaneously and more-or-less independently. AF Huxley won the Nobel Prize in 1963 and was knighted in 1974.

Milers initially produce lactate, but then activate PDH by the end of the first lap and cruise for the next two laps, burning glycogen aerobically with a small contribution from muscle fat; they experience large increases in breathing that require effort, but are supportable. During the final lap anaerobic glycolysis is recruited again, and they breast the tape with muscle glycogen depleted, muscles burning and breathing to their limit the systems have all reached their maximum.

Marathon runners experience an initial breathing effort that declines after a few minutes as lactate production stops and they get their second wind. They adjust their pace so that they are running easily, and breathing goes into "cruise control". Muscle glycogen is burnt aerobically, glucose is delivered from the liver and fat in muscle is also used. At about 20 to 30 minutes into the race, fatty acids have been mobilized from fat stores and CO_2 output reaches an optimum level; a "third wind" is experienced. Through the next two hours fat is metabolized at its maximum rate, sufficient to provide about 50% of the needed energy with the remaining 50% coming from glycogen in muscle and glucose from the liver. From then on, there is a risk of running out of muscle glycogen, and more crucially of running out of liver glycogen, leading to a fall in blood sugar. Both muscle and brain are at risk of failing.

Many attributes contribute to an athlete's success, but it is often impossible to say what makes one more successful than others. To some extent we can put this down to how well all the attributes are coordinated together. One of the first scientists to really get to grips with the integration that has to occur between the body's essential functions was the eminent physiologist Sir Joseph Barcroft, who wrote his seminal text *Features in the Architecture of Physiological Function* in 1934, a wonderful

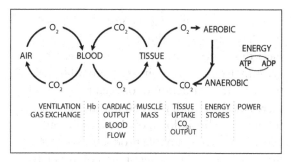

Figure 33 The transport lines for O_2 and CO_2

example of intuitive and scientific thinking. Not only did he make it clear the energy load had to be shared, but also that spare capacity in a system would not necessarily improve overall function. For example, a marathoner will not benefit from large, strong leg muscles, if the heart and circulation cannot supply the additional oxygen that they are capable of taking up. Of course, the closer the sport is dependent on muscle alone, the less important become the support systems; a weightlifter needs large muscles coupled with the nervous system's ability to recruit a large proportion of their motor units. The explosive and coordinated muscle contraction lasts for only a second or two, and thus barely needs the support of the cardiovascular system. A sprinter similarly needs leg muscle strength and the ability to breakdown glycogen rapidly to achieve maximum speed for 10 or 20 seconds; the heart and lungs are called into play mainly during recovery, as much for the removal of lactate and CO_2 as for the supply of oxygen to muscle.

When we come to Roger Bannister, the support systems become more important and at the end of 4 minutes, they will all have been taxed to the maximum. We can actually put approximate numbers to them all, because in the year before he broke the four minute barrier he took part in a research study, whilst a physiology student at Oxford. His running speed of 403m/min,

119

is equivalent to an oxygen consumption of 4.5 litres/min, almost 20 times the resting rate. To meet this demand, cardiac output increases six-fold, from 5 litres/min at rest to 30 litres/min, and the extraction of oxygen from blood increases three-fold, from 50 ml/litre to 150 ml/litre. The breakdown of glycogen in muscle leads to a carbon dioxide production of 4.4 litres/min, requiring a ventilation of about 105 litres/min. The final burst of energy during the last lap of the race increases lactate production, which is associated with an increase in blood acidity, further increasing the drive to breathe. Ventilation is then up to 125 litres/min. Bearing in mind that breathing at rest amounts to only 5 or 6 litres/min, the roughly 20-fold increase in breathing is hard for the respiratory muscles to keep up for more than 3 or 4 minutes.

We may compare these values with those of a world class marathoner, whose running speed is 323 m/min (42 km in 130 mins), requiring an energy expenditure, equivalent to an oxygen consumption of 3.6 litres/min. These energy demands, sustained for over two hours, cannot be met by burning glycogen alone, which would be depleted within the first hour; free fatty acids are mobilized, and at 1 hour into the race will account for at least 50% of the demands; little or no lactate will be produced. Carbon dioxide output will then be about 3.0 litres/min, requiring a ventilation of 70 litres/min. The accompanying effort in breathing will be well within the athlete's capacity to sustain for the rest of the race. Cardiac output will increase to 23 litres/min, also easily sustainable for a well-trained individual.

We could analyze performance in any sport in similar terms, and in each we could assess the contributions of a given system to the overall achievement. In all, the brain and central nervous system, and muscles will be at times be taxed to their capacity. The supply of metabolic fuel and oxygen becomes increasingly critical as the duration of activity increases, and breathing is called into play to remove CO_2 and help in controlling changes in acidity (hydrogen ion concentration). The mile (or 1500 m) race has for years been considered the ultimate test of athletic performance, and for good reason because it is the event requiring all the systems to respond more-or-less to their limit, and to integrate, or cooperate, perfectly. Before May 6th 1954 many thought a four-minute mile was beyond man's capacity; the previous record time of 4:1.4, by Gundar Haegg of Sweden, had stood for 8 years. However, on August 7th of the same year Bannister repeated the feat in winning the Empire Games Mile in Vancouver. This has remained a classic race, as Bannister overtook the Australian runner John Landy with only 80 yards to go, to win in a time of 3 min 58.8 sec; Landy's time was also under the 4 min mark at 3:59.6. Everyone knows that since 1954 innumerable athletes have bettered 4 mins for the mile; the world record of 3 mins 41.3 sec, by the Moroccan Hicham El Guierruj has stood since 1999. His pace of 440 m/min implies that Bannister would have trailed him by more than 120 m!

On the same day as the Empire Games mile another classic moment occurred, but remembered for the agony of defeat. The British runner Jim Peters staggered into the stadium at the end of the marathon in first position, but was unable to reach the finish because of extreme exhaustion of both brain and body: he had run out of glucose.

We all sense the effort involved in breathing with great precision—we know whether the effort is "appropriate" for the level of exercise. In heavy exercise, such as hurrying up several flights of stairs, we may not experience breathlessness until after we get to the top—the flood of lactic acid from our muscles generates lots of CO_2, to greatly stimulate breathing. During exercise that lasts for longer than a few minutes, a greater breathing effort than we expect provides an important signal that we are relying on glycogen for fuel and blood lactate concentration is increasing. If the exercise lasts for longer than an hour, increased breathing effort warns us that we are running out of glycogen and urgently need to moderate our pace in order to avoid the devastating effects of a lowered blood sugar.

A question that may remain in many reader's minds, is what <u>does</u> limit exercise in performance athletes? A conclusion that we are left with is that any one of a number of factors may separate the winner from the one that comes last, some fairly obvious and some that remain indefinable. Because of the emphasis placed on oxygen supply, maximal oxygen uptake is often identified as the most important defining measurement. In the past few decades this belief has led to the practice of blood doping. By taking an athlete's blood, storing it for a few weeks until the bone marrow has restored the subject's red cells and blood hemoglobin, and then re-infusing the taken blood, a boost is achieved in the blood's oxygen carrying capacity. It sounds easy, but can be tricky, because too many red cells increase the viscosity of blood that muscle perfusion is compromised. However, the process can increase maximal oxygen uptake and running speed. This would seem to settle the case in favor of oxygen delivery being a limiting factor in performance. Perhaps, but it is equally possible that increased performance is the result of improved buffering and greater carriage of CO_2 offered by the increased hemoglobin concentration. I say this because some 30 years ago Robert Taylor, a graduate student working in my laboratory, showed similar improvements when subjects were given sodium bicarbonate to improve their ability to buffer lactic acid during exercise.

CHAPTER 11

THOUGHTFUL BREATHS

*"And now I see with eye serene
The very pulse of the machine
A being breathing thoughtful breath,
A traveler between life and death…"*

William Wordsworth (1770-1850), *Perfect
Woman*

We don't have to think hard to perceive our breathing, whether easy or full of effort, and normally we give it no thought. However, when breathing does become difficult it can take on a very life-threatening quality, whether it occurs on our way upstairs, or during an attack of asthma, or even in a stressful situation. The perception of difficulty in breathing, called dyspnea by the doctors, or shortness of breath by lesser mortals, has been surprisingly difficult to understand. In part, we can trace this difficulty (an editorial in *The Lancet* a few years ago called it an "enigma") to the fact that the sensation is "subjective". This designation immediately leads to two conclusions; first that it is coloured by personality, leading to the pejorative label of "psychosomatic" being applied to many patients who might have benefited from more thought; and second, that being subjective it could not be quantified. Both these notions have proved incorrect, and we now know a lot about it.

DYSPNEA

The symptom of shortness of breath was recognized as a harbinger of death in Grecian times, and ascribed to an imbalance between the humors; centuries later the advent of pathological studies led to the identification

of structural change in essential organs. In pulmonary diseases no one was quicker to apply the new pathological information than the inventor of the stethoscope, the French physician Réné-Théophile-Hyacinthe Laënnec (as someone pointed out "pronounced Le Neck, and not because of the anatomical site where it is hung by aspiring physicians!"). Laënnec wrote his *Treatise on Diseases of the Chest* in 1821, in which there is the first description of emphysema; dyspnea is recognized as an important symptom of the condition, and of asthma, bronchitis, pneumonia and tuberculosis. When the role was established of changes in blood oxygen and carbon dioxide in the control of breathing, through reflexes acting on the midbrain, low oxygen (hypoxia) and high carbon dioxide (hypercapnia) were put forward as the main causes of dyspnea. Similarly, the demonstration by Breuer and Hering that obstruction of inspiration led to increased force of the next inspiration, mediated by the vagus nerve, gave rise to the theory that stimulation of the vagus was responsible. However, even Breuer and Hering found it hard to explain the symptom, which could arise in different situations, many of which were not associated with hypoxia, hypercapnia or vagal stimulation. In 1938, Ronald Christie, a physician at the London Hospital, who had carried out landmark studies on breathing in emphysema, commented—"Though the conditions under which dyspnea occurs are various and manifold, giving rise to an impression of complexity, the fundamental causes are few and relatively simple. They consist of chemical and reflex disturbances." Jonathan Campbell Meakins, who had been Professor of Therapeutics at the Edinburgh Royal Infirmary but later moved to McGill University in Montreal, was also interested in dyspnea, and in 1930 persuaded Christie to join him. Although Christie went back to the UK after a few years, he returned to McGill in 1955; thus began the tradition for respiratory research that eventually became the Meakins-Christie Institute, the source of many advances made in this field in succeeding decades, up to present times. Meakins, in a lecture to a local branch of the British Medical Association in 1923, accepted the importance of oxygen lack and CO_2 excess in stimulating breathing, but presented a definition that was broader than previously proposed—"Dyspnea is the consciousness of the necessity for increased respiratory effort". The definition represented a fundamental shift in reasoning, moving dyspnea out of the purely reflex domain into that of sensory physiology. Thus, stimuli and reflexes contributed to increases in breathing and recruitment of respiratory muscles; these changes in turn generated the sensation of effort that was consciously perceived.

Dickinson W Richards, the great chest physician at Bellevue Hospital in New York (and with André Cournand winner of the 1956 Nobel Prize for Medicine) popularized the concept of dyspnea as representing the balance between the demand for breathing and the maximum breathing capacity. Dyspnea could be due to increased ventilation (demand), increased mechanical hindrance to breathing (reduced capacity) or, commonly, a combination of the two. Both factors contributed to the effort expended, and sensed during breathing.

PSYCHOPHYSICS

Investigation into the function of sense organs was in its infancy during the latter half of the nineteenth century, when the anatomy of the sensory nervous system was defined. At the same time it was obvious that there were large differences in the quality of different sensations, such as between taste and sight, and that within a given sense there were differences related to quality as well as quantity, such as the appreciation of different colours and hues as well as their intensities.

Scientists first became intrigued about the possibility of measuring the intensity of sensations, later known as the field of psychophysics. The first sensation to be measured was that of light appreciation by the ancient Greeks, when Hipparchus used a six-point scale to follow the brightness of the stars. Much later, the perception of brightness could be compared to brightness measured with a photometer. Initially, although it was conceded that one could detect differences in intensity ("this light is brighter than that"), the perception was thought to be too personal to be able to quantify intensity (such as "this light is twice as bright as that"). The problem was how to create units of sensory intensity, and in 1834, the professor of anatomy and physiology at Leipzig, Ernst Heinrich Weber, put forward the concept of the "just noticeable difference" (JND). Weber, since known as the father of experimental psychology, found that when the stimulus (such as brightness) was small, only a small increase in intensity was needed for the increase to be perceived, but when the starting intensity was high, it needed a much greater added increase to be noticed. "Weber's Law" states that the JND increases in proportion to the intensity of the stimulus. In the 1860, Gustav Theodor Fechner, professor of physics at Leipzig, applied the mathematics of physics to the problem; he proposed that sensation increased as a logarithmic function of the stimulus—as the stimulus increases geometrically (say, by a doubling) the sensation increases by a constant amount. Later, he used Weber's concept of the JND to quantify the intensity of a given sensation by adding up JNDs, and the resulting relationship is known as the Weber-Fechner Law. Thus, the Law expressed the concept that a doubling of the stimulus, whether small or large, led to the same increase in sensory intensity. Fechner performed countless studies on sensations from skin and muscle (he left records of nearly 25,000 estimates of weights), and clearly felt that his law was scientifically and philosophically pre-eminent, for "it bears that that simple character that we are accustomed to find in fundamental laws of nature". However, the ability to measure sensation was widely questioned, no more strongly and lucidly than by the American pragmatist philosopher William James. James had a remarkable career, graduating in medicine at Harvard and remaining there as lecturer in anatomy and physiology, then as professor of philosophy and finally as professor of psychology, to achieve similar fame in his field as his brother Henry, the great novelist. Of the field of psychophysics he had much to say, including—"the whole notion of measuring sensations numerically remains, in short, mere mathematical speculation" and "in the humble opinion of the present writer, the proper psychological outcome is just *nothing*". Such opinions seem to have held considerable sway, and even in the 1930s, a distinguished committee appointed by the British Association for the Advancement of Science argued for many years, without resolving the question of sensory measurement. However, doubt about this conjecture was dispelled by the extraordinary work of Stanley Smith Stevens in his Harvard laboratory over four decades; he applied mathematical insight and rigorous experimental techniques to make modern psychophysics his own. His book *Psychophysics* was published in 1975, two years after his death; in it he summarizes the extensive evidence that led him to state a law that has similar attractions, in its rigor and simplicity, as that put forward by Fechner. The Psychophysical Law states that equal stimulus *ratios* produce equal sensation *ratios*. Stevens' psychophysical law is a power function.[1] Mathematically this means that any sensation capable of being scaled could be expressed in terms of the stimulus intensity raised to an exponent (power) whose value was an attribute of the quality of the sensation. To take two examples—first, the sense of effort experienced during a measured hand grip has a power of 1.7; this means that for a doubling of the applied force the sense of effort increases by 2 raised to the power 1.7, or 3.2 times; loudness has a power function exponent of 0.67, so that a doubling of sound pressure is appreciated as a 1.6 ($2^{0.67}$) increase in loudness.

With regard to the sensations experienced in the act of breathing, some of the qualities we can recognize relate to the depth of the breath (volume), the pressure we generate in the thorax (tension), pain that may be experienced during breathing, and the effort or discomfort in breathing. Each of these sensations may vary from zero to intolerable, and may lead to the adoption of patterns of breathing that help to minimize discomfort. In addition to sensations experienced during breathing, there are others that are less easily related to the act of breathing and remain controversial in their origin; one is a feeling best understood as a "drive" to breathe and another as a feeling of "breathing enough", analogous to satiety or "eating enough".

The sensation of a drive to breathe is most intense when we hold our breath—we reach a point when we "break" and have to take a breath. This might be interpreted as due to carbon dioxide increasing or oxygen falling

---

1   In mathematical terms, the sensation magnitude (ψ) is a power function of the stimulus magnitude (φ)-$\psi = \kappa\varphi^{\beta}$

sufficiently to stimulate breathing reflexly; however, in a famous experiment in 1954, Ward Fowler showed that the feeling could be instantly relieved by breathing a mixture of CO_2 and O_2 identical to that present at the end of the breath-hold. Thus, the sensation was abolished without any change in the gas concentrations, and needed to be explained in some other way.

Most of the sensations associated with breathing, especially those causing discomfort, have their origin in the respiratory muscles. Sensory receptors and nerve endings in muscle were demonstrated at the end of the 19th century, notably by the Spanish histologist Santiago Ramón y Cajal, winner of the Nobel Prize in 1906 for his seminal work on the organization and function of the nervous system. The receptors are actuated by changes in respiratory muscle length, the tension developed by them, and the extent to which the muscle is stretched, so generating nerve impulses which are relayed to the brain.

The first person to systematically investigate the sensations associated with breathing Moran Campbell, who with his colleague Jack Howell at the Middlesex Hospital in London, decided to study the ability of people to detect applied loads to breathing. In the early 1960s they interested a number of medical students in the problem and together they developed an experimental set-up worthy of the eccentric cartoonist Heath Robinson. The "loads" were generated by breathing from closed canisters, leading to an "elastic" load, and through perforated tubes covered with porous paper, which provided "resistive" loads. The canisters were of varying volumes, from the size of a bucket through to several large oil drums connected together. The smaller the volume the more pressure was required to obtain a breath, and the resistive loads could be varied in a similar way. The

pressure required to breathe was measured, and loads were presented randomly, with the subject being asked to indicate when a change in load was detected; this was a similar concept to Weber's JND, and it was found that a change of about 20% was required over the natural load to breathing, for the load to be detected. Campbell and Howell found that the stimulus for detection did not seem to be any change in lung volume or pressure achieved, and they argued that detection had to be related to the interaction between the two. Applying known stress-strain relationships found in muscle, and the fact that changes in lung volume were associated with changes in respiratory muscle length, and changes in the pressure with changes in muscle tension, they proposed the concept of "length-tension inappropriateness" as the signal for the sensation of breathlessness. Moran Campbell always carried a rubber band to illustrate the concept; it was analogous to judging the stiffness of the band—"To do this one normally pulls the band in and out, noting the sensation. One neither fixes one end and observes the change in length for a given pull, nor the pull required to obtain a given length." On this relatively simple concept was built a complex neurophysiological edifice to explain how changes in length *versus* tension were sensed. This expansion made the concept more difficult to grasp, and it proved difficult to use in a quantitative way to measure the sensation of breathlessness in the many situations where it was experienced. At one level, however, inappropriateness remains a useful notion: breathlessness is sensed when the effort associated with breathing is greater than we expect, and thus inappropriate, for a given level of activity.

The Swedish psychologist Gunnar Borg was a student of S.S. Stevens in the 1950's, and applied his mentor's scaling techniques to quantify perceived effort during exercise. He was able to show that effort satisfied Stevens' power law: an increase in work intensity was associated with an increase in effort raised to a power of 1.6. This means, for example that a doubling of work intensity increased effort by $2^{1.6}$, or 3-fold.

In the 1970's Borg turned this finding into a scale of practical utility by fixing the two ends of the scale (0-10), and linking the intervening numbers to verbal descriptions (such as "light", "moderate", "somewhat hard") that, through many studies, he showed preserved the ratio qualities. He tested the scale in populations of varying educational levels and languages to test its general validity. The "Borg Scale" has proved to be a remarkably useful tool for assessing symptom intensity, particularly during progressive exercise, in which symptoms may increase from zero to intolerable.

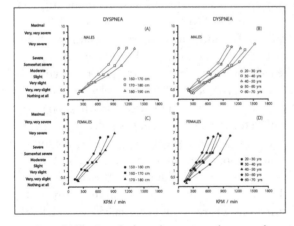

Figure 34 The Borg Scale used to measure the sense of effort in breathing during progressive exercise (work intensity is expressed in kpm/min) in healthy males (top) and females, related to their height (left) and age. For a given exercise load effort is higher in females, and increases less in taller and younger individuals.

It was not long before its usefulness in quantifying the sense of effort in breathing became apparent to clinical physiologists, and it was a Godsend to our own group. It meant that the intensity of dyspnea could be measured under the loading conditions used by Moran Campbell to detect loading, under exercising as well as resting conditions, during rebreathing, in simulated altitude, with asthma provocation, and in dyspneic patients. Briefly, the most important factor contributing to the effort of breathing was the pressure (tension) achieved by the respiratory muscles, expressed as a fraction of the muscle strength; differences between individuals' perceptions are often related to differences in strength. Perhaps it should not have come as a surprise that the maximum inspiratory pressure (how hard you can suck) was very variable, from 50 to 250 cm H_2O- a five-fold range. Respiratory muscle weakness is a common cause of shortness of breath, especially in the elderly and any patient with a chronic respiratory disease. Other factors included the total ventilation, the size of each breath, the frequency of breathing and the rapidity of inspiration. Increased loads to breathing acted through the increases in pressure required to breathe against them.

WHAT IS IT THAT WE FEEL, WHEN WE'RE "SHORT OF BREATH"?

The sensation of effort in breathing thus turned out to be closely similar to the sense of effort experienced in any other muscular task, which depends on the load (tension) as a proportion of the muscle strength, the extent of the muscle contraction (size of breath), the frequency of contraction, and the velocity of contraction (speed of inspiration or flow). The sense of effort also increases if breathing is initiated at a high lung volume, because the respiratory muscles start from a shortened position—analogous to trying to lift a weight with your elbow already bent. The independent role of changes in oxygen and carbon dioxide, other than their role in

126

stimulating an increase in breathing, remains quite controversial.

One of the more heroic experiments that I have been involved in was a study of the effect of paralysis on breathlessness. Moran Campbell decided that the only way to discover whether dyspnea was sensed through receptors in the respiratory muscles signalling tension to the brain, was to eliminate them, and see if the sensation resulted from increases in CO_2 in the lungs and blood. To do this required the administration of curare, the poison used by South American tribes to paralyze their prey by tipping their arrows with the stuff; it is routinely used in operations to achieve muscle relaxation. Not many of us were keen to undergo this study, and in the end only two subjects took part, one of whom was Moran. The curare was administered by the Chief of Anaesthesia at the Royal Postgraduate Medical School, Gordon Robson, and his colleague John Norman looked after the adequacy of ventilation; a blood pressure cuff prevented paralysis of the hand, so that Moran could signal with his thumb in response to regular questions. During the study Moran was able to tolerate a 4-minute long suspension of his breathing, during which the CO_2 pressure increased from 36 to 60 mmHg—a level that is usually intolerable—without feeling any distress or "drive" to breathe. It was also certainly less than the distress of the team looking after the study, as we collectively "held our breath" until it was all safely over. A second subject, Mark Noble, underwent the procedure, with similar results. This seemed to "prove" that the drive to breathe, at least during a breathhold, was mainly an impression of an intolerable tension in respiratory muscles prevented from contracting.

As often happens in science, when the study was repeated by others, including two of Moran's protégés, different results were obtained; Kieran Killian and Simon Gandevia concluded that "dyspnea is preserved following neuromuscular blockade. This suggests that chemoreceptor activity, via the central neuronal activity which it evokes, can lead to discomfort in the absence of any contraction of respiratory muscles". It will prove difficult to resolve arguments, because Gandevia has shown that stimuli arising in the higher brain, whether to initiate a movement voluntarily or as part of a reflex, are sensed through what is termed "corollary discharge".

Pinned to Kieran Killian's wall is Lord Kelvin's aphorism "When description gives way to measurement, calculation replaces debate"; the Borg scale has provided the measurement, and helped to move dyspnea from its initial subjective uncertainty. There is still debate, but it need not worry us because the system normally works to maintain PCO_2 constant, and the drive to breathing is provided by the amount of CO_2 that the body produces. Anyone who allows their PCO_2 to rise is almost by definition unresponsive to it, and is actually *less* short of breath than someone who maintains a normal or low PCO_2. We will think about this again in the context of severe chronic airflow limitation, chronic obstructive pulmonary disease (COPD), where chronic increases in PCO_2 are common.

In the Cardiorespiratory Unit at McMaster one of our main aims during the 1970's was to develop an exercise testing system that could be used in all situations—healthy adults and children, and patients with cardiac, respiratory and neurological disorders. Simple non-invasive measurements were made during exercise, on a cycle ergometer, that progressed in steps from rest to a symptom-limited maximum in 10-20 minutes. Limiting symptoms in a test of this sort usually consist of severe leg muscle fatigue, shortness of breath, or chest pain. All of these symptoms may be quantified with the Borg scale, and examined in relation to such responses as the heart rate and blood pressure, electrocardiogram, and respiratory measurements. This allows us to identify the factors that contribute to a patient's limitation: almost invariably there are several of these acting in concert. This helps to decide what may be done to improve function. We now have a data base that exceeds 25,000 studies, and allows us to generalize on the main factors that limit exercise. Kieran Killian has made imaginative use of the data, to help tease out these factors and assess their contribution to an individual's disability. Breathlessness, then, can be seen to result from an imbalance between the demand for breathing and the ability to achieve the demand.

We now know that the demand for breathing is primarily metabolic, related to CO_2 production, and secondarily reflex, related to stimuli arising in receptors that respond to increased CO_2, increased acidity (hydrogen ion concentration) and reduced blood O_2 saturation, and to stimuli in higher brain centres. The ability to achieve the demand in comfort is reduced by increases in lung stiffness (elastic recoil) and resistance to airflow (airway narrowing), and by weakness of the respiratory muscles. In addition to reduced strength of the muscles, they are weakened when required to work at a shortened length (ie. at high lung volume), at a high velocity (shortened time for inspiration), high frequency and long duration. We shall come across these factors again when we consider such situations as exercise, going to altitude, lung disorders and mind-body interactions. All these situations may provoke an increase in the effort of breathing. Whether they are perceived as an inability to achieve a satisfactory breath, breathing much

more than we expect, not enough to satisfy the drive to breathe, all these feelings are appreciated as a threat to life.

128

CHAPTER 12

BREATHING AT ALTITUDE Man's quest to go ever higher

"Our pace was wretched. My ambition was to do twenty consecutive paces uphill without a pause to rest and pant, elbow on bent knee; yet I never remember achieving it—thirteen was nearer the mark. The process of breathing in the intensely cold dry air, which caught the back of the larynx, had a disastrous effect on poor Somervell's already very bad sore throat and he had constantly to stop and cough".

"I still believe that there is nothing in the atmospheric conditions even between 28,000 and 29,000 feet to prevent a fresh and fit party from achieving the top of Mount Everest without oxygen"

Lieutenant-Colonel E.F. Norton, The fight for Everest, 1924.

"After every few steps, we huddle over our ice axes, mouths agape, struggling for sufficient breath to keep our muscles going. I have the feeling I am about to burst apart. As we get higher, it becomes necessary to lie down to recover our breath".

Reinhold Messner, Everest. Expedition to the Ultimate, (1978)

Edward Norton and Reinhold Messner both believed that Everest, 8848 metres above sea-level, could be climbed without the use of supplemental oxygen. Norton was a member of the ill-fated 1924 expedition in which

George Leigh Mallory and Andrew Ervine lost their lives; although less famous than they, he reached almost 8600 metres without oxygen. A photograph of Norton and Mallory on their climb, shows them in trilby hats and plus-fours, as if going out on a grouse shoot. The day after Norton's failed attempt with Somervell, Mallory chose Ervine in preference to the much more experienced Noel Odell for a final attempt, because Ervine had more faith in the oxygen equipment they were to use, and because he "had a peculiar genius for mechanical expedients". More than 50 years was to pass before Norton's achievement was surpassed by Messner and his colleague Peter Habeler, who climbed to the summit without the aid of oxygen on May 8th, 1978; they had the benefit of many technological and scientific advances that had accrued in the intervening years.

In spite of Norton's belief and achievement, most mountaineers were convinced that Everest could not be climbed without the help of oxygen, and they persisted in carrying the bulky and temperamental oxygen equipment. The first successful climb, by Edmund Hillary and the Sherpa Tenzing Norgay on May 29th 1953, was achieved with the use of oxygen, although their account details many problems with the equipment, including kinked tubing, leaking connecters and faulty gauges. That said, there is no doubt that oxygen breathing lessened fatigue and breathlessness and improved brain function at that extreme altitude.

Norton realized that oxygen lack was not the only problem that faced mountaineers at extreme altitude; when he arrived back to Camp IV after his record climb, he was met by a colleague carrying an oxygen cylinder, but "I remember shouting again and again, 'We don't want the damned oxygen, we want drink'". It was many years before the reasons for their extreme thirst was investigated by the great British altitude physiologist LGCE (Griff) Pugh during several Himalayan expeditions in the 1950s and 60s. An imposing, charismatic man with tousled red hair, Griff Pugh became a legend in his own time: he insisted that comfort was important if good experimental work was to be done: in addition to fragile glass analytical apparatus and a cycle ergometer, his luggage—carried by the indefatigable Sherpas—included a Persian carpet, chest of drawers, bed and chairs. His careful studies, especially on water and calorie intake, became crucial information that allowed the oxygen-free ascents of Messner and Habeler. Hr found that large losses of water and heat occurred from the lungs at the extreme altitude and low temperature of Everest. His findings led to very large increases in calorie and water intake. It had become clear that survival at extreme altitude is a complex affair involving all body systems as they adapt not only to low oxygen (hypoxia), but also to water and fuel depletion. But let's go back to the beginning.

ALTITUDE AND PRESSURE

The realization that pressure declines with altitude and air becomes thin, dates back to 1644, when Evangelista Torricelli, a pupil of Galileo in Pisa, found that a closed glass tube with its open end in a bowl of mercury (Hg) could support a column 760 millimeters (mm) high. He argued that "the force which holds up that quicksilver is external" and due to the weight of the air pressing down on its exposed surface. Shortly after, in 1648, the young French physicist Blaise Pascal took the thought further with the idea that the weight of air would become progressively less with altitude. With his

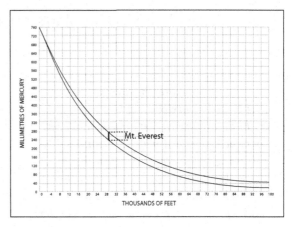

Figure 35 The relation between altitude and pressure, from Haldane and Priestley's *Respiration* (1935)

brother-in-law Peter, Pascal took his Torricellian barometer up the Puy-de-Dôme mountain to confirm the observation. Since then, pressure has been measured using three main, and related, units—millimeters of mercury (mm Hg), Torr (for Torricelli, equals mm Hg) and kiloPascals (kPa, equals [mm Hg ÷ 760] x 100); we will use mm Hg. Also, in situations of great pressure, such as occur underwater, atmospheres (A) are used, multiples of the sea-level pressure.

Studies in the 19th century showed that pressure declined with altitude in a gentle curve. The relationship predicted that at the summit of Everest (8848 m) the pressure was 230 mm Hg.[1] When John West was planning studies to be made on the American Medical Research Expedition to Everest in 1981, I was surprised to hear that one of the most important measures was to be pressure. He explained to me that although pressure on the earth's sea-level surface is latitude independent, at altitudes

---

1   Like many so-called "laws of nature" the relationship is a power function. Approximately, at constant temperature, pressure halves for every 20,000 ft (6500 m) increase in altitude, falling from its sea-level value of 760 mm Hg to 380 at 20,000 ft, and 190 at 40,000 ft.

between 4 and 16 km there is a marked effect of latitude due to a huge mass of very cold air in the stratosphere above the equator. On his expedition one recording was made at the summit, of 253 mm Hg. Also, temperature exerts an effect by increasing molecular motion; balloon measurements have shown that average pressure at the Everest summit's altitude varies between 243 mm Hg in January and 255 in July. It seems strange that such small differences in pressure may mean the difference between life and death, but the effect of pressure on the oxygen in air (and lungs) is very sensitive to these changes.

EARLY ALTITUDE STUDIES

Interest in taking off from the earth's surface began with the Montgolfier brothers, Joseph and Etienne; they made a balloon 18 m in diameter, and on June 5th, 1783, filled it with hot air and watched it rise 2000 m into the air, to the rapturous applause of a large crowd and the later plaudits of the French Academy of Sciences. Six months later, a member of the Academy, François Pilâtre de Rozier and the Marquis d'Arlandes made the first human ascent in a Montgolfier balloon. Two young, later to be famous, scientists—Jean Baptiste Biot and Louis Gay-Lussac—ascended to 7000 m in 1804, and suffered no ill-effects. They may have been lucky, for in 1842, the Britons James Glaisher and Henry Tracy Coxwell did not fare as well when their balloon reached over 8000 m. At around this height, Glaisher was unable to read the barometer or his watch, and soon after became paralyzed and unable to speak, then became blind and finally he lost consciousness. Coxwell suddenly became paralyzed in his arms; by a superhuman effort he pulled the emergency release valve with his teeth, and the balloon descended, both balloonists recovering on the way down. Not so lucky were the two colleagues

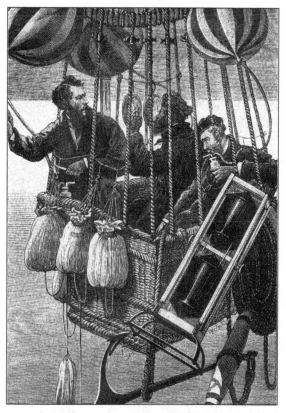

Figure 36 The famous etching of the ascent of the Zenith, showing (l-r) Sivel about to cut the ballast free, Tissandier reading the barometer and Croce-Spinelli with the oxygen supply

of Gaston Tissandier, Joseph Croce-Spinelli and Théodor Sibel, who ascended with him in the balloon *Zenith* to 8600 m on April 15th, 1875. Although they had undergone tests conducted by Paul Bert in low pressure (hypobaric) tanks, and were supplied with bags of oxygen, they became paralyzed without warning, and lost consciousness, just as Coxwell had. Only Tissandier regained consciousness on the way down, and he later observed "one does not suffer in any way, on the contrary. One experiences inner joy, as if it were an effect of the inundating flood of light. One becomes indifferent; one no longer thinks of the perilous situation or of the danger; one rises and is happy to rise". The suddenness and insidiousness of brain hypoxia and the surprising absence of breathlessness, are due mainly to the shape of the oxygen dissociation curve.

IS THE PROBLEM DUE TO LOW PRESSURE, OR LOW OXYGEN?

This question was debated only briefly, before the "father of aviation medicine" answered it definitively in 1878, in his massive book *La pression barometrique*. Paul Bert had been appointed by the Academy as the principal investigator of altitude effects, and he set about the question with unparalleled skill. In his book he gives credit to Robert Boyle, who through the 1660s performed many experiments (or rather his assistant Robert Hooke did) with his pneumatic pump, which allowed him to expose animals to a partial vacuum; among his novel findings were the longer survival of frogs and snakes than small mammals, and of new born kittens compared to mature animals. Bert used tanks that could be pressurized at will, and gas mixtures in which oxygen concentration could be varied from zero to 100%; he demonstrated conclusively in animals and later in man that it was low oxygen pressure that determined the occurrence of the dangerous symptoms experienced at altitude. He also showed that high oxygen pressures were toxic to animals, resulting in convulsions and death, but that's another story.

Paul Bert was a pupil of Claude Bernard at the Sorbonne, and succeeded him as professor of physiology; Bernard had realized the importance of measurements of oxygen and carbon dioxide in blood, and Bert developed methods to measure pressure and content of the two gases in blood. He showed that the relationship between oxygen pressure and content was curved; as pressure fell from its normal sea level

value of 100 mm Hg, there was little change in blood oxygen content until pressure fell below 60 mm Hg. Although his methods were crude and not very reproducible, his findings paved the way for later investigators, such as the Danish trio of Christian Harald Bohr, Karl Albert Hasselbalch and August Steenberg Krogh, who demonstrated in 1904 the S-shaped (sigmoid) nature of the oxygen "dissociation curve", and the effects of carbon dioxide on it. Basically, the sigmoid hemoglobin oxygen dissociation curve means that little change in blood oxygen content occurs as you ascend from sea-level to about half way up Everest but higher up you can expect large falls, which in a rising balloon can occur very rapidly. The reduction in oxygen pressure as you go higher parallels atmospheric pressure, but the amount (content) of oxygen in arterial blood, which is what affects the brain and the respiratory control centre, is more like a cliff than a gentle curve. Thus, as you rise from sea-level to 7000 m, pressure falls to about 330 mm Hg: the ambient oxygen pressure is about 70 mm Hg, and arterial oxygen pressure about 60 mm Hg, compared to about 100 mm Hg at sea-level. Although the PO_2 has fallen by 40%, the oxygen content has only fallen by 5%, from 95% to 90%. This fall has little effect on the brain or breathing. However, ascend another 1000 m and arterial PO_2 will be close to 40 mm Hg, with arterial oxygen content 75%: brain function will be impaired and breathing markedly stimulated. The records of the intrepid Glaisher and Coxwell revealed that they ascended to the height of Everest in 48 minutes: at this rate of climb, little time will elapse between feeling elated to feeling nothing at all!

ADAPTING TO LOW OXYGEN PRESSURE

Many physiological changes occur when man is exposed to low oxygen pressure in inspired air (hypoxia). The great British physiologist Joseph Barcroft conceived of oxygen supply to the tissues, such as muscles and brain, as a linked transport chain, in which oxygen pressure provided the driving force between the atmosphere and tissues; also to be considered is the amount of oxygen being delivered down the chain. Thus, the adaptation to altitude consist of changes that attempt to maintain oxygen pressure (PO_2), but also increase the amount (or content) of oxygen as it is being transported. As we consider the adaptations we will need to switch between pressure and content, as we have already done in considering the oxygen hemoglobin dissociation curve, in which blood oxygen content, or the percentage saturation of hemoglobin with oxygen, is plotted against PO_2. Nearly all the adaptations were recognized by Barcroft in his classic work, *Features in the Architecture of Physiological Function*, particularly in a section titled *Every Adaptation is an Integration*. We can summarize the changes by proceeding down the oxygen transport line. The first change is an increase in breathing; this reduces the carbon dioxide pressure in the lung alveoli leaving more space for oxygen and thus increasing alveolar PO_2 and the amount of oxygen delivered to alveoli. Increases in alveolar PO_2 aid the diffusion of oxygen across the alveolar walls into the lung capillary blood within a given time. Complete diffusion leads to equality between the alveolar PO_2 and the PO_2 of blood at the end of the lung capillary, but if the driving pressure (alveolar PO_2) falls, equilibration will not occur in time—a definite problem on the summit of Everest.

Changes in the hemoglobin dissociation curve come next; a "shift in the curve to the left" indicates that the oxygen content (or hemoglobin O_2 saturation) increases for a given PO_2. Reductions in carbon dioxide pressure (PCO_2), increases in blood pH (more alkaline), and

the binding of a glucose derived phosphate to the hemoglobin, all contribute to increases in blood O_2 saturation. The content of oxygen in blood is also increased by an increase in blood hemoglobin, due to increased production of blood cells by bone marrow, and sometimes by movement of water from blood plasma. The flow of blood is increased; cardiac output is increased through secretion of adrenal hormones.

There are downsides to most of these adaptations, and some are time dependent, either taking time to develop during acclimatization or becoming less effective as time goes on. Furthermore they may help the development of the two major high-altitude illnesses—cerebral edema and pulmonary edema, in which fluid accumulates in the brain and the lung alveoli—conditions in which emergency evacuation to lower altitude is vital.

THE EFFECTS OF LOW OXYGEN ON BREATHING

Everyone knows that you breathe more at altitude than at sea level, and the effect becomes relatively greater with each increasing meter. Also, it is common knowledge that the acute effect of altitude exposure on breathing lessens after a few days at altitude, and is far less in people who live permanently at altitude.

The mechanisms involved have already been touched on in Chapter 2; the physiological changes were established between 1910 and 1940, by physiologists on both sides of the Atlantic. JS Haldane, AV Hill and Joseph Barcroft in the UK, and Arlie Vernon Bock and Yandell Henderson at the Harvard Fatigue Laboratory in the US, often worked in collaboration.

The first adaptation to the reduced PO_2 of altitude is a stimulus to breathing related to reduced arterial PO_2 acting on chemoreceptors in the aortic and carotid bodies. If this reflex is tested by reducing PO_2 and keeping PCO_2 constant, ventilation increases linearly in relation to the fall in oxygen <u>saturation</u>. As mentioned above, this means that substantial increases in breathing do not occur until the PO_2 has fallen below 60 mm Hg.

Increases in breathing reduce arterial PCO_2 and tend to minimize the reduction in PO_2 in the alveoli, by reducing the space occupied by CO_2. Careful measurements of alveolar PO_2 and PCO_2 (as well as blood hemoglobin) were made by an unsung colleague of Haldane's, Mabel Purefoy FitzGerald. The present Professor of Physiology at Oxford, Frances Ashcroft, recounts that when the group went to Pike's Peak in Colorado in 1913, to the meteorological station also used by the Harvard Fatigue Laboratory, Mabel did not stay with the men, but "was dispatched on a mule to lower altitude to examine the hemoglobin content of the blood, and the carbon dioxide concentration in the expired air, of the local mining population". She collected an impressive amount of data in subjects living at altitude, and in the members of the expedition; she found that the average alveolar PCO_2 fell from 40 mm Hg at sea level to 28 at 4300 m, where barometric pressure was 440 mm Hg. In the scientific group the adaptation took 2-5 days to reach a stable state. Alveolar oxygen pressure fell from 105 to 55 mm Hg. The change in PCO_2 indicated that alveolar ventilation increased by 43% (40÷28), but if it had not occurred and PCO_2 had remained at 40 mm Hg, we can calculate that alveolar PO_2 would have been only 32 mm Hg. This difference has a potentially huge effect on the saturation of hemoglobin in the pulmonary capillaries.[2] Mabel FitzGerald's

2   Oxygen saturation at a PO2 of 55 mm Hg is 83%, but
    at 32 mm Hg only 58%

results remain valid to this day, but she appears to have been lost from scientific view after 1920. She lived a secluded life in Oxford, but in 1963 attended the Symposium held to honour the centenary of Haldane's birth, when she herself was 91 years old.

Measurements of arterial blood gases (PO_2 and PCO_2) are hard to do at extreme altitude, which is why alveolar gas sampling has been preferred on scientific expeditions. Measurements of arterial blood gases performed to heights comparable to Miss FitzGerald's have shown that arterial blood PO_2 and PCO_2 show similar trends to the alveolar levels. Now, people have never chosen to live at altitudes that are much higher than 4300 m—that is at half the altitude of Everest. Andean miners have always lived at about this altitude and traveled each day to the higher altitudes of the mines, because of the difficulty in sleeping at the higher levels and the long term effects. More recent altitude expeditions have shown that above 4500 m the relative increase in breathing, and reduction in PCO_2, become progressively greater. Alveolar ventilation increases to 143% of its sea level value with a reduction in atmospheric pressure from 760 mm Hg to 440 mm Hg, to 200% (alveolar PCO_2 20 mm Hg) at 350 mm Hg (an altitude of 6500 m), and 270% (PCO_2 15) at 300 mm Hg (7900 m). Finally, on the summit of Everest (8848 m) Dr Christopher Pizzo, who had climbed without oxygen on October 24, 1981, used an automatic alveolar gas sampler to find his PCO_2 to be only 7.5 mm Hg, indicating an alveolar ventilation that was 530% of the sea level value. The implications of the findings at extreme altitude are that alveolar PO_2 is defended, at the expense of greatly increased ventilation, at around 35 mm Hg at altitudes between 6500 m and 8848 m. The ability to increase ventilation appears to be an important contributor to success in high altitude climbing, in that studies of ventilatory response to CO_2 have shown that climbers showing a high responsiveness are able to climb higher than their less responsive colleagues.

As we have already seen, respiratory physiology received a large boost during the World War II, mainly in order to solve problems facing aviators. A number of superb scientists put their previous interests on hold and turned their attention to altitude physiology. The Rochester group of Wallace Fenn, Hermann Rahn and Arthur Otis got together in 1941. All three later admitted that at the time they knew little more than "human beings like many other organisms consumed oxygen and gave off carbon dioxide", but during the succeeding decade they established themselves as the leading researchers in the field. Literally taking a leaf out of Paul Bert's book, they constructed an altitude chamber and amassed a large range of equipment by begging, borrowing and improvising, because their equipment budget amounted to only $500. The altitude chamber was a master stroke; it was a steel tank made for transporting large quantities of beer, and thus capable of withstanding high pressures. A small circular entry hatch was cut into one end, and a pump normally used to spray trees, was borrowed from the University Grounds Department and used to reduce the pressure inside. In this way the subjects in the tank could be rapidly taken to "altitude"—the "summit of Everest" could be reached in six minutes! The chamber could accommodate two subjects who kept in touch with the outside experimenters by microphone; "when the outside observer no longer obtained from a subject a reasonable response to his interrogation over the loudspeaker, he would open a valve to admit air to the chamber until the subject demonstrated satisfactory activity". Experiments progressed well until one day the Dean of the Medical

School chanced by at an inopportune time to see Dr Fenn pass out at, and ordered that he should not be allowed in the tank again.

Wallace Fenn was a lot more than an innovative problem solver and intrepid self-experimenter; his was a mind capable of beautiful ideas, one of which was the "O_2/CO_2 diagram", first published by his junior colleague Hermann Rahn in 1949.[3] The diagram was not only useful as a mathematical aid, but also provided a map that showed the path taken by the alveolar gases when a change occurred in any of the defining parameters, such as atmospheric pressure, inspired oxygen concentration, and ventilation. Finally, it proved to be useful in predicting what might happen during an ascent to altitude, or

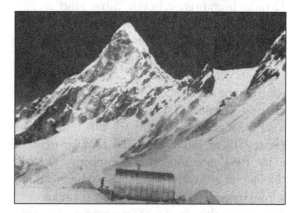

Figure 37 The Silver Hut, below the peak of Ama Dablam

some other event such as sudden decompression in an aircraft. It also demonstrated that when the increase in ventilation had occurred at altitude, you failed to maintain it at your peril; reduction in ventilation at this point led to a severe worsening in the low alveolar oxygen, to a point far worse than when you began. If, for example your respiratory muscles fatigued on

---

3   "O2/CO2 diagram", first published by his junior colleague Hermann Rahn in 1949

135

the summit of Everest, the oxygen pressure was likely to fall rapidly to below 20 mm Hg; loss of consciousness would be bound to follow.

Of course, in order to survive you have to be able to move, and to this point we have considered only what happens to the individual at rest. What happens when you exercise? Measurements of breathing during exercise have been made on Himalayan expeditions, the findings being amplified by more complex studies at sea level, some in pressure chambers and some during the breathing of gas mixtures having low oxygen concentrations. For its time, the British expedition of 1960-61, led by Griff Pugh was the most elegant. A laboratory was sited at a height of 5,800 m on the Mingbo Glacier, only 12 miles from Everest. In this "Silver Hut" difficult gas analysis measurements were made at rest and exercise. Pugh showed that maximum exercise, measured as the maximal oxygen intake (VO_2max), fell by 20% as the atmospheric PO_2 fell from the sea-level of 150 mm Hg to 100 mm Hg, and a further 40% to only 40% of the sea level VO_2max with a further fall in PO_2 to 50 mm Hg at 7500 m. John West found a similar trend in the 1981 expedition; the atmospheric PO_2 on the summit of Everest was simulated by breathing a low oxygen concentration (14% instead of 21%) at an altitude of 6300 m; maximal oxygen intake was only 25% of sea-level capacity. As you need about 10% just to survive in an inactive state, this does not leave much in reserve for the final push to the summit. It helps if you are very fit and light in weight—you need a very high power/weight ratio to get to the summit without oxygen. Reinhold Messner and his companion Peter Habeler are outstanding examples of this combination; they weighed 56 and 64 kg, compared with Hillary at 84. Also, their maximal oxygen intake was estimated at nearly 5 litres/min, some 30-60% greater than members of British expeditions of the 1950s to 1980s.

The demands on breathing in achieving even the reduced oxygen intakes of altitude are huge. The clearest information on this aspect of altitude physiology were obtained in Operation Everest II, in which the time profile and ambient pressure exposure experienced on an Everest climb were simulated in the large pressure chamber at the US Army Research Institute of Environmental Medicine in 1985, by a team of eminent physiologists coordinated by John Robert Sutton and Charles Houston. Maximal oxygen intake fell from 4 litres/min at sea level to 1 litre at the "summit"; the ventilation needed to achieve these values was 125 litres/min and 175 litres/min respectively. More breathing was required to achieve an exercise level that was only a quarter of what it had been at sea level; put in another way, six times the breathing was needed at the summit for the same amount of work! Given this fact, the sensations experienced by Norton, Messner and countless other mountaineers come as no surprise.

At this point I have to come clean and say that I am only an armchair mountaineer; the highest I ventured is about 3000 m, when I cross-country skied above Aspen, Colorado. However, I have been fortunate to work with two of the most productive altitude researchers, John West and John Sutton. John Sutton, who came to work with us at McMaster in 1972, was one of the few people who can be said to have been "a legend in his time". A charismatic Australian, by the time he arrived he had already climbed in the Andes, trekked in northern India improbably disguised as a monk, and worked in the Flying Doctor service in remote parts of Australia. His interests in high altitude physiology were soon obvious, and before long he learnt of the Arctic Institute of North America's High Altitude Physiology Study which had begun in the 1960's and had established a High Camp Laboratory 5400 m (17600t ft) up Canada's

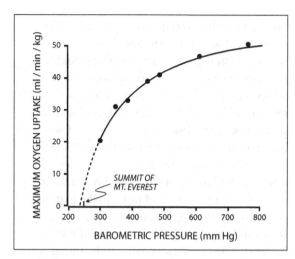

Figure 38 The fall in maximal oxygen uptake with increasing altitude, as a function of barometric pressure

highest mountain, Mount Logan, in the St Elias mountain range of the Canadian Yukon. The leader of the project was Dr Charles S Houston, an American scientist-climber who had first reconnoitered an approach to Everest from the Nepalese side. With the Briton H.W. Tillman he reached the Khumbu icefall (6100 m) in 1951. The Mt Logan multinational group carried out many studies on high altitude physiology and medicine, investigating high altitude pulmonary and cerebral edema—two potentially lethal conditions in which excess fluid accumulates in the lungs and brain—and the less deadly problems of bleeding into the retina of the eye and sleep disturbances. The studies took place in mid-summer, when John Sutton was able to commandeer analytical equipment without incurring the wrath of other members of the department who did not share his urge to climb into thin air. Although very successful, the studies were often difficult or impossible to complete due to problems with the weather on Mount Logan, and the altitude of the laboratory was not high enough to provide data relevant to the top of Everest. So they devised the most elaborate and well-designed study yet achieved

by simulating the climb in the large environmental chamber at the US Army and Research Institute of Environmental Medicine at Natick, Massachusetts in the Fall of 1985.[4] Eight subjects lived in the chamber for six weeks, whilst the pressure was gradually reduced at exactly the same rate as on an actual expedition; during the last five days the pressure was dropped to 247 mm Hg during the day and the recompressed at night, to simulate attempts on the summit. Of course, purists would point out that certain aspects of an Everest climb were not simulated—the sub-zero temperature, howling wind, deep snow, limited fluid and calorie intake, but the absence of these problems also allowed many more and better quality measurements than could have been achieved on the mountain. We can summarize the findings during maximal exercise as follows—Maximal oxygen intake capacity was 5.6 litres per minute at sea level, and 1.5 "at the summit"; arterial blood oxygen saturation was close to 100% at rest and maximal exercise at sea level, but only 60% and 40% respectively at the summit. This severe degree of oxygen desaturation, was in spite of huge increases in breathing; ventilation at maximum capacity was 130 litres/minute at sea level and 220 l/min at altitude, beyond the breathing capacity in the less rarified sea level air. The extent of this adaptation is underscored by the fact that at sea level, only 45 l/min of ventilation were required for the oxygen uptake attained at altitude. The pressure of carbon dioxide in arterial blood was 36 mm Hg at sea level and 10 mm Hg at the summit barometric pressure; this compares with Dr Pizzo's alveolar gas PCO_2 of 7.5 mm Hg on the actual summit. The low blood oxygen at extreme altitude is not solely due to the low inspired oxygen; when we

137

---

4   The size and scope of this scientific effort may be gauged from the number of senior scientists (26), institutions (10) and technical staff (70) that took part.

exercise at sea level we can maintain an oxygen saturation of close to 100%, but at altitude oxygen falls dramatically during exercise from 60% to a potentially lethal 40%, in spite of very high levels of alveolar ventilation. The cause of this reduction is the limited capacity for diffusion of oxygen when the alveolar pressure is very low. Gas diffusion is directly influenced by the pressure difference between the alveoli and blood; at extreme altitude, the reduced "driving" pressure means that there is not enough time for oxygen to diffuse into the blood, especially when the demands are increased and blood is flowing rapidly through the lungs. Similarly, when the blood reaches the tissues there is a much reduced pressure available to allow oxygen to diffuse into the muscles and heart. In order to achieve an oxygen uptake of 1.0 to 1.5 litres/min, necessary for climbing, with an arterial oxygen that is less than half what it is at sea level, the heart's output has to increase by at least twice; instead of a cardiac output of 10-13 litres/min, 20-30 litres/min are required. Because blood pressure in both the lung and systemic circulation is also increased in hypoxia, the heart is at its capacity in this situation.

Always at the end of experimental altitude studies the question is asked "what <u>does</u> limit the ability of humans to climb Everest without oxygen?" Even with monumental increases in breathing, with reductions in carbon dioxide pressure that few would have thought possible, the amount of oxygen in blood cannot be defended sufficiently to prevent brain hypoxia. The history of Everest climbing is replete with descriptions of the disabling effects of low oxygen supply to the brain; Hillary described failing sight when he removed his oxygen mask for only a few minutes, and many climbers have made disastrous decisions that led to their deaths. Reinhold Messner's colleague and expedition

doctor, Oswald Oelz, describes staying a few moments alone on the summit, leaving his colleagues to begin the descent; then, "suddenly, I was not alone. A tall, German-speaking fellow whom I had never seen before walked beside me and told me to leave the track and take a shortcut straight down a steeper route. I was by no means surprised to meet this gentleman here, and I followed his reasonable advice." As a result, Dr Oelz spent the night bivouacking in -40°C temperature, had more hallucinations, of his friends coming to build a cable car, and then was swept down for hundreds of metres by an avalanche. He was lucky to be found by his colleagues with "only" severe frostbite as his worst ill-effect. This leads to the conclusion that in addition to the lungs and heart reaching their capacity, brain hypoxia and severe muscle fatigue also appear to reach critical limits. The most intriguing fact remains—that all the mechanisms that integrate to supply oxygen to the brain, heart and muscles, appear to reach their limits on the world's tallest mountain.

TOO LITTLE CARBON DIOXIDE?

Some of us contend that carbon dioxide is at least as important as oxygen in the physiological scheme of things, and for at least a century there has been a suspicion that some of altitude's deleterious effects may be due to reductions in carbon dioxide due to increased breathing. The colourful Italian physiologist Angelo Mosso, performed many high altitude studies at his laboratory in the Capanna Regina Margherita on Monte Rosa, a 4600 m peak in the Alps. In 1898 he published his magnum opus *Life of Man in the High Alps,* in which he put forward the view that most altitude disorders were due to "acapnia" (low CO_2). The theory was supported by studies that showed improved oxygenation when a mixture of oxygen and CO_2 was breathed at altitude, but was

138

roundly dismissed by Haldane and Priestley in *Respiration* (1935). However, both high and low deviations in CO_2 pressure from its normal value in arterial blood of 35-45 mm Hg, do have profound effects on many body systems.

Oxygen and CO_2 share some properties, such as their effects on breathing control, but the differences between them are more striking. The body has only a small store of oxygen, of about a litre, whereas the storage capacity for CO_2 is at least 40 litres, without taking into account all the carbonate present in bone. When someone overbreathes, CO_2 leaves arterial blood very rapidly and the low CO_2 pressure leads to CO_2 leaving body tissues; as it is in equilibrium with its acid form, carbonic acid, blood and tissues become alkaline. The body responds by retaining acid (mainly chloride) and excreting alkali (mainly sodium), but this may take several days. Very low CO_2 in blood and brain tissue has a number of effects: it causes narrowing of the blood vessels to the brain, thus compromising oxygen and glucose delivery, and the biochemical processes in brain cells become inhibited. Also in situations of low CO_2 muscles become very twitchy—a condition known as tetany.

TOO LITTLE WATER?

Water exists as a gas that behaves rather differently to the other gases that we breathe; unlike CO_2 (at 0.03%) and O_2 (at 20.93%), water in the air around us varies with climatic conditions, and in the extreme cold of the mountains is almost absent. However, once air reaches the lungs it becomes saturated with water at the temperature of the body, exerting a pressure of 47 mm Hg, whatever the pressure of the atmosphere is. Haldane and Priestley write of their surprise when they calculated that an airman breathing pure oxygen at a height of about 45,000 ft, would be at risk of having

almost no oxygen in the lungs at the end of a breath, because at an atmospheric pressure of around 100 mm Hg, almost half would be water (47 mm Hg) and half CO_2 (40 mm Hg). In practical terms, however, what this means is that very large amounts of water are lost to the body just in breathing loss. In his physiological studies on Everest, Griff Pugh calculated this water loss, which combined with sweating and inadequate intake, could amount to as much as 10% of body fluid volume; although this will lead to ill effects such as a fall in blood pressure in untrained individuals, trained marathon runners regularly loose this much water without ill-effect. Marathoners also burn fat as a fuel, which leads to less CO_2 being generated for a given oxygen consumption. The training effect appears to be one reason for Messner and Habeler's success. However, the ability of the brain to function normally when seriously deprived of oxygen is more important; during the preparation for their ascent, Messner and Habeler flew over Everest at a height 9,000 meters without using oxygen, whereas Hillary lost consciousness when subjected to a pressure equivalent to 8,000 meters in a decompression chamber before the 1953 expedition. Even so, it must have been a close run thing, for Messner described how he felt over the last 50 meters "We can no longer keep on our feet while we rest... Every 10 to 15 steps we collapse into the snow to rest, then crawl on again".

Although many will be tempted to emulate their achievement or climb one of the other 8,000 + meters peaks, they should first reflect on Messner and Habeler's preparation, superb fitness, skill and judgment, to say nothing of their overarching motivation, and possibly, luck.

LIVING AT ALTITUDE PERMANENTLY

Paul Bert, in his seminal book *Barometric Pressure*, notes that Europeans were awed by the peaks of the Alps, which at the time appeared inaccessible, although few were higher than 4,000 meters high. In contrast, much of the ancient Mayan civilization had for centuries lived at above this height, and there were many ancient Andean cities built at about this altitude. The main adaptations that allow people to live at this altitude are collectively known as acclimatization, and mainly consist of a chronic increase in breathing associated with a reduced PCO_2, and increases in blood hemoglobin concentration and red cell count (polycythemia), a change noted by Bert. Other changes seen in high altitude natives are increases in the small blood vessels (capillaries) in muscle, and in muscle oxidative enzymes; these changes may occur mainly before and soon after birth and serve to increase oxygen supply and its utilization. It is clear that adaptation to oxygen lack (hypoxia) is extremely complex and involves many systems. In common with other problems involving adaptive changes in several systems, much has been learnt during the past two decades, when studies on isolated cells (molecular biology) and the application of cloning techniques have revealed the pathways by which they are regulated.

The main acclimatization processes take up to a week in the case of PCO_2 and up to 6 weeks for hemoglobin. In 1913, Miss FitzGerald found that hemoglobin concentration rose linearly by 30% from sea level to 16,000 feet (4,500 meters), and as barometric pressure fell from 760 to 450 mm Hg. She also found in permanent altitude dwellers that PCO_2 fell from 40 to 28 mm Hg over the same change in altitude. Crucially she showed that quite small changes in altitude were associated with increases in blood red cells,

indicating a very sensitive control of red blood cell formation by the bone marrow through changes in circulating oxygen.

The mechanism underlying red cell production (erythropoesis) at altitude remained obscure until the 1950s, when a young Danish researcher, working first at Yale and then at Harvard, showed that the effect was due to a factor carried in plasma. Alan Erslev performed the key experiments and went on to isolate a protein hormone secreted by the kidney, naming it "erythropoietin". In 1987 it became possible to clone the gene responsible for its production, and soon after it was produced commercially by recombinant genetic methods. In medicine, erythropoietin (EPO) has been used extensively in conditions where blood cell formation is poor, leading to anaemia, notably in kidney failure and cancer. More recently EPO has gained notoriety through its use by athletes to boost their blood's oxygen carrying capacity, and so increase their maximal oxygen intake by up to 15%. The production of red cells in conditions of hypoxia through the action of EPO is tightly regulated, which is just as well because increases in the number of red cells increases the viscosity of blood, potentially making it more difficult for blood to circulate, predisposing to clot formation in veins and the lungs, and raising blood pressure. Increases in viscosity usually occur when the red cell concentration (hematocrit) rises to above 60% of the blood volume; the usual sea level hematocrit is 45%, and this may rise to 55% or higher at altitude. Sometimes, acclimatized people get into serious trouble from these side effects when they become dehydrated; dehydration may acutely increase red cell concentration further, due to a reduction in blood water.

Recently a revolution has occurred in our understanding of how the body responds to oxygen lack. Surprisingly this happened during investigations into the molecular mechanisms that regulate expression of the EPO gene. A hypoxia inducible factor (HIF) was identified in hypoxic cells, not only in the kidney—where it stimulated EPO production, but also in many other cells. Thus, this factor is now recognized as being important in the developing small blood vessels of the fetus. It is even implicated in the formation of the carotid body, the microscopic organ in the neck responsible for increases in ventilation and heart rate during hypoxia. HIF appears to be the master controller of the responses to oxygen lack.

GOING EVER HIGHER

Few of us climb 8,000 meter peaks, but most of us fly at higher altitudes without feeling much. To begin with, aeroplanes had unpressurized cabins, and kept well below 5,000 meters. Modern commercial propeller driven planes are limited to 10,000 meters because they need the air resistance to fly. Modern jets make use of the decreased friction of higher altitudes but still require some atmospheric oxygen and are limited to 20,000 meters, Concorde's cruising altitude. Unpressurized planes are still limited to about 3,000 meters; theoretically they might fly at higher altitudes if everyone was supplied with oxygen, but maintaining an adequate supply carries some risk. Many studies have shown that there are few effects of flying at an altitude of 3,000 meters, and cabin pressure in modern commercial aircraft is maintained at that equivalent height (barometric pressure around 550 mm Hg). This means that the oxygen pressure (PO_2) in inspired air is around 110 mm Hg (instead of 150 at sea level), and in lung alveoli between 65 and 70 (instead of 100), ensuring that in healthy individuals the hemoglobin in arterial blood will be 90% saturated with oxygen (instead of 95%). This seems to have few effects, although some

impairment of higher brain function has been measured. Of course, in individuals with lung or heart disease, impaired gas exchange may lead to a lowering of oxygen saturation in this environment, with several effects such as breathlessness or poor vision, which are readily reversed by oxygen administration. Airline personnel are well trained to take care of such problems.

Does anyone want to think about what might happen if the cabin suddenly loses pressure? Probably only if you are considering joining the Air Force, when this problem may arise more frequently than being struck by lightning. Briefly, if your plane is cruising at 15,000 metres and cabin pressure is lost, you will be exposed to an oxygen pressure of only 25 mm Hg or less; you have only 10-20 seconds to use the oxygen mask that drops down automatically. The gas in your lungs immediately expands by about fourfold, so be sure you breathe out as hard as possible, and expect a dense fog as the water vapour in the cabin condenses. In military aircraft, personnel are trained to expect such events, and measures are automatically taken to protect them against damage from large pressure changes and aid in leaving the aircraft safely.

Fighter pilots face unique problems as the aircraft are light and only pressurized to 7-8,000 metres, so they have to breathe oxygen mixtures. Computer chips control oxygen supply and pressurized suits that combat the large gravity (G) forces that act on the body during steep banks and at the end of dives. The effects of gravity forces on the lungs were identified in fighter pilots in World War II, who experienced coughing and shortness of breath and in whom chest X-rays revealed areas of airless lung at the bottom of the lungs. The explanation was a combination of G-forces and oxygen breathing. Oxygen breathing meant that nitrogen was lost from the lungs, and the G-forces caused blood to flood into the lower parts of the lungs and airways to close; the trapped oxygen and carbon dioxide became completely absorbed and the alveoli collapsed and became airless. Normally nitrogen prevents this from happening as it is poorly absorbed and acts to stabilize the alveoli. Once the mechanism had been understood, airmen were taught to take a few full breaths after G-forces had been experienced, readily expanding the affected areas of the lung.

All the cells of the body rely on oxygen to turn the potential energy in sugars and fats into the chemical energy required for the processes that sustain life. When oxygen supply is compromised, as at altitude and in many other life-threatening situations, the body adapts, both rapidly and in the longer term. The adaptations may be local, such as the widening of small blood vessels, or affect the body as a whole, as in increases in ventilation. This is a tricky balancing act, because excessive oxygen is damaging to large molecules in the cells, so it comes as no surprise that the adaptations are complex and extensive. However, in some situations such as a severe heart attack, you may need all of them. In the case of altitude exposure, immediate responses include increases in breathing, heart rate and blood pressure, and a partial switch in metabolism to lactate production. Other responses may take several days as they involve the production of molecules involved in erythropoietin secretion. In some individuals the responses may be slowed, leaving them at risk of acute mountain sickness, in which fluid accumulates in the brain and lungs, a truly life-threatening emergency.

Sooner or later, we are all likely to be exposed to a low blood oxygen, whether because of exposure to high altitude or perhaps as a result of a heart or lung complaint. As the early balloomers found out to their cost, the effects

may appear with great rapidity because we store very little spare oxygen. The brain effects also make it difficult for us to appreciate the seriousness of the situation, and to respond appropriately. Fortunately, the provision of oxygen and access to individuals trained in cardio-pulmonary resuscitation has improved outcome in these life-threatening situations.

142

CHAPTER 13

BREATHING AT DEPTH Underwater adventures

"I descended equipped with an apparatus into a little circular basin 3 meters deep... the water was very muddy, and vision was almost completely obscured...I had lost my bearings...and could not find the ladder...air suddenly failed me...I succeeded easily in detaching one of the weights but the second was still attached by a cord when all effort became impossible...I was perspiring abundantly. I had a sensation of intense heat...and a feeling that I could not exhale...my ears rang and luminous circles appeared before my eyes..."

Paul Bert, 1898

In his monumental work *Atmospheric Pressure* Paul Bert describes his experiences, and those of others before him, of ascending to great heights and descending underwater, of being subjected to low and high pressure. He observed that there is little discomfort in climbing to 5,000 metres, but you can almost taste his panic when he submerged a mere 3 metres below the surface. As he well understood, the difficulties in breathing underwater are due to the fact that water is 770 times as heavy as air; if we measure pressure relative to sea-level (760 mm Hg, or 1 *atmosphere*, A), it increases by an atmosphere every 10 m we descend. At 10 metres it is 2 A, at 20, 3A and so on.[1] There are two main effects

that we need to think about. The first is Robert Boyle's (17th century) Law, that the product of pressure and volume is always constant for a gas. This means that, for example, gas volume halves as pressure doubles in diving to a depth of 10 metres. Second, by Dalton's Law of partial pressures, the pressure of each gas increases by the same proportional amount; if one is breathing air (20% oxygen and 80% nitrogen), the pressure of oxygen increases from 150 mm Hg (760 x 0.2) to 300 at 10 metres, and that of nitrogen from 600 to 1200 mm Hg. At greater depths the increases become very large, and greater quantities of both gases dissolve in blood and other body tissues. Interestingly, the effects are of greater importance during the return to the surface than during the dive itself, as we shall see.

WORKING UNDERWATER

Water covers some 75% of the Earth's surface and contains many resources—animal, vegetable and mineral; also it may form a barrier to movement, requiring the building of ships and bridges. For all these reasons humans for centuries have worked beneath its surface in many occupations, and have devised ways of overcoming the effects of great pressures in a variety of ways, but often at great risk to themselves. Some merely hold their breath and dive; the depth they reach depends on their diving technique and the time they are able to work for depends on their breath-holding time. Probably the most famous are the pearl diving women of Korea, known as Ama, who begin diving in their teens and frequently continue well into their seventies. Over centuries they evolved a diving pattern that has proved safe

143

---

1   Because sea water is heavier than pure water (by 2-5%) the increase in pressure is 2-5% higher in sea water; however, the difference is small and we will use the round number for pure water. It is also the reason that we are more buoyant in sea water.

and effective in allowing them to dive to a depth of 10-20 metres and collect pearls, abalone and seaweed. What happens to them during their dive was established in the mid-1960s by Dr Hermann Rahn, one of the true geniuses of modern respiratory physiology, working with Dr S.K. Hong of Yonsei University, by obtaining samples of lung gas from Ama diving in the Yellow Sea. Perhaps the most revealing fact was the uniformity of the diving patterns and gas pressures, indicating that the Amas had all learnt what the safe limits were in diving to a depth of 20 metres. The dives lasted 80 seconds, 20 to reach the sea floor, 40 for their work and 20 to reach the surface again. We can use the study as a basis for a discussion of breath-hold dives.

On the surface, you float or sink depending on the density of your body and the volume of air in the lungs. Body density, the relation between weight and volume, is mainly dependent on the proportion of fat to lean body tissues, as the latter have a lower density; indeed, the technique of underwater weighing has always been used as the "gold standard" for body composition analysis. On average, body density is higher than water so that if you breathe out fully you will sink—you are then 3 kg "negatively buoyant"; breathe fully in to increase the volume of air in the lungs by 5 or 6 litres, equivalent to 5-6 kg, and you become 2-3 kg buoyant. Most people take a deep breath before they dive, which increases the amount of oxygen available to them at the expense, unless they carry weights, of having to swim actively down. The Amas attach weights to their belts to reduce this effect; once on the sea-floor these are detached; at 20 metres below the surface, the 3-fold increase in pressure has reduced the lung volume to a third, eliminating buoyancy. After 40 seconds on the sea-bed they signal to their (male) partner, who pulls them up in a final 20 seconds.

During a dive the air in the lungs is compressed, so that below about 10 meters, their volume is halved and buoyancy is lost. The reduction in lung volume is one limiting factor in achieving depth in a dive; the ribs and diaphragm are not infinitely deformable and will eventually crush; most regular divers do not exceed 30 metres, where the lung volume is reduced to a quarter. It is not easy to find the record for the depth achieved during an unassisted dive; some of the records were obtained using weights and fins to speed up both descent and ascent—not that these aids make the depth any less impressive. That impeccable source of information on human achievement, *The Guiness World Records 2005*, accords the honour to the British woman Tanya Streeter who on August 17th, 2002 "took a single breath" and descended to the astonishing depth of 160 metres. The achievement is astonishing for two main reasons; first, her body was subjected to a pressure 16 times that at sea level, and her lung volume will have been squeezed down to only 1/16th, or less than a pint in size. This could only have been accomplished by allowing the pressure exerted on her abdomen to push the diaphragm up to almost the top of her lungs—a real case of her heart being in her mouth! Second, the time she took to accomplish the dive of 160 metres down and then back up is not provided, but even if she was capable of staying under for 4 minutes has to imply a swimming speed that was also of Olympic quality. Of course she was assisted probably by very heavy weights for the descent, and compressed air for the subsequent rise back to the surface, but the *GWR* does not record this.[2]

---

2 Tanya Streeter has been described as "the world's most perfect athlete"—with lungs that are twice the size predicted for a male of the same stature, very little body fat, and extremely strong abdominal muscles; a devotee of yoga, she can slow her heart rate to 15 beats/

144

The extent to which these aids help in achieving great depth may be gauged by the records for "constant weight without fins" which are less than half as deep—86 m by New Zealander William Trubridge and 60 m by the Russian, Natalia Molchanova. All accounts of the "sport" of competitive deep diving include a sad statement regarding the number of contestants that die during their attempts. In an interview with Tanya Streeter contained in the *GWR* she is asked "Is it fair to say that free diving is an extreme sport", to which Streeter replies "No, absolutely not", an answer that reveals more about herself than about the sport, though later she admits that it is all about attempting what is "on the extreme of human potential". We should mention snorkeling here; if you breathe underwater through a tube you have to generate enough pressure to overcome the pressure of the water surrounding the chest; this depends on the strength of the respiratory muscles, which interestingly is measured in centimeters of water and normally 100-200 cms H_2O. This means that no one can maintain such breathing at depths below one metre, which accounts for the normal length of snorkel tubes of about half a metre; it may also mean that fugitives who famously eluded capture by submerging and breathing through a tube, must also have been helped by seriously murky water.

In studying the Korean Ama, Drs. Rahn and Hong found that they did not overbreathe (hyperventilate) before the dive, merely taking a couple of deep breaths; as they descended 10 metres the oxygen pressure in the lungs doubled

to 200 mm Hg, but carbon dioxide increased by only a few mm Hg, being stored in body tissues. During the 40 seconds on the sea bed the oxygen steadily fell, but on the ascent the fall in oxygen slowed. This was surprising, because as the surrounding pressure lessens, so will the oxygen pressure in the lungs; what happened was that for a short time the oxygen pressure in the lungs fell to below that of the venous blood entering the lungs, and oxygen is released into the lungs. This can be seen as fortuitous, because it prevents the oxygen pressure in arterial blood falling below the level at which brain function is compromised; even so, the final oxygen pressure in the lungs was only 25 mm Hg. The Ama, with the accumulated experience of over 2000 years, seem to have got their timing just right.

One cannot say the same for the pearl divers of the Tuamoto archipelago in the South Pacific. The Tuamoto divers go deeper and stay under for longer than the Amas, and their occupation carries a much higher risk, and appreciable mortality. About 20% of them suffer from the "taravana syndrome"; *taravana* means "to fall about wildly", but the syndrome consists of visual disturbances, blindness and unconsciousness as well as staggering; death occurs in about 10% of those experiencing severe symptoms. In contrast to the Ama, the pearl divers hyperventilate before diving to reduce their carbon dioxide pressure, which prolongs their breath-holding time but does nothing for their oxygen. They dive to 40 meters where pressure is 5 times what it is on the surface, so their oxygen pressure is high in spite of its dwindling amount in the lungs; then as they ascend they become very hypoxic. The symptoms of taravana are mainly due to low oxygen in the brain; as they remain below the surface for 2 minutes or longer, the oxygen in arterial blood can fall as low as 30%. Many tissues will be short of oxygen and produce

min, and hold her breath for over 6 minutes. Add to these attributes a very high pain threshold that allows her to withstand the chest discomfort at depth ("like an elephant on your chest") and the feeling that eardrums will burst, and you have some inkling on what it takes to dive to below 150 metres—probably more than it takes to ascend Everest.

lactic acid; the acidosis means that less oxygen is carried in blood in subsequent dives. And here the third difference between them and the Ama becomes important; they spend less time on the surface between dives; at least 10-15 minutes is required for the blood lactate to fall sufficiently, meaning that greater than 5 or 6 dives in an hour will prove dangerous; many pearl divers achieve 15 dives in an hour. Finally, frequent dives to great depth carry the risk of nitrogen accumulating in the tissues, to cause the "bends" as the diver ascends or "decompresses".

We can appreciate that diving to great depths depends on the size of your lungs, the length of time you can hold your breath, and the rate at which you consume oxygen (your "metabolic rate"). If your lungs contain 7.5 litres (you are a tall man), of which one fifth is oxygen (1.5 litres), you will have about 2.5 litres to live on (body stores of oxygen are about a litre). Then, if you weigh 70 kg (you are also very lean!), your oxygen consumption in a completely inert state may be as low as 0.25 litres per minute. So you have 10 minutes' worth of oxygen if you are lying at the bottom of a swimming pool trying to break the "apnea" (Greek for "no breathing") record. World records for apnea are 10 min 12 sec by Tom Sietas of Germany and 8 min 0 sec by Natalia Molchanova; to achieve such times you must be good at resisting the stimulus to breathe from the increase in carbon dioxide pressure, which amounts to about 6 mm Hg per minute; most divers and elite swimmers are relatively insensitive to increases in PCO_2. Of course, any activity increases oxygen consumption, to reduce breath holding time. Typically, pearl divers use about 1 litre of oxygen per minute; a fourfold increase over resting levels will reduce breath hold time to a quarter.

Obviously, a way to counteract some of the problems met in free-diving is to replace the nitrogen in the lungs with pure oxygen, thereby increasing the amount of oxygen available by 4-5 times. The breath can then be held for more than 15 minutes, the possibility of the bends is reduced by eliminating nitrogen from the lungs. However, the great drawback of this seemingly useful measure is that oxygen is toxic to the lungs and nervous system at high pressure. Oxygen is one of the most reactive elements known, as it has the property of removing electrons and thus oxidizing compounds that are in contact with it, such as water. The oxidations produce "active" oxygen species, such as superoxide (O_2^-), hydrogen peroxide (H_2O_2) and hydroxyl (OH^-). Active oxygen species are capable of causing molecular damage to a number of cell components, including DNA. Pure oxygen is not used in diving to depths greater than 20 meters; below 30 m., where ambient pressure exceeds 4 atmospheres, convulsions occur after only a few minutes. Oxygen enrichment of air is a safe alternative, especially in clinical practice; this may be achieved by supplying oxygen at a low flow, or through mixtures of oxygen and nitrogen (nitrox). Such mixtures do not usually exceed 40% O_2.

OTHER DIVING MAMMALS

Because of the problems experienced by humans during diving, there has been great interest in diving mammals, such as the Antarctic Weddell seal, which is capable of diving to 600 meters and staying under for longer than an hour. The late Peter Hochachka, a brilliant biologist at the University of British Columbia, worked out the "self-sustaining life support system" that allowed the Weddell seal to be such a prodigious diver. Interestingly, unlike less intelligent humans, it does not hyperventilate, but may actually breathe out before diving. Then as it dives, the lungs almost completely empty; the airways are reinforced, allowing the alveoli to collapse. A number of reflexes shut down the circulation, including the so-called diving reflex, which dramatically reduces heart rate (from 60 to 15 beats/min) and cardiac output (from 40 to 6 litres/min). Other reflexes cause narrowing of the blood vessels, so that central blood pressure is maintained. Blood flow to all organs other than the heart, lungs and the nervous system is greatly reduced. These changes are not enough to explain the seal's diving capabilities; the seal's brain is small, and requires less than 1% of its total metabolic activity, compared with at least 15% in humans; also its blood volume is relatively greater, affording a much larger storage capacity for oxygen and glucose. Finally, during activity in the course of a dive the active tissues produce large amounts of lactic acid; because of the shut-down of the circulation the lactic acid remains in the tissues until the seal surfaces, when it floods into the blood and is taken up by the heart, liver and muscles and either turned back into glycogen or oxidized to carbon dioxide. Lactate acts as a strong acid having many deleterious effects which probably explains why the Weddel seal usually dives to less than 20 meters in depth and 20 minutes in duration, saving its marathon dives for exploration or emergencies.

DEVICES TO HELP DIVERS

An abiding memory of my childhood is that of playing in the rock pools by the seaside with a toy submarine, in the summer of 1939. My parents became distraught as they heard of the tragedy of the British submarine *Thetis* which on her maiden voyage underwent compartmental flooding and fell back onto the sea bed, at a depth of 46 m, in Liverpool Bay. Only four members of the crew were able to escape, before the remaining 99 were overcome by a lethal rise in carbon dioxide pressure, due to its inadequate removal, overcrowding and the sudden rise in pressure that accompanied its descent. One of

the supreme failures of the British Navy, the tragedy could have been avoided if the principles established decades before by John Scott Haldane had been properly implemented.

In the beginning, the limitations to breath-hold diving in terms of depth and duration meant that man had to devise ways in which air might be delivered at depth, to allow longer, and thus more productive work under water. This development had to wait for the invention of pumps that could overcome the pressure at depth and deliver air to metal domes or helmets. Paul Bert credits Edmund Halley, seafarer, astronomer and friend of Isaac Newton, with the invention of a bell and helmet that allowed someone to work at depth. Halley was an associate of Robert Hooke and Robert Boyle, who demonstrated their pressure chamber and pump at the meetings of the Royal Society. Halley rose to become president of the Society in 1728. The invention of caissons, huge cast-iron tubes that were sunk below a river bed for the construction of bridge foundations, followed soon after. Bert describes the symptoms experienced by workers after surfacing— excruciating itching of the skin, painful joints and painful muscle swelling—noting that they were rapidly reversed by recompression.

The problems associated with diving became a major concern for the great Oxford physiologist JS Haldane, who was asked by the British Admiralty in 1907 to research methods for lessening the hazards of working at depth; the results of his work were applied during World War I, and the work was continued by his son JBS Haldane in the late 1930s and through World War II. Father and son made inestimable contributions, often at great personal risk, to such naval operations as the "human torpedoes", frogmen, mini-submarines, the

147

clearance of mines from harbours, as well as in helping escape from disabled submarines.

At the time JS Haldane began his research, air was pumped down to the copper helmet of the diver at a pressure slightly greater than the water surrounding him, escaping through an exhaust valve.[3] The setting of the valve governed both the supply of fresh air and removal of carbon dioxide, and also the amount of air in the upper part of his suit, which helped to reduce the effort of breathing. At depths below 20 m. and during hard work, these divers became exhausted, showed errors of judgment and even lost consciousness; on resurfacing they frequently suffered from decompression sickness, or the "bends". Robert Boyle had noted the presence of bubbles in the eyes of snakes that underwent sudden reductions in pressure, and Paul Bert found tiny bubbles in small blood vessels and a variety of other tissues including the nervous system; he showed that these were bubbles of nitrogen that dissolved in these tissues at high pressure, and were then released when the pressure was rapidly reduced, similar to what happens when you uncork a bottle of champagne, to use Bill Bryson's analogy. Bert was, however, more interested in changes in pressure occurring during rapid ascent in balloons rather than the joint pains of caisson workers, and it was left to Haldane to provide an experimental approach to these problems. Haldane initially believed most of the symptoms were caused by the action of high pressures of carbon dioxide, which accumulated in the divers' helmets because of insufficient venting. He found that carbon dioxide could increase to 3% or higher in the helmet; at a depth of 20m. (3 atmospheres of pressure) this is equivalent to 9%. Carbon dioxide was known to be a narcotic at high pressure; indeed, for many

148

years it was used for procedures requiring only brief anesthesia, such as electro-convulsion therapy for psychiatric disorders. Haldane improved the pumps and established rules for the delivery of air in different situations to ensure that all the carbon dioxide produced would be cleared; for dives at greater depths, he devised a method for absorbing carbon dioxide to eliminate its accumulation. His colleague Sir Robert Davis, who was the proprietor of the largest manufacturer of diving equipment (Siebe Gorman & Co), invented a submarine escape apparatus that incorporated a cylinder of oxygen and a canister containing a carbon dioxide absorber. The *pièce de resistance* was the valve that controlled the flow of oxygen so that the pressure in the apparatus equalled the pressure surrounding the submariner. Very importantly, submariners were trained to continuously breathe freely during a rapid ascent, to prevent lung damage from the rapid expansion of lung volume that occurs as the surrounding water pressure lessens. Famously, the Davis apparatus saved several members of the crew of the submarine HMS *Poseidon* in 1931, which sank after a collision in the China Sea. Similar valves to those in the Davis escape apparatus that supply oxygen on demand and at a pressure equal to that of the surroundings, became more sophisticated in World War II, enabling frogmen to dive safely, and later incorporated into SCUBA (self-contained underwater breathing apparatus) equipment that is now used for recreational diving. The safe limit for the use of compressed air in diving is 30m., due to all the problems encountered at greater depths; chief among the rules that must be followed in recreational diving are adequate education and certification, and never to dive alone.

JS Haldane, with Professor AE Boycott and a Royal Naval officer, Lieutenant GCC Damant, set about solving the problem of decompression illness, associated with the liberation of nitrogen

---

3   The same principle is used in modern SCUBA diving.

bubbles, in the first decade of the 20th century. They started with a number of facts—that decompression sickness only occurred after dives to a depth greater than 13 m. (pressure greater than 2¼ atmospheres); that the amount of nitrogen held in tissues varied (fat held six times as much as blood); and that the rate of entry and release of nitrogen was a function of the tissue's blood flow. Finally, Haldane came up with the deceptively simple concept that the volume of nitrogen liberated was always the same as the pressure was halved, no matter what the absolute pressures were. Paul Bert had advised that ascent from a dive should be slow and the time spent should be greater the longer the duration of the dive. Haldane worked out specific times to be taken, depending on depth and duration, but more importantly his brilliant concept indicated that ascent could be initially rapid, and then slower as the surface was approached. The times and depths were provided in tables that became standard practice ever since; although some of the rates of clearance of nitrogen were later shown to be erroneous, no one has been able to improve on the tables in any significant way. The key physiological tissue in the problem is fat, which has the greatest capacity to store nitrogen, yet has a poor blood flow; and specifically, the fat that surrounds nerves. The liberation of nitrogen bubbles leads to nerve compression and distortion, accounting for many of the neurological features of decompression sickness—pain, itching, weakness, paralysis and loss of consciousness.

The data used to construct Haldane's Stoppages during the ascent of a diver after ordinary limits of time from the surface" were obtained from studies on goats in the pressure chambers at the Siebe Gorman plant. Goats were chosen because similar physiological function and body composition (lean vs. fat mass) as humans, and

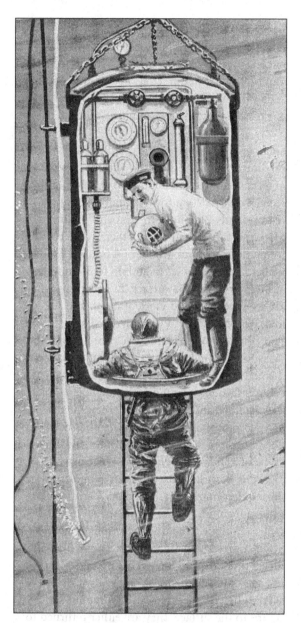

Figure 39 Davies' decompression chamber

service to the Navy, one of the most experienced of them being nicknamed "Lord Nelson", and they provided the essential information needed before human studies could be begun. The main subjects for these studies in pressure chambers and at sea were Captain (later Commander) Damant and Lieutenant AY Catto, who in

149

retrospect exposed themselves to many uncertain risks in dives of up to 100 m in depth and of 3 hours in duration. The monumental achievement of Haldane's decompression tables is a testament to their commitment and bravery.

Some brief examples of the use of the tables may provide an indication of how specific they are in terms of times and depths. At one end of the scale, a dive to 20 m for less than 20 minutes requires only 2 minutes to be spent at 10m, before surfacing; and at the other, a dive to 60 m for an hour requires a total of 4 hours, beginning with 15 minutes at 25 m and up to 30 minutes at 30 intervals to the surface. In situations where divers were having to work at depth and for long periods, Robert Davis invented a chamber that could accommodate three people under pressurized conditions at a depth required for the first stage of decompression; the divers entered through a trap door at the bottom of the chamber, and could remove their helmet and sit comfortably whist the chamber was positioned for the appropriate times and depths. Some of Haldane's ideas, such as the use of vigorous exercise and of oxygen administration during decompression, have since been found to be unhelpful, but the regimes shown in the tables continue to be used by commercial and SCUBA divers ever since. Recreational SCUBA divers do not spend long at great depths, and use a simplified scheme to render their dives safe. When divers experience symptoms on return to the surface, they are either returned to a depth where symptoms subside, or they are placed in a hyperbaric chamber. These measures are immediately effective; Haldane recounts a sequence of events experienced by one diver, whose ascent from 80 m was delayed because he "got foul and it took 3 hours before he could be liberated". On reaching the surface he spoke a few words and then became unconscious; the diving suit was "quickly ripped off and he was

hurried into the recompression chamber…by this time he was black in the face, his breathing had ceased, and no pulse could be felt"; the pressure "was run up to 75 lb. in 3½ minutes, which ruptured both the ear drums of one of the doctors. As 75 lb. pressure was reached the patient suddenly recovered and sat up, feeling alright again." However, it took some 12 hours in the chamber before he could tolerate the outside atmospheric pressure, without developing severe symptoms. There are indications that even divers who do not experience symptoms will later show evidence of the effects of bubble formation in bones and the brain.

In some situations, such as escapes from submarines at great depths, extremely rapid decompression may occur. This leads to extensive bubble formation, even in arterial blood going to tissues, and venous blood arriving in the lungs. The bubbles coalesce and lead to blockage of the capillaries (emboli). Bubbles in the lungs cause severe shortness of breath ("the chokes"), and the deformation of the lung may lead to tears in the airways with escape of air into the pleural space (pneumothorax). The only treatment is rapid recompression.

The symptoms of "the bends" occur on the ascent from dives; there are also symptoms experienced by divers during long dives at great depth, that include various behavioural abnormalities such as mood swings, poor judgment and bizarre actions, such as "offering their air tube to a passing fish". Although initially thought to be due to the stress of deep diving, researchers of the US Navy showed that these effects are due to a direct effect of large quantities of nitrogen becoming dissolved in the brain.

Paul Bert's experiences, described more than a century ago after he submerged a mere 3 metres below the surface, and quoted at the start of this chapter, stand as a dramatic reminder that diving to any depth carries risk. Several studies have documented the risks as being greater than in other recreational activities. Things can go wrong very suddenly and become life-threatening within seconds. At such times rapid reactions are needed, and there is no substitute for adequate training and meticulous preparation. Recreational SCUBA diving had its origins in the frogmen of World War II and the pioneering work of the renowned marine explorer Jacques-Yves Cousteau in the late 1940s. The apparatus for delivering oxygen and nitrox mixtures is now sophisticated and reliable, and there are many diving schools that offer expert training, to make the sport safe.

CHAPTER 14

THE FIRST, OFTEN DIFFICULT, BREATH

"The lung is probably unique among the tissues in its extraordinary ability to expand and contract. So far, this has been regarded as due to the elasticity of the tissue itself, and particularly that of the elastic fibres...one force has not been taken into account that definitely merits consideration in this context. This is surface tension."

Kurt von Neergaard, 1929.

There are few events more miraculous in our life than the first breath we take. Think of it: we are forcibly ejected from a liquid environment and have to breathe, on pain of death. But when we do, we find our lungs are full of a watery mucus, which has to be cleared, to make way for life-supporting air. Our immature brains have to signal our infantile breathing muscles to generate sufficient pressure to pop open the air sacs and provide oxygen to the blood circulating through the lung capillaries and onward to the heart's left ventricle and so to the rest of the body. If we are born prematurely, as occurs in about 10% of us, it may all be too much for us—our brains may not provide a signal, our diaphragm may be too weak, our lungs may remain unexpanded. The result may be what used to be called, more descriptively than many medical terms, the neonatal *Respiratory Distress Syndrome*. The story of how this problem became to be understood and finally managed, so that even infants born many weeks premature and weighing less than one kg have a good chance of making it, is of one of the greatest achievements of medical science.

But let's go back to the beginning. Actually, the breath we take shortly after birth is not our first; breathing movements in utero were noticed by doctors in the 19th century merely by examining abdominal movements in pregnant women. However, the movements were erratic and many physicians did not believe they represented breathing. Once pregnancy and fetal development came under scientific scrutiny in the 1930s, the early observations were confirmed in experimental animals; clearly, invasive studies could not be carried out in human foetus, and the experiments gave new meaning to the term "sacrificial lamb".

One of a number of activities that I now regret during my days as a medical student at St. Mary's Hospital in the late 1940s, was the treatment of our Professor of Physiology by the students. Short and thickset, and sporting thick glasses, waistcoat and gold watch chain, Professor Arthur St. George Joseph McCarthy Huggett became an object of derision; he was not the department's best lecturer, and things tended to go hilariously wrong with his demonstrations of animal physiology. Perhaps if we had known of his scientific breakthrough 20 years previously we might have treated him with more respect. In 1927, Huggett had shown that a fetal goat could be delivered by Caesarean section and kept attached to the mother, allowing observations to be made on fetal blood gases and pressures. Later the fetal lamb became the preferred experimental subject, and successively sophisticated techniques (such as cine-radiography of blood vessels) were applied. In the 1970s Geoffrey Dawes, who later became Director of the Nuffield Institute of Medical Research at the University Oxford, used the preparation to make landmark studies that helped to understand how breathing control developed, and what happened following division of the umbilical cord. Breathing is first observed at around 10 weeks of gestation, about a quarter of the way through our intra-uterine life; at first they are continuous and regular, but later they become less regular and are associated with slow wave activity in the developing baby's brain. Of course, breathing doesn't "do" anything because all that is being moved is the (amniotic) fluid in the uterus; gas exchange in the baby is through the placenta, with the mother doing all the work. However, the foetus responds to the mother's oxygen and carbon dioxide pressures; increases in maternal CO_2 pressure lead to "appropriate" increased breathing movements in the foetus, but falls in O_2 pressure are associated with cessation of breathing. This finding has always been difficult to understand—it is usually "explained" as a protective mechanism—and can pose a problem in early life. The control centre in the brain stem seems to gradually develop in the first few months of life so that a fall in O_2 pressure leads to "appropriate" increases in breathing.

During intra-uterine life the lung develops its branching system of airways leading to alveoli, and blood vessels leading to capillaries, to become an efficient gas-exchanging organ ready to perform its vital function. However, the dual and parallel circulation of blood, through the lungs and the rest of the body, does not occur, due to the effect of two bypasses—one in the heart between the right and left atrium (the foramen ovale) and one between the pulmonary artery and aorta (the ductus arteriosus). If we consider the total circulating fetal blood flow, 55% goes through the placenta to take up O_2 from, and transfer CO_2 to the mother. This oxygenated blood joins with the 20% returning from the lower body; of this 75% of total flow,

45% flows through the foramen ovale into the left atrium. The remaining 30% enters the right heart to join blood from the upper body (15%) and flows on into the pulmonary artery; only 15% enters the lungs, with the rest (30%) going through the ductus arteriosus into the lower aorta, and thence to the lower body and placenta. The blood going through the lungs joins the 45% in the left ventricle and flows into the upper aorta; this arrangement carries the benefit of the best-oxygenated blood from the placenta being delivered to the head (15% of total flow); the remainder (30%) joins the rest of the flow below the ductus (45%). These flows, which still seem complex even when rounded off and summarized like this, took decades of work and scientific debate to establish, and there are still questions to be answered. One point that, perhaps surprisingly, is still debated is the saturation of oxygen in human fetal blood going, for example, to the brain. Estimates have varied between 10 and 50%; Joseph Barcroft, a contemporary of Huggett but more famous as a physiologist, coined the phrase "Mount Everest in utero" to describe the situation. Barcroft made extensive studies of fetal hemoglobin, whose molecular structure allows it to carry more oxygen for a given pressure; however, this still leaves the foetus quite short of oxygen.

Studies in the lamb also established the complex changes that occur in the circulation and breathing when the umbilical cord is cut. These changes appear to be set in motion by the stoppage in flow from the placenta, leading to a fall in the pressures on the right side of the heart, and increases in left heart pressures that involve nerve reflexes, hormones and chemicals that change the calibre of blood vessels. Again, a complete account of what happens at birth remains in the future, at least in part because there is no such thing as an average birth—each is unique in terms of duration, difficulty and

153

the stress imposed on the baby. However, when the cord is cut there are increases in heart rate and blood pressure; blood oxygen falls and CO_2 rises, so that after a couple of minutes, an inspiratory gasp is provoked. There are forcible contractions of the inspiratory muscles and the lung expands with air; proper breathing has really begun.

Just before the first breath of air the lungs are dense and airless; after, they are light and spongy. In premature infants, however, inspiratory struggles continue as they attempt to expand the non-expandable; the lung may remain dense and poorly aerated. As the chest wall is not rigid in the newborn it becomes pulled in with every breath; this is the neonatal respiratory distress syndrome (RDS). The distress of the infant is matched by that of onlooking parents, and also doctors, who until recently believed that it was due to immaturity of the lungs and breathing controls, and had few approaches, either conceptual or therapeutic, to bring to bear on the problem. The story of the development of understanding and improved outlook in the condition has some parallels to other medical advances of the last century, such as the discovery and development of penicillin.

THE DISCOVERY OF SURFACTANT

Benjamin Franklin, the influential Bostonian who, amongst many achievements contributed to the drawing up of the Declaration of Independence, often went to London on diplomatic visits in the mid-18th century. On one visit, he became intrigued with oily films on water. The phrase "pouring oil on troubled waters" was already in use, perhaps originating from descriptions of early whalers, who observed the effect of whale oil as it spread around their boats. But Franklin was interested in how little oil was needed: he went to the pond on Clapham Common in south London and dropped some oil "not more than a teaspoonful" on the surface of the water. He watched it gradually spread until "it reached the lea side, making all that quarter of the pond, perhaps half an acre, as smooth as a looking glass"—the layer was only one molecule thick, but each molecule was attached to the next so as to form an unbroken film. Two centuries were to pass before the molecular basis for his observation and its relevance to the lung were fully realized. We all know that our bodies are mainly composed of water, and the ways in which water is handled dominate the workings of our bodies. Water has featured prominently in nearly all the chapters of this book, and usually its chemistry is what concerns us most. However, in the lung where water meets air, its physics is seen to be equally important, and at birth, when the lungs change from being full of water to being full of air.

Water seems such a simple substance, composed of only two elements, and seemingly without structure, that it comes as a surprise to find this is far from the truth. The molecular structure of water provides it with a cohesive force that is particularly evident at its surface: this is known as surface tension. In a liquid such as water there are forces of attraction between the molecules; on the surface, these forces cannot be equal in all directions but are aligned in the plane of the surface, leading to an elastic force that resists expansion; the force is measured as surface tension. The high surface tension of water is due the effect of "hydrogen bonds"; these are unlike the usual "covalent" bonds between atoms in a molecule: they are due to electrostatic forces between the positively charged proton in hydrogen and the strong electrons of oxygen. The forces at the surface of water are directed into the bulk of water producing a retractive force. In the lung such a

154

force would make it difficult to expand the fluid-lined alveoli. The discovery of the substance that lines alveoli and counteracts the retractive force of water, known as surfactant, is one of the most exciting in modern medical research.

The story of surfactant's discovery is similar to another transforming medical breakthrough, that of penicillin. There was an initial chance observation by a scientist who realized its theoretical importance: the theory was tested by a researcher and then applied clinically, to fully realize its medical importance.

The initial observation was made in 1955 by a "boffin" working in the top secret Chemical Defence Experimental Establishment on Porton Down in the West of England; Richard Pattle trained as a physicist and joined the Physics Section of the Establishment in 1953. Doing work on nerve impulses he became frustrated with small bubbles in microscopical tubes, and realized that they were due to surface tension effects. Pattle devised a method of estimating surface tension from the rate at which the bubbles shrank; the faster the shrinkage, the greater the tension acting on the bubble wall. In another section at Porton Down, physiologists were studying the foam that is produced in lungs exposed to the poisonous gas phosgene, and Pattle was consulted; the foam was composed of minute bubbles that would not disperse or break up. He realized that the surface tension of the liquid that formed the bubbles must be low, approaching zero, and that it came from the alveoli of the lung. In a famous, and very brief paper to the journal *Nature* Pattle describes how the bubbles contracted by about 25% and then remained stable almost indefinitely; the liquid forming the bubbles reduced surface tension and "a layer of some form of mucus, secreted in the depths of the lung, is the source of the insoluble alveolar lining layer".

Clearly, this was an example of an observation impacting a prepared mind, as was the clear area observed by Alexander Fleming in the culture of staphylococci, which eventually led to use of penicillin. By 1958 Pattle was able to write a longer paper dealing with the properties of the layer which acted "by reducing the surface tension to nearly zero". He also observed that "the finding that the lung lining substance appears only late in the fetal life of the guinea pig suggests that absence of the lining substance may sometimes be one of the difficulties with which a premature baby has to contend". He cited the Canadian anatomist Charles C Macklin, who in 1954 on the basis of careful microscopical studies had shown a "layer of mucus lining the alveoli; he suggests that its function is in some way concerned with surface tension". Macklin also postulated that the origin of the film was the granular "pneumonocyte", cells of very characteristic structure, found only in the alveoli and their walls, whose function to that time was unknown; they contained granules that stained similarly to the alveolar "mucus" and suggested they were fatty acid compounds. By that time, 1958, two "breathing giants" were on the scene, taking Pattle's initial discovery of a surface active lung liquid, and Macklin's observations, to new levels; they were John Clements and Mary Ellen Avery, and together they elucidated the composition and function, and clinical implications of the alveolar lining fluid.

In 1950, around the time that Richard Pattle joined the British chemical warfare group at Porton Down, John Clements reported for his National Service duties at the US Army Chemical Center at Edgewood, Maryland. Respiratory physiology had been made a military priority, and an unparalleled group of physiology geniuses dating back to the 1940s had made great strides in understanding lung function. A group at Harvard, including James

Whittenberger, Jere Mead and Edward Radford, had provided the framework for present understanding of the elastic forces—relationships between pressure and volume changes—and Clements went to see them at a time that surface active forces were being discussed.

One of the real puzzles in the story of surface activity in the lung is that a paper by the Swiss physiologist Kurt von Neergaard written as long before as 1929, and quoted at the start of this chapter, did not come to the attention of people working in this field until after 1954. Whilst investigating changes in lung volume produced by changes in pressure, von Neergaard had the insight that increases in volume were less than one might expect from the known structure of the lung and might be due to the surface tension exerted by liquid lining the alveoli. With wonderful imagination and intuition he reasoned that if surface forces were important they might be abolished experimentally by filling the lung with fluid—thus eliminating an air-liquid interface—and comparing the pressure-volume characteristics with those of the air-filled lung. The results were described in a paper which even 75 years later seems breathtaking in its scope, blending classical physics with new physiological understanding. Suspending a pig's lung in a large bell-jar, von Neergaard inflated it fully and then allowed it to deflate; he found that the recoil pressure was far less when the lung was filled with fluid than with air. Because the abolition of an air-liquid boundary reduced alveolar tension, the results indicated that surface tension was a major contributor to the lungs' elasticity. Crucially, von Neergaard also calculated that the fluid lining the alveoli was not water or plasma, but a substance having a surface tension that was less than half that of water. Finally, he provided an analysis for lung expansive forces that was based on established physical laws as they apply to spheres; he compared the alveoli

to bubbles on the end of tubes (mimicking small airways); the surface tension effects varied as a function of the radius of the spheres. In the last sentence of his paper, von Neergaard alluded to surface tension playing a role in the poor lung expansion in the newborn.

In the early 1950s, the Harvard group had more-or-less repeated von Neergaard's work, without realizing it, and had come to similar conclusions. However, they clearly had not realized that the alveolar lining liquid had a low surface tension. In 1954, Edward Radford, at Harvard, published calculations of lung surface area based on a surface tension equal to that of plasma; von Neergaard had already shown that this was too high, accounting for Radford's anomalous surface area estimates that were too low. Even though he was not actively working in this field yet, John Clements was intrigued by the discrepancy, and determined to understand surface forces and their action in the lung. The start of his career commitment to what became to be called "lung surfactant" was boosted by two events; first, the appearance of Pattle's note in Nature, and second, the opportunity to escort the German physical chemist Hans Trurnit to Niagara Falls. As they were driving top the Falls Trurnit described his work on liquid films that were one molecule thick (monomolecular layers), and the physical balance that he used to study their behaviour. In 1955, Clements and Elwyn Brown, a postgraduate research fellow, reworked the data in Radford's paper using Pattle's estimates of surface tension, set about studies of pressure and volume changes in the lung during both phases of breathing, and began measuring the surface properties of liquid obtained from animal lungs in a balance similar to that used by Trurnit,. John Clements was able to measure the attraction between molecules in his balance. The balance was composed of a shallow trough (analogous to Franklin's pond) whose area could be varied by a barrier that extended across the tray. A very thin platinum plate was suspended vertically so that its edge that just dipped into the surface; a very sensitive transducer measured the retractive tension on this plate as the film was expanded, and the resistive force as it was compressed. As Clements later put it "There remained little doubt that the surfactant was working as advertised in the lungs", contributing to lung recoil as the lungs expanded, and preventing lung collapse during expiration by reducing surface tension to almost zero.

The studies rapidly bore fruit, and extended von Neergaard's results for two main reasons. First, his measurements had been carried out during falls in volume—that is in expiration only. Second, the physical balance could measure the surface tension of the alveolar fluid as it expanded and contracted, in both phases of "breathing". Both the Harvard group and a similar group of outstanding physiologists at the University of Rochester (Wallace Fenn, Hermann Rahn and Arthur Otis) had recently shown that the pressure required to expand alveoli during inspiration is greater than that required to maintain alveolar volume during the expiratory phase of breathing. Clements and Brown showed theoretically that this behaviour could be due to *changes* in surface tension and that the alveolar fluid had exactly the same property—it could both resist expansion at high lung volume *and* resist alveolar collapse at low lung volume. Thus the lung lining fluid provided stability when stretched while breathing in and when compressed while breathing out; it had the property of reducing its surface tension during compression; this was a major advance since von Neergaard had measured a single value for its surface tension.

THE RESPIRATORY DISTRESS SYNDROME, FINALLY UNMASKED

It has taken us some time to reach Mary Ellen Avery, who in 1952 developed pulmonary tuberculosis whilst beginning her training in paediatrics at Johns Hopkins. She spent six months in a sanatorium, and in common with a number of physicians in the same situation, spent the time thinking about lung problems and deciding her future career in this field of medicine. She completed her training, becoming increasingly interested in "hyaline membrane disease"—as Respiratory Distress Syndrome was then known, a relatively common disease in the newborn, especially premature infants, in which severe respiratory difficulty occurring soon after birth usually progressed to death in a few days from lung failure. Following her bliss, Avery decided that she needed training in lung mechanics with Jere Mead, who in 1957 was the clear leader in this field. By then, Pattle's note, Macklin's observations on the alveolar lining, and papers by Clements had all appeared and von Neergard's work had finally reached the light of day. However, in spite of suggestions by all these researchers, that the airless lungs of new born infants with respiratory distress might be due to high surface tension, no one had followed the clues actively. Mary Ellen Avery was the one to do so; intriguingly, she soon found evidence to support this contention, but so difficult was it to change current thinking in the condition, that it was not until the fourth edition of her book *The Lung and its Disorders in the Newborn Infant* in 1981, that she could state unequivocally that the disorder was due to lack of surfactant production. A number of factors can be seen to have prevented a change of mind (a "paradigm shift") in our understanding of the condition. At the time it went under at least a dozen different names, with as many theories being held regarding

157

its cause, from prematurity of various organs, heart failure and asphyxia, to disorders of the nervous system. The term hyaline membrane refers to the formless (hyaline) substance found in the airless lungs *post mortem*; the lungs were solid, but contained large spaces that gave them a Swiss cheese appearance. Avery soon ascribed this appearance to the Law of Laplace, which states that pressure in a sphere (such as the alveolus) increases directly with surface tension and inversely to its radius.[1] This means that where bubbles connect, smaller bubbles empty into larger ones, to account for the Swiss cheese appearance. Also, fluid from the lungs of infants dying from hyaline membrane disease would not form bubbles. So when she went to visit John Clements during her Christmas vacation in 1957 to find out how to measure surface tension of the fluid, Mar-Ellen Avery was already convinced that it would be abnormally high. Clements recalled that the Christmas gift he gave her was a demonstration of his home made surface balance, and "an exposition of everything I knew about lung physiology. It only took four hours". Avery returned to the Boston Lying-In Hospital where she was a research fellow in the Newborn Service; with the cooperation of the pathology department and working with Jere Mead at Harvard, she measured the dynamic properties of films made from the lung fluid obtained from children that had died from a number of conditions. Within an exceptionally short time she had gathered data from 50 infants, 5 children and 4 adults. The results were submitted for publication in less than a year, and clearly impressed the Editor of the American Medical Association's

158

Journal of Diseases in Childhood, as they were published within 6 months. Avery and Mead showed that in adults, children and infants weighing more than 1200 grams maximum tensions obtained during expansion of the film ("inspiration") were lower than plasma, and fell markedly (by 85%) during compression ("expiration"). In contrast 9 infants weighing less than 12oo grams, and 10 infants dying from hyaline membrane disease showed much less fall in surface tension (by 50%) during compression—their minimum tension was 3-4 times greater than the other groups.

The work of Clements and Brown, and of Avery and Mead, marked a huge turning point in the management of neonatal respiratory distress and set in motion research that has culminated in a dramatic lowering in its incidence and mortality; in the US the number of deaths has been cut from about 20,000 to 1,000 per year during this time.

WHAT IS SURFACTANT, AND WHERE DOES IT COME FROM?

In the early 1960s Clements joined an elite group of scientists at the Cardiovascular Research Institute (CVRI) at the University of California in San Francisco. The CVRI occupied the 13th floor of the UCSF Medical Center, deemed unsuitable for a medical ward by reason of superstition, and directed by Julius H Comroe, Jr. "Uncle Julius" believed that many innovative scientists were neither good managers nor entrepreneurs, and sometimes even were very poor at describing their work and slow at writing papers, which could mean that they "published and/or perished". Thus, Dr Comroe took the responsibility for writing grant applications from their shoulders, successfully gaining multi-million dollar funding for the Institute as a whole, administering the whole operation, and imaginatively providing such

---

1   The 18th century French mathematician Pierre Simon de Laplace derived the Law, which is usually written as $P = 2T / r$. Simply put, the pressure in a sphere is directly related to its surface tension (T) and inversely to the radius of curvature.

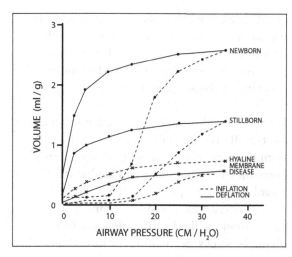

Figure 40 Mary Ellen Avery found that the lungs of babies with hyaline membrane disease (RDS) required a greater inflation pressure than healthy newborn infants, and maintained a greater volume during deflation.

services as a Scientific Editor to ensure that high quality publications flowed regularly from it. John Clements found himself in an environment where in addition to carrying on with his physiological research, there was expertise in modern biochemical analysis, electron microscopy and neonatal intensive care. Working with the lipid biochemist Richard Havel, a lipoprotein was isolated from beef lungs with surfactant properties, and Michel Campiche, a Swiss research fellow, employed new techniques of electron microscopy to show that "lamellar bodies" in type II alveolar cells (Charles Macklin's "granular pneumonocytes") contained phospholipid strands. Later, Mary C Williams was able to show these strands exiting the lamellar body onto the alveolar wall as a single layer that could form a lattice structure. Finally, as previously noted in Chapter 3, in 1977 Ewald Weibel and Joan Gil were able to demonstrate the lipid lining to alveoli in electron micrographs. Once the constituents of surfactant had been identified, the door was opened for their use

in babies with RDS. Here John Clements was joined by Dr William Tooley and Dr Marshall Klaus in the pediatrics department, and together they investigated clinical approaches to neonatal RDS. They had found that several factors might influence surfactant production, in addition to lung immaturity. Poor blood flow to a lung reduced surfactant production, just as poor blood flow to any organ impairs its metabolism; also poor ventilation of a local lung area had a similar effect—alveoli had to be expanded for surfactant to be made. This led to the concept of a vicious cycle in which a number of factors might contribute to poor surfactant function; the cycle might be broken at any one of a number of points, but of course complicated the management of these sick infants. To improve lung blood flow and ventilation and administer surfactant required a well-trained team and modern technology; the neonatal intensive care unit was born. Clements and his clinical colleagues conceived the idea of a clinical trial of one of the surfactant lipoproteins, dipalmytoil lecithin (DPL), carried out in a hospital with a large obstetrics department. Thus it was that in early 1964 they set out for the Kandang Kerbau Hospital in Singapore, where there were over 3,000 deliveries every year. When I arrived in the CVRI later in that year as a research fellow with Dick Havel, there was great excitement and anticipation of the results, and when they returned in the fall, their presentations were standing room only affairs. In the event, it was a case of "good news, bad news"; whilst the general approach to treatment was shown to improve outcome, the surfactant aerosol did not confer significant benefit. The problem with surfactant was two-fold; first, it was difficult to get the DPL down to the alveoli, especially where the changes of hyaline membrane disease were present; and second, an aerosol proved not the best form of administration—direct instillation of DPL into the airway via a tube, was more

159

successful. However, the total approach based on their concept of a vicious cycle, had borne fruit; this applied especially to changes in the mode of assisted breathing. Up to that time it had been the practice to increase the expanding pressure used by ventilators attached to a tube extending into the main airway, but such high pressures were required that lung and tracheal damage was frequent. Their new approach was to maintain a much lower pressure at the end of expiration (positive end-expiratory pressure, PEEP) to keep alveoli from collapsing due to the absence of surfactant. This was later shown to improve survival of infants with RDS from around 10% to over 80%. The interdisciplinary approach used in the CVRI was ahead of its time, and by the late 1960s had achieved spectacular breakthroughs on several fronts.

Chemical analysis showed that surfactant is composed of about a dozen phospholipids, that all have the same basic chemical structure but differ slightly in their properties; the dominant (80%) molecule is phosphotidylcholine. The phospholipids consist of a protein head and long chain fatty acid tail; they are "polar" molecules, with an electrically charged head that combines loosely with electrical charges (H^+ and OH^-) in water—it thereby attracts water (is hydrophilic). The long chain fatty acid tail is uncharged and repels water (it is hydrophobic). This polar structure allows the molecules to arrange themselves in a sheet, with the polar heads in contact with water molecules on the alveolar walls and the tails projecting out into the gas phase. The charged heads link together to form the insoluble alveolar lining layer. As well as reducing surface tension and maintain alveolar volume, this layer also acts to reduce evaporation of water from the alveoli, acting in the same way as oil layers are used to reduce evaporation from reservoirs in very hot dry climates. During compression of the lipid layer

phospholipids with smaller charges tend to be forced out, into the small airways and back into alveolar cells to be recycled. The whole process is very dynamic, with surfactant being constantly produced and recycled.

Formation and storage of surfactant occurs in the type II alveolar cells, and is controlled by hormones (mainly corticosteroids and thyroid hormone), nerve impulses and mediators. The alveolar cell first appears at about 28 weeks of fetal development and surfactant is found in the amniotic fluid surrounding the foetus at about 34 weeks, accounting for its deficiency in premature infants.

The basic research into surfactant and its function, contributed to modern prevention and treatment of neonatal respiratory distress syndrome (or hyaline membrane disease). Preventive measures include delaying birth in mothers going into premature labour, to allow the type 2 alveolar cells to mature; identifying infants at risk by analysing amniotic fluid for phospholipids; and administering corticosteroids to the mothers in the days preceding birth to boost surfactant production. Treatment includes the use of constant positive pressure ventilation, and the administration of synthetic surfactant to affected infants; this sounds easier than it proved in practice. Everyone thought that once the structure of surfactant became known it would be easy to synthesize the molecules and give them as an aerosol. However, synthetic phospholipids tend to form balls with the polar groups in the middle, so making them unavailable to the alveoli. An alternative was to obtain surfactant from animal lungs, but reactions to foreign protein were feared. Now, problems have been overcome; effective synthetic preparations and surfactant from cow lungs are available, and both have been shown to improve outcome.

One of the benefits of surfactant and modern techniques to support ventilation, is to reduce the need for oxygen. This is important because high concentrations of oxygen are damaging to several developing organs. In the immature eye oxygen contributes to retrolental hyperplasia, also known as retinopathy of prematurity, a condition in which there is disorganized overgrowth of the small blood vessels of the retina. This may progress to blindness, which used to be a tragic problem in babies who survived hyaline membrane disease.

Surfactant is one of those products of the body that seem now almost magically developed during evolution. Once it was found in snakes, which do not have alveoli, all sorts of functions have been attributed to it in addition to the stabilization of the lung surface and loss of water from it. The insoluble layer provides a barrier against bacteria, and surfactant production in the lung is increased when noxious fumes, such as ozone, are inhaled.

Many people were involved in the research that culminated in the dramatic improvements in prevention and management of hyaline membrane disease in the newborn. Although Richard Pattle, John Clements and Mary Ellen Avery were prime movers in changing views of the lung and treatment of a deadly condition, the whole story can be seen as a triumph of modern clinical science, in which researchers from many fields were able to contribute their own bricks in building the final edifice. Finally, the lessons learnt from treatment of neonatal respiratory distress have been successfully applied to a similar condition in adults—adult respiratory distress syndrome (ARDS), or shock lung—which is caused by a variety of injuries, from near-drowning to massive infection. Maintenance of pulmonary ventilation (by PEEP) and blood flow (by fluid replacement and drugs), and use of surfactant, are now all mainstays of treatment.

CHAPTER 15

BODY, MIND, SPIRIT, BREATH

"Breathing is truly a strange phenomenon of life, caught midway between the conscious and the unconscious, and peculiarly sensitive to both".

Dickinson W Richards, Jr, 1953.

The link between our mind and breathing is self evident; we all feel short of breath in tense situations, and for some people the sensation is intolerable, when they may be labelled as suffering from "psychogenic dyspnea", or less pejoratively "behavioural breathlessness". The advice to "take a breather" suggests that if we control our breathing, tension will lessen. Breathing control features prominently in Yoga techniques, both as a part of relaxation and to achieve trance-like states, and there are many descriptions of Yogis suspending breathing for long periods. The English playwright Christopher Isherwood was a committed devotee of Yoga, and practiced Yogic breathing to control his "obstinate" hangovers. Thus the corollary to breathing being largely an unconscious act, is that a conscious focus on breathing "clears the mind"; you cannot think about much else if you focus on, and consciously appreciate, air being drawn in and out of your lungs.

Abnormal breathing patterns in psychiatric disorders were identified by Ronald Christie in 1935, and more recently controlled yogic breathing has been shown to be effective in their management. All this confirms the opinion, quoted above, of Dickinson Richards, the outstanding clinical physiologist of the 1930s and winner of the 1956 Nobel Prize. Changes in breathing have profound influences on the function of nearly all organs in the body; these influences may be exerted directly, mainly through changes in pressure within the chest, or indirectly, through nervous reflexes or by the changes in blood that accompany increases or decreases in breathing. Needless to say, the effects, direct and indirect, are often combined, leading to quite complex and sometimes serious clinical situations.

EFFECTS OF PRESSURE CHANGES IN THE CHEST

First, let's consider mechanical effects of pressure changes occurring in and around the lungs during breathing. As the small blood vessels in the lung offer less resistance to blood flow than elsewhere in the body, and also are quite distensible, the amount of blood in them varies during breathing, as they are subjected to the changes in pressure that occur in the chest. Richard Lower, in the mid-17th century, was the first to observe that the flow of blood from the lungs changed with the phase of breathing, and the observation has been confirmed many times, to the point of describing the lung as an "accessory heart". During inspiration the negative pressure in the chest provides a pressure gradient that promotes movement of blood into the lungs and expands the small pulmonary blood vessels to accommodate the change in volume. The presence of uni-directional valves in the heart and venous circulation also helps this flow. Greater pressure swings in more forceful breathing will increase this effect up to a point; as the lungs expand close to their full volume the capacity of the blood vessels lessens, as the alveoli expand

and compete for the volume. However, very large pressure swings of up to 300 mmHg, almost three times the normal arterial blood pressure, can be obtained with repeated forceful coughing, and are enough to maintain a cardiac output without the help of the heart; patients who are known to experience episodes of severely disturbed cardiac rhythm (ventricular fibrillation) have been trained to cough rhythmically while they are awaiting treatment to take effect.

Large changes in pressure in the chest can have large effects on the heart and circulation. If you close off your glottis (larynx) and suck in hard, there is a large fall in intrathoracic pressure—this is known as *Müller's Maneuver*.[1] This has two main effects—blood flows into the lungs and heart rate increases. The left ventricle faces the problem of contracting against a greatly increased pressure difference between the negative pressure in the surrounding lung and the atmosphere surrounding the arteries to the body. Blood pressure falls, and there is a reflex increase in heart rate due to stimulation of sympathetic nerves to the heart. The situation may occur where large negative pressures have to be generated, for example because of a growth in the larynx; the left ventricle may fail and fluid accumulates in the lungs (pulmonary edema). The opposite situation may occur in the *Valsalva Maneuver*.[2] In this breathing gymnastic, one closes the glottis and strains to breathe

out, leading to a great increase in pressure in the chest; blood is forced out and also impeded from entering the lungs, and the heart becomes smaller. There is a brief increase in arterial pressure, followed by a fall; this stimulates pressure receptors in the aortic body, leading to a reflex increase in heart rate. Then, when breathing is recommenced, there is an increase in blood pressure and a fall in heart rate, due to stimulation of the vagus nerve. Pressure changes in the chest thus cause the autonomic nervous system to be activated; indeed, these two maneuvers are used to test autonomic function.

The autonomic nervous system has two arms, parasympathetic and sympathetic. "Autonomic" indicates nerve impulses that are generated reflexly—you don't have to think about these functions, the system takes care of them; not only that, but the system takes care of matters on a split-second basis. The system works by having receptors that respond to a variety of stimuli, such as pressure (called baroreceptors), or changes in the pressure of O_2 and CO_2 (called chemoreceptors), with transmission of the nerve impulses to centres in the part of the brain known as the medulla, or brain stem (sometimes even, hind-brain). These inflowing (or afferent) impulses lead in turn to outflowing (or efferent) impulses in nerves that are widely distributed through the body. The networks of nerves are classified as sympathetic (not because they look after you sympathetically) and parasympathetic (or vagus nerves). Anatomically, the distribution of the two networks is very complex and integrated with the rest of the central nervous system, with close integration between them in the spinal cord. Outside of the spinal cord the nerves are organized into a chain of nerve connections (ganglia) running down each side of the spinal column. The parasympathetic's main extension is the vagus nerve (the name having the same Latin root as "vagabond"), which runs

163

---

1   Johannes Peter Müller became professor of physiology at the University of Bonn in 1826, and later chair of anatomy and physiology at the University of Berlin; in these positions he was enormously effective and influential, becoming known as the father of modern German physiology.

2   Antonio Maria Valsalva (1666-1723) was a famous pupil of Marcellus Malpighi in Bologna.

down from the neck into the back of the chest to the heart and into the abdomen. Both networks have extensive nerve branches going to blood vessels, airways, organs such as the eye, heart, stomach and intestines, and even hormonal glands. To a large extent the two networks have opposing actions that are determined by the chemical transmitters that are released at the nerve endings. Their actions have widespread effects which are broadly related to effective control of the internal environment and proper functioning of all the body's organs, extending as far as behaviour. To simplify the contrasting influences of the two, we can say that the sympathetic activity leads to narrowing of blood vessels (vaso-constriction) and increases in heart rate and the force with which the left ventricle contracts; adrenaline secretion; release of glucose from the liver; sweating; and shivering. As all these reactions usually accompany sudden activity, they are often termed "fight or flight" responses. Parasympathetic, or vagal, activity leads to slowing of the heart rate and relaxation of small blood vessels (vaso-dilation); acid secretion in the stomach; secretion of saliva; and secretion of insulin by the pancreas. It would be nice to think that the wisdom of the body keeps these actions entirely separate, but there is some overlap so that in some situations both are activated and the result is a tug of war, with the stronger stimulus winning.

BREATHING AND THE AUTONOMIC NERVOUS SYSTEMS

The autonomic nervous systems, sympathetic and parasympathetic, both influence and are influenced by breathing. Everyone has experienced the stress-related increase in breathing that occurs when the sympathetic nervous system is activated. Impulses travel in both the vagus and sympathetic nerves with each breath, passing up the sympathetic nerves at the same time as impulses are traveling down the phrenic nerve during inspiration. At the peak of inspiration and during expiration impulses travel up the vagus nerves (the Hering-Breuer reflex). The effects of this nervous traffic can be easily appreciated by feeling one's own pulse, and breathing slowly; when you slowly breathe out (expiration) the heart rate slows, whilst in inspiration it quickens. In quiet breathing the vagus predominates, so that by consciously controlling the breath sympathetic activity can be lessened and the vagus is allowed to have its effect on an a number of cardiac and metabolic functions, as we'll see when we consider Yoga. The variation in heart rate with breathing is known as sinus arrhythmia (or sinus bradycardia), and is more prominent in well trained individuals than their less fit counterparts.

In the last decade there has been increased interest in the autonomic control of heart rate; heart rate can be monitored through long periods (Holter monitoring), and computer analysis is used to record trends in the variation of beat-to-beat intervals, known as the power spectrum of heart rate variability. Two peaks are observed in this analysis—at low and high frequency; the high frequency is linked to breathing and represents the effect of the vagus on the heart pacemaker, and is especially evident in athletes. When the low frequency peak dominates, heart rate changes are being controlled mainly by sympathetic activation. The analysis has found a number of clinical applications, of which the most striking has been in patients studied following a heart attack. Lack of heart rate variability, with loss of the high frequency component, is associated with a poor outlook—only 70% of patients are alive 3 years after the heart attack, in contrast to 93% in those with a normal variability. The extent to which your breathing controls your heart seems to have an important bearing on how long you live! Many other research studies have established that abnormal heart rate variability may be seen in many chronic disorders, such as diabetes and Parkinson's disease, and reflects impaired autonomic nervous system control of cardiovascular function. The autonomic nervous systems have such a widespread distribution, that it is easy to appreciate that they exert widespread influences on many aspects of health. The Belgian, Corneille Heymans, the 1938 Nobel Prize winner, was the first to produce evidence of the influence of the autonomic nervous system on breathing. In his experiments, discussed in more detail in Chapter 7, he showed that a fall in blood pressure stimulated the respiratory center in the medulla, leading to an increase in breathing. Increases in blood pressure had the opposite effect; injection of adrenaline into the aorta could lead to a complete cessation of breathing.

An extreme example of the links between breathing and the heart is the "diving reflex". Since the time of Claudius Galen in the 2nd century CE, this has been seen as a defensive reflex to shut down breathing when the face is immersed in water, and it was scientifically investigated by Florian Kratschmer in 1870. When the face is immersed there is a marked slowing of heart rate, partly related to breath-holding and partly to stimuli from the face and nose. In 1933 Edgar Adrian, winner of the Nobel Prize with Charles Sherrington in the year before, showed increased traffic in the vagus nerve associated with the maneuver. Not surprisingly, it is seen in its most dramatic form in diving mammals. In the Weddell seal, one of the most accomplished divers ever to be studied—with dives lasting in excess of one hour, the heart rate falls almost immediately at the start of a dive, and eventually reaches 10-15 beats/min. At the same time various parts of the circulation shut down, so that only the circulation to the brain is defended. The same reflex is seen in humans, when the face is immersed; Neil Oldridge showed that when healthy subjects cycling on an ergometer placed their faces in water, heart rate fell by 50% in trained synchronized swimmers and by 30% in untrained subjects; breath-holding (apnea) alone was associated with reductions of 37 and 25%. The greatest slowing was from 130 to 28 beats/min in one of the trained individuals; the slowing increased with the duration of apnea. The effect of training on heart rate slowing with apnea is particularly marked in yogis, who practice controlled breathing with apnea on a daily basis.

EFFECTS OF CHANGES IN BREATHING ON BLOOD AND OTHER TISSUES

Considering that breathing exerts important changes on the composition of blood and body fluids, it comes as no surprise that changes in breathing have important effects on many of the body's vital organs, but to some extent these are counter-intuitive. We might think that a reduction in breathing, leading to an increase in carbon dioxide pressure (PCO_2), has more serious effects than over-breathing, but the reverse is the case, especially in the short term. Of course, relative under-breathing is less common than over-breathing, because normally our reflexes cut in to maintain a constant PCO_2, and it is hard for anyone to voluntarily reduce their breathing appreciably. Some people naturally tend to under-breathe (they have a "high set-point for CO_2"), and some may develop the tendency because of their occupation as divers or through yoga, but in people who are otherwise healthy, keeping PCO_2 at 50 mm Hg instead of 40 seems not to have any ill effects. Higher levels, seen in patients with a primary absence of respiratory control

("Ondine's curse" described in Chapter 7), and also patients severe lung disease (see Chapter 18), lead to increases in blood acidity, which the body counteracts by water and sodium retention by the kidney, but eventually this may lead to heart failure. Over-breathing is another matter—it may be distinctly uncomfortable and can be very dangerous. The problem is that it is easily produced either unconsciously or volitionally, and there are no reflexes that are activated to limit it. It is easy to breathe deeply and frequently, and within less than a minute blood PCO_2 may drop to below 20 mm Hg, from its usual level of 40 mmHg; there are no changes to counteract this fall and you become alkalotic—blood hydrogen ion concentration falls, and pH rises from its normal value of 7.4 to over 7.6. A major effect of the lowered PCO_2 is to cause narrowing of the small arteries in the brain, and brain blood flow falls, leading to dizziness, weakness and weird psychological effects that are similar to some psychoactive drugs. The high pH and low PCO_2 leads to binding of calcium ions, and a fall in blood calcium; this may lead to muscle pain and muscle contractions—tetany—and even to fits. There is also an effect on enzymes that regulate sugar metabolism, leading to lactic acid production. At this point we have all the features of "behavioral (or psychogenic) hyperventilation", "panic attack", even the "fatigue syndrome". The victims of this behaviour often become panic-stricken due to the sensation that they "cannot breathe", ironic in that they are over-breathing, but the feeling is due to incomplete expiration, leading them to breathe at a higher and higher lung volume. This leads to an intense feeling of effort. The sufferers of this syndrome are often perfectionists, although some may be hysterical, or even manipulative; attacks may be provoked by such life stresses as bereavement. Often the condition is misdiagnosed as asthma or heart disease; to the anxiety associated with such labels is added the failure of treatment, leading to frustration and resentment. If symptoms are due to hyperventilation, they should be corrected by rebreathing into a plastic bag, which corrects the low PCO_2 within a few minutes.

Over-breathing is often consciously used by track athletes and swimmers, and dangerously by breath-hold divers, in the mistaken belief that they become charged with oxygen that will help them perform. The body is unable to store much oxygen, and the increase is in any case marginal. In the case of divers who over-breathe, oxygen in the lungs becomes depleted rapidly at depth, and before CO_2 has had any chance of building back up to the point that provides a drive to breathe; profound oxygen lack (hypoxia) follows, leading to unconsciousness and death. Death in uninjured swimmers and divers is almost always due to hyperventilation before immersion.

Mental activity, such as the performance of mental arithmetic, increases breathing, probably through nerve links between the higher (cortical) areas in the brain and the lower respiratory control centres. Many other body functions are linked to breathing through changes in metabolism and secretion of hormones, accounting for increases in breathing after meals and during the progesterone phase of the menstrual cycle, for example.

BREATHING CONTROL IN YOGA AND OTHER MEDITATIVE STATES

Conscious manipulation of breathing is an important part of Yoga and other meditative and even psychodynamic experiences. The techniques are in the most part easily understood in physiological terms, although often the results and benefits are explained in terms that a physiologist finds bizarre, mainly because they emphasize spiritual benefits established centuries ago in ayurvedic writings. One important concept in such schemes is that breathing is a rhythmic act and as such links to many other rhythms, both within the body (such as the rhythmic beating of the heart) and in the environment (daily, or diurnal, rhythms). At the extreme of the concept is the linkage of breathing to all the rhythms and vibrations (light, sound, radiation) that constitute "cosmic energy". In the yogic literature the act of breathing brings into the body the vital charge of *chee*, a Chinese word meaning "breath", "energy" and "air". Chee (energy) is distributed to the vital centers along lines of energy radiation: and chee (breath) moves the energy into the body. Sometimes, this concept is taken to the extreme, where the most important element associated with breathing is not oxygen or any other gas, but the negative charge in the atmosphere, equivalent to an electron. Modern science, in the absence of evidence, can make nothing of such concepts. Be that as it may, we can appreciate the effects of breathing and relaxation techniques, in conventional, physiological, terms. Throughout its history yogic breathing control has been seen as only one part of the philosophy, knowledge and practice that have as their ultimate goal a healthy life-style and self-awareness.

In various Yoga regimes, "pranayama" is an important component of meditation and other regularly practiced disciplines of living; its importance may be gauged by the fact that prana as well as meaning "breath", is also used for "life principle", "energy", and "cosmic electrical currents". Yama indicates "pause" and "control", and the principle of pranayama in its various types of breath control consists of a four-phase breathing cycle (in, pause, out, pause). Usually, there is a conscious effort to spend about twice as long in expiration as in inspiration. There is also emphasis on body position (cross-legged sitting, or horizontal), a quiet mind, and near-fasting state. Visualization and concentration are important components; the practitioner visualizes the oxygen drawn in with inspiration (the nourishing phase), the oxygenated blood moving to the tissues, and picking up carbon dioxide to return to the lungs and expelling it on expiration (the cleansing phase). These preconditions help to achieve a minimal metabolic state, with relaxed muscles and a low cardiac output (the cross-leg position virtually shuts down circulation to the lower body). During the training, there is an emphasis on diaphragmatic breathing, allowing the abdomen to relax outward, followed by rib cage expansion. Most forms of pranayama emphasize full expiration, with abdominal muscle contraction to achieve the smallest possible residual lung volume; physiologically this makes good sense because it minimizes the residual volume in the lungs so that the ensuing inspiration of fresh air is minimally changed; also it eases the load on the inspiratory muscles. Increased time of expiration also means that vagal influences dominate sympathetic effects— heart rate and blood pressure are lessened. Experienced yogis attain heart rates as low as 30 per minute. Emphasis is also placed on slow breathing, and most experienced subjects attain breathing rates of 2-3 per minute, compared to the usual rate of 8-12; slow breathing reduces the fluctuations in CO_2 with each breath, thus reducing chemoreceptor "drive". Regular practice has been shown to lead to a slow and efficient breathing pattern in all activities, a reduced CO_2 responsiveness, improved lung capacity and stronger respiratory muscles. Although the detailed respiratory pattern suggests that a lot of concentration and effort is required, the object is to adopt a breathing strategy that is satisfying, relaxed and effort-free. It then becomes possible for controlled, relaxed breathing to be adopted in stressful situations in daily life, inducing calmness and focused concentration.

Studies in asthma patients who have practiced pranayama, for as little as 15 minutes twice daily for two weeks, have shown reductions in airway reactivity (a laboratory test of airway irritability or "twitchiness"), reduced inhaler use and fewer symptoms compared to controls on regular treatment.

Among the variations of the basic pranayama, are a number of more advanced practices, which have been less well studied. Kumbhak is a type of very slow breathing with a period of breath holding at the end of inspiration that can last as long as half the total breathing cycle. A long end-inspiratory pause (apnea) may be associated with a greater reduction in oxygen consumption than a short pause. Bhastrika, or "bellows" breathing is a more explosive practice employing full inspiration and expiration, which may help to train respiratory muscles. Nadisuddhi, is a technique of breathing through alternate nostrils, with the other kept closed by gentle pressure from a thumb; this has its traditional basis in a concept that was close to that of the contrast between yin and yang; "breath is both positive and negative, that flowing into the right nostril is *hot*, and known as the sun breath; that through the left is *cold* and known as the moon breath". Whatever we may feel about this notion, the technique has been used successfully to improve concentration and visualization; theoretically, it provides an increased resistance to inspiration that may help to train inspiratory muscles.[3] Kapalabhati ("recharge breathing") employs high frequency breathing with forceful expiration through pursed lips; this type of

168

maneuver is quite different to other forms of pranayama in that the sympathetic system is stimulated, with increases in heart rate and blood pressure; an end-inspiratory breath-hold may be added. This type of breathing may help before meditation or physical exertion.

Many yogis are able to suspend breathing whilst practicing meditation for prolonged periods, and at first sight it may be difficult to see how they can breathhold for 15 minutes without any sign of distress. However, in deep trance states muscular activity is absent, heart rate is slowed and metabolism at a minimum. Carbon dioxide production falls to less than 30% of the usual resting value and distributed in a relatively large lung volume in an individual with a blunted carbon dioxide responsiveness; a combination of factors that reduce the need to breathe and allow the breath to be held for several times as long as normal.

Hyperventilation, overbreathing, has for centuries been known to lead to changes in the conscious state, and has been used as an aid in psychotherapy. Stanislav and Christina Grof at the Esalen Institute in California developed the technique, since known as "Grof breathing", as an aid in psychotherapy and for self-exploration. Short periods of fast deep breathing, together with music lead, in Fritjof Capra's words, to "surprisingly intense sensations, related to unconscious emotions and memories, [which] emerge and may trigger a wide range of revealing experiences". Capra, famed author of *The Tao of Physics*, saw parallels to experiences under the influence of psychedelic drugs, with the advantage that one remained in control, knowing that over-breathing could be stopped at will.

Finally, in a discussion of the importance of breathing control in the ancient Hatha Yoga disciplines, we should mention chanting. The

3   I am reminded of a story told by a present day respiratory guru, Dr Sol Permutt of Johns Hopkins—"a man comes to a scientist's workbench, sees a horseshoe nailed above it, and asks "My God, you don't believe in that do you?" To which the scientist replies "No, I certainly don't, but you don't have to believe in it, for it to work".

singing of deep resonant notes (such as the OM, or AUM, in Buddhist practice) requires great breathing control and training. The ancient sacred syllable resonates through all the body cavities, aiding meditation and prayer, or when used as a mantra.

Having established links between breathing, the brain, and the autonomic nervous system we are ready explore some more interactions between the mind and the body, obvious in human experience since the beginning of time, but until recently largely ignored in scientific medicine.

BREATHING AND THE IMMUNE SYSTEM

Interactions between nerves, chemical transmitters and the body's immune responses have been receiving increasing attention since the early 1990s. Not surprisingly, because the immune system is incredibly complex, these linkages have proved difficult to establish; some of the initial impetus for research were observations that chronic stress could predispose people to a variety of infectious illnesses.

As a junior doctor at St Mary's Hospital in London in the mid-1950s, the safe and effective use of sulphonamides and early antibiotics for the treatment of infections was a frequent topic of discussion at ward rounds. The need to "stimulate the phagocytes" became a joke phrase used by the consultant in patients with severe infections; a joke, because no one knew how to do it, and mainly it referred to supportive care. Later, I found out that the phrase was first used (in 1906) by a character in George Bernard Shaw's play, *The Doctor's Dilemma*; the character was Sir Colenso Ridgeon, and he was based on one of Shaw's friends, Sir Edward Almroth Wright. Almroth Wright had founded the Inoculation Department at St Mary's at the

turn of the century, and was still its director in 1945, when Alexander Fleming, a member of his department since 1907, was awarded the Nobel Prize for Medicine and was knighted himself. It seems that he deserved to be lampooned by Shaw; the Department's Director for over a half-century, he expected everyone to work a twelve-hour day, never employed a woman, even as a secretary (although he was always at pains to impress them!), considered male supporters of women's rights to be not masculine, and was insufferably pompous.[4] At tea time on the day when Fleming returned from his investiture by the King in Buckingham Palace, Wright studiously ignored him, and did not attend the evening's celebration (no doubt to everyone's relief). His overbearing behaviour earned him a few derogatory nicknames, including "Sir Almost Right" and "Sir Always Wrong". Before Fleming, However, at the time, Almroth Wright was St Mary's most famous medical scientist; he followed up the ideas of Metchnikoff on the body's responses to infection, by applying careful quantitative observations of white blood cells engulfing bacteria.

Ilia Ilyich Metchnikoff was a Russian pathologist, who in 1887 was surprisingly appointed the sub-director of Pasteur's Institute in Paris; he observed that white blood cells were attracted to sites of infection where they ingested the germs. He called the cells "phagocytes" from the Greek words for "eat" and "cells", thus providing the first model of cellular immunity. Almroth Wright's studies of the white cell response to bacteria led to a theory of chemicals

169

---

4 In his bafflingly titled book "Alethetropic Logic" are the following choice opinions—"Women belong to the logical underworld"; "Man is the prototype of the human species, woman the aberration"; "Women object to definitions. They don't consider it an advantage to know what they are talking about".

influencing their ability to take up bacteria; he called the proposed chemicals "opsonins" (from the Greek word "to prepare food"), and devised the "opsonic index" to measure the factors that influenced the number of bacteria taken up. Later, the theory was replaced by one that emphasized circulating antibodies, and the role of antigen-antibody reactions. Metchnikoff and Wright focused on the macrophages and granulocytes, or "polymorphs", in blood, known to be produced in the bone marrow. The function of blood lymphocytes, smaller and fewer in number, although known to originate in lymphoid tissue (lymph nodes scattered through the body, in the spleen and in patches of tissue in the lungs and gut), was not clearly understood until the work of the American paediatrician, Robert Good. He identified children subject to severe infections who lacked an immune response, and often had a congenital absence of the thymus gland, situated at the base of the neck. Later work showed that thymus-derived lymphocytes (T-lymphocytes) acted to coordinate the immune response, different groups of them having helper and suppressor effects on the growth and function of the B-lymphocytes (B for "bursa", a structure in birds where they were first identified); a final type of the T-cell has the capacity to kill "foreign" cells. It was also shown that lymphocytes derive from primitive cells in the bone marrow and later migrate to the thymus and lymphoid tissues, where they differentiate into their various types and develop their specific functions. As the role of the white blood cells became clearer, attention became focused on how they were produced and what controlled their ability to "recognize" harmful agents, antigens such as bacteria and viruses, and what allowed them to produce antibodies that acted to reduce their effects and help phagocytosis.

The brain has the capacity to influence the immune system through two main mechanisms—the autonomic nervous system and a variety of hormones whose production is influenced by the pituitary gland. Nerve endings produce chemicals known as neurotransmitters, including noradrenaline, which influence function of the target organ by activating enzymes to turn on chemical processes. During the past 20 years the nerve supply to lymphoid tissue has been recognized as important to the growth and function of lymphocytes; chemically specific nerve fibres have been identified and the mediators released interact with receptors on the surface of the lymphocytes to influence antibody production. Many animal experiments and clinical studies have shown how important the mediators released by nerves are to the whole process of inflammation. An intriguing example is afforded by patients with a paralyzed limb, who later develop joint inflammation (rheumatoid arthritis, RA); although this condition is usually characterized by a symmetrical inflammation of many small joints, the joints of the paralyzed limb often are not involved. The cause of RA is a lasting medical puzzle, but immune mechanisms involving interactions between T- and B-lymphocytes appear to cause an "autoimmune" process, whereby the body's immune system misidentifies parts of the body as "foreign". Mediators released by local nerve endings are just one part of the puzzle.

There are many conditions in which psychological factors appear to loom large, and a few, such as the irritable bowel syndrome and chronic fatigue syndrome, are considered by many physicians consider to be *caused* by them. Often, these conditions are termed psychogenic, but this label is not helpful. The simplistic designation changes a physician's approach to the patient from then on, leading them to dismiss symptoms that might otherwise be taken at face value and investigated. Furthermore, the psychogenic label can seldom be based on firm evidence, being made after other causes have been excluded, and without understanding the physiology underlying not non-specific symptoms of anxiety, fatigue and breathlessness. Many of these conditions show features of an immune disorder, such as susceptibility to infection, and an autonomic nervous system disorder—overactive gut, high heart rate, sweating and faintness. Hyperventilation— overbreathing—is also common. Assessing the autonomic nervous system is not rocket science, but is seldom part of the investigation, which is a pity, because at least it affords an explanation of symptoms that may be accessible to patients as part of their management.

Associations between psychological disturbances and many organic disorders involving immune mechanisms, such as asthma, ulcerative colitis and inflammatory skin disorders, may eventually be explained in terms of molecular biology, but the role of the autonomic nervous system, controlling smooth muscle contraction in the airways and gut and the micro-circulation, cannot be ignored. At that time the role that breath awareness and control may play in the management of such chronic and disabling illnesses will be ripe for research.

The interactions of nerves, hormones and the immune system have recently been clarified; the systems produce similar sets of chemicals that allow "communication" between them. Cells of the immune system produce a variety of peptides—small protein molecules that can diffuse in body fluids and attach to specific "receptors" on inflammatory cells to modify their growth and action. These molecules are called "cytokines" from the Greek words for "cells" and "movement". Sub-groups of cytokines have other names, such as "leukotrienes" (affecting white blood cells),

and "interferon" (a chemical produced by lymphocytes activated by viruses and other external agents). Receptors are chemicals on the outer cell surface membrane which have a structure that allows them to bind with molecules having a specific structure—the analogy is often made to a lock-and-key system. The structure of both the lock and the key ensure that only one key can open the lock; the analogy may be taken further because binding influences chemical reactions in the cell. Part of the receptor extends into the interior of the cell thereby "opening" it to outside influences. In the endocrine system, hormones such as cortisol act on cells by binding to receptors, and similarly "neurotransmitters" act on nervous tissue receptors, such as the "opioid" receptors in the brain. The first clues to the linkages between systems came from animal studies that showed hormonal and brain effects following administration of cytokines such as interferon. One of the effects suggested that the adrenocorticotrophic hormone (ACTH) was acting on the adrenal glands to produce cortisone; this effect was due to lymphocytes of the immune system producing a molecule that contained the chemical sequence for ACTH. The molecule also contained the sequence for a hormone called β-endorphin, that binds to opioid receptors in the brain to produce a pain-killing (analgesic) effect. In these and other ways the immune system produces chemicals that stimulate hormonal and analgesic effects. Then in the 1980s it was discovered that lymphocytes had ACTH receptors; thus, when the pituitary gland was stimulated to produce ACTH, lymphocytes were stimulated to grow. Furthermore, chemical transmitters released by nerves were shown to influence lymphocytes, helping to explain how the nervous responses to stress could also impair immune function. The chemical transmitters include adrenaline from the sympathetic nerves, and acetylcholine

171

from vagal nerve endings. It was found that lymphocytes, macrophages and other cells of the immune system contain receptors for acetylcholine, and that its release from the vagus helps to block inflammation and reduce shock.

Our new knowledge regarding chemical messengers and receptors has allowed scientists to construct and test hypotheses related to the neuro-immuno-hormonal interactions, which will doubtless eventually explain the health effects of many measures used in complementary medicine, such as yoga, massage, acupuncture, and the placebo effect. It remains to be seen if our views will change to the extent of considering the immune system as a "sixth sense", as some researchers, such as Dr Edwin Blalock of the University of Alabama, believe. Dr Blalock, a longtime researcher in this field, feels that the cells of the immune system continuously sample the circulation for infective agents like viruses and other toxic agents. The liberation of cytokines and neurotransmitters may then alert the central nervous system, allowing us to sense the presence of things that should not be in our "internal environment". At a more trivial level, we can begin to understand why influenza, for example, causes fatigue, muscle soreness and a decline in energy.

The links between breathing and the rest of the body are myriad, complex and based on well founded scientific evidence. Breathing is affected in all serious medical problems, but the other side of the coin is that controlled breathing contributes to healthy function of most systems, including the brain, autonomic nervous system and the immune system. Some of the beneficial effects of regular exercise may be mediated through the controlled increase in breathing that accompanies exertion, and contributes to the sense of well being so often described by runners. Siegfried Sassoon, in *Memoirs*

of an Infantry Officer relates his improbable elation experienced in World War I—"I've felt extraordinarily happy, even in the trenches … it's probably something to do with being in the open air so much, and getting a lot of exercise."

Breathing is susceptible to voluntary control to an extent that is far greater than any other essential body function. Controlled breathing is a feature of most alternative medicine techniques that employ meditation and visualization, in yoga and martial arts, as well as mainstream disciplines in treating conditions, including asthma and other respiratory complaints. It is helpful in so-called psychosomatic disorders, such as chronic fatigue syndrome, panic disorders and irritable bowel syndrome. In all these situations it has the added advantage of providing a way for the patient to exert a degree of control over their symptoms, with benefit to their quality of life.

CHAPTER 16

SLEEPING BREATHS

"How wonderful is Death,
Death and his brother Sleep!
One pale as the yonder pale and horned moon,
With lips of lurid blue,
The other glowing like the vital morn,
When throned on ocean's wave
It breathes over the world:
Yet both so passing strange and wonderful!"

Percy Bysshe Shelley, The Daemon of the world, 1820.

For centuries sleep was thought of as a necessary state, midway between waking activity and the total shutdown of all living functions. There was little change in this view until the advent of electroencephalography in the early 20th century, and still we know relatively little what causes its onset. We accept it as a periodic reduction in metabolism, activity and awareness. We thank our lucky stars that breathing goes on automatically, however deeply we sleep; in a very few of us this automatic control is absent, leading to a number of serious effects including heart failure. That's not to say that we breathe as perfectly in sleep as when we merely rest in the awake state; probably all of us breathe quite noisily when asleep, and many of us snore loudly enough to make the windows rattle (intensities of 100 decibels have been recorded!), or at least cause our bed-partner to give us a swift kick.

Up to 30 or 40 years ago, no one took much notice of snoring and breathing was always assumed to be perfectly regulated in sleep. The source of all knowledge regarding breathing, the American Physiology Society's Handbook on Respiration Physiology, published in 1965

contained only a few lines on breathing in sleep (in a chapter devoted to anaesthesia). Then, within a few years this all changed, with many books and journals devoted to the subject, and disordered nocturnal breathing was recognized as common and clinically important. Nowadays, any general hospital worth its salt will have a sleep clinic and laboratory, run by a physician who is kept very busy doing nothing else. Actually it's quite hard to know what set off this train of events. Possibly, it was the recognition in 1965, by Gastaut, Tussinari and Duron, that patients with the "Pickwickian Syndrome" showed many episodes of breathing cessation (apneas) during sleep.

Sir William Osler, the most famous physician of the late 19th and early 20th centuries, wrote the first edition of his classic textbook *The Principles of Medicine* in 1892; in the 8th edition of 1918 he refers to a syndrome of obesity and excessive daytime sleepiness.[1] A character in Charles Dickens' *The Posthumous Papers of*

---

1   Sir William Osler (1849-1919) was brought up in Dundas, a small town close to Hamilton, Ontario; he was a medical student in nearby Toronto, and after faculty positions at McGill and Philadelphia, in 1889 became the first Professor of Medicine at Johns Hopkins University in Baltimore and first Chief of Medicine at the University Hospital. Soon after, he took just a year to write the hugely successful *Principles*—a book of over 1000 pages, published in 1892. In 1905 he was invited to become Regius Professor of Physic at the University of Oxford, where he remained until his death in 1919. Many medical institutions have been named after him, especially in Canada. He was a prolific source of aphorisms, of which my favorite is "The physician without physiology and chemistry flounders along in an aimless fashion, never able to gain any accurate conception of disease, practicing a sort of popgun pharmacy".

the *Pickwick Club*, Mr Weller's son Joe, was extremely fat and often fell asleep during the day as he ran errands or did odd jobs; Dickens refers to him as the "fat boy", and provides many instances of his day time somnolence. Osler found this description fitted patients that he had seen, and being of a literary bent (this is probably an understatement), he wrote two sentences about them—"A remarkable phenomenon associated with excessive fat is an uncontrollable tendency to sleep—like the fat boy in Pickwick. It is probable that this narcolepsy is a manifestation of disturbed pituitary function." Thus, he named the syndrome after the book; not after Mr Pickwick or his fellow club members ("Pickwickians"), who were neither fatter nor sleepier than other well off Londoners of their time. It is remarkable that such a brief note was picked up much later (1956), and the term "Pickwickian Syndrome" was used to denote obese, somnolent patients who breathed less than they should (they were hypercapnic, with elevated blood carbon dioxide levels), and had a bluish complexion due to low blood oxygen and high levels of hemoglobin. Although obese, they had normal lungs but often showed evidence of heart disease, with high blood pressure and heart failure. Henri Gastaut and his colleagues, from the French Institut National de la Santé et de la Recherche Médicale (INSERM) investigated their patients with "le syndrome de Pickwick" from a new standpoint; they shifted the focus from the heart and lungs to what was happening during sleep, and found that they experienced numerous episodes when breathing ceased (apnea). The breathing pauses led to severe decreases in arterial O_2, disturbing sleep and accounting for the increased sleepiness during the day.[2] We're not talking here about having a snooze after dinner; there is an overwhelming and irresistible desire to sleep; patients fall asleep in the outpatient clinic, whilst driving, and even when holding a Royal Flush at poker.

SLEEP PHYSIOLOGY AND BRAINWAVES

Patients with daytime somnolence began to be investigated in sleep studies, and a huge Pandora's Box was opened. Sleep induced apnea was found to be common, not necessarily associated with obesity, and the sufferers might show no abnormality when seen in the day. Snoring suddenly became as important to physicians as it was to the other occupants of the snorer's household. The Sleep Disorders Clinic was born.

Sleep studies are now more-or-less routine; obviously, they involve observation and measurements made during the night, although sleep during the day (so-called nap studies) may yield sufficient information. At their simplest, the studies involve observation of the subject, with recordings of heart rate and the saturation of hemoglobin with oxygen (using an oximeter which measures the absorption of light wave lengths appropriate to reduced and oxygenated hemoglobin through the skin). However, our present understanding of breathing, and its cessation, during sleep was obtained in studies that additionally included recordings of brain waves with skin electrodes (electroencephalography, EEG), movements of the chest, contraction of eye and throat muscles, sensors for air flow and CO_2 pressure at the nose, and blood pressure. The process is called polysomnography (multiple recordings in sleep).

2   In their report at a séance of the Société Française de Neurologie they presented their studies in one patient whose arterial oxygen saturation fell to as low as 65% during apnea, equivalent to being flown up to the top of Everest.

The change in thinking that identified sleep as an entirely separate state from that of complete relaxation in the awake state began with the work of the German psychiatrist Hans Berger who, unlike his compatriot Hans Krebs, did not win a deserved Nobel Prize because of the Third Reich. Born in 1873, he decided to study psychiatry after receiving a telegram sent by his sister, who had a premonition that he was in danger. Berger was in the army, and unknown to his sister had slipped down an embankment on his horse, a potentially dangerous accident; from then on, extra-sensory perception was an abiding interest for him. Berger received his doctorate in 1897 at the University of Jena, where he remained for the rest of his life. He became interested in the hypothetical problem of "psychical energy", in which the brain was thought to greatly increase its metabolism in various forms of mania. Berger came across the work of a Liverpool physician, Richard Caton, who in 1875 had managed to record electrical currents in the exposed brains of rabbits and monkeys, noting that alterations in activity occurred when limbs moved or when the animals were exposed to a bright light. This was a remarkable achievement as the currents were tiny and the measurement of small voltages was crude, in the order on thousandths of a volt. This fact makes Berger's achievements even more remarkable because "he was completely ignorant of the technical and physical basis of his method"—a comment by Dr William Grey Walter, a British neurologist who accepted his work, unlike his compatriots who considered him a crank. In the 1920s, Berger began by recording brain electrical activity from the exposed brain of patients undergoing brain surgery, and then systematically studied normal subjects—initially himself and his son—using silver wires inserted in the scalp. With technical improvements recordings were obtained from silver foil electrodes stuck on to the scalp,

enabling Berger to collect a vast amount of data. In brief, he showed that several brain wave patterns could be distinguished. The normal resting, eyes closed, rhythm he termed alpha waves, at 8-12 cycles/sec (Hz); on opening the eyes alpha waves were replaced by more frequent, less regular beta waves at 15-30 Hz; this change also occurred if the subject undertook mental tasks or was subjected to noise and painful stimuli. The leading British neurophysiologist of the time, Edgar Douglas Adrian (winner of the 1932 Nobel Prize), accepted Berger's work and confirmed it with the use of the cathode ray oscilloscope in the mid-1930s. Berger's pioneering work led to new concepts of brain function, which after some 50 years of technical and physiological progress, were applied to the sleeping state.

BREATHING AND SLEEP STAGE

During sleep, brain activity changes, and brain waves become progressively slower as it becomes progressively more difficult to rouse the subject—this is often divided into four stages, with stage IV being deep slow wave sleep, but each stage merges indistinctly into the next. Breathing becomes less, by about 10%, but normally any pauses are short and the CO_2 pressure hardly rises; the reduction in breathing is related to a reduction in the central drive to ventilation, associated with changes in brain activity.

A leading Canadian researcher, Dr John Remmers of the University of Calgary, was one of the first to investigate "accessory" muscles of breathing in the neck, whilst working at the University of Texas in Galveston in the early 1970s. He found that in the awake state, the muscles of the throat and larynx contract in phase with breathing; the larynx opens and other muscles act to stiffen and open the otherwise floppy tissue of the upper airway. With deepening sleep the central drive to these muscles lessens and the upper airway may be drawn in by the negative pressure to cause vibration, heard as snoring, and eventually closure (apnea). These effects, due to inhibition of the muscles of the upper airway, are more likely to cause apnea if the airway is narrowed by an anatomical, or structural reason. Thus, obese individuals with fat deposits in the neck, children with large adenoids and tonsils, and patients with less common obstructive conditions, are all at risk for sleep apneas.

Added to deepening slow wave sleep are episodes in which the brain becomes more active, and we experience the dreams that are most remembered later; the eyes are seen to move under their lids, leading to the term *rapid eye movement*, or REM sleep. The episodes last about 30 minutes and occur about four times a night, and during these times there is a virtual paralysis of all muscles, including the intercostals muscles, but excepting (luckily) the diaphragm; sometimes the paralysis is interrupted by muscle jerking (this is especially common in dogs, as any dog lover knows). In REM sleep breathing becomes irregular, perhaps because of all the other activity going on in the brain. Because of the paralysis of upper airway muscles, the upper airway narrows and if the diaphragm is weak, as it may be in the elderly, breathing may fall off and some reduction in blood oxygen may occur. Bearing these facts in mind, it comes as no surprise that patients with muscle disorders such as amyotrophic lateral sclerosis (ALS, or Lou Gehrig's disease), or obstructions in the upper airway such as large tonsils and adenoids, may experience serious reductions in breathing at night.

On this background of "normal" sleep, we can return to the "Pickwickians", who were found to have numerous episodes in which breathing stops and blood oxygen saturation plummets, the so-called sleep apnea syndromes. By far the majority suffer from obstruction of the upper airway—they have *obstructive sleep apnea*. In a minority, the problem is related to a disorder of the central brain drive to breathing—*central sleep apnea*; and, not surprisingly, mixed central and obstructive apneas may be seen.

In obstructive sleep apnea, airflow at the mouth is greatly reduced or stops, but there is continued contraction of the diaphragm, which becomes increasingly violent with successive contractions; arterial oxygen saturation (SaO_2) falls progressively and may reach very low levels; finally, the diaphragmatic contractions overcome the airway obstruction, usually with an explosive snore, and the subject often wakes up. The episodes, of snoring, followed by silence and a final convulsive snore or gasp, last up to a minute and may occur several times an hour.

As everybody's pharyngeal muscles become inactive in REM sleep, this is only part of the problem, and usually there are additional causes for narrowing of the airway. In obese individuals it is the fat deposits surrounding the airway in the neck: sleep apnea becomes increasingly common in people having a neck circumference of over 45 cm. In others it may be due to a number of causes, from an underset jaw to large tonsils. Any narrowing of the upper airway means that during inspiration a negative pressure is developed just below the narrowing, becoming much lower than the pressure surrounding the neck and leading to narrowing of the floppy segment in the pharynx; the pressure fluctuates and leads to vibration. The ensuing snoring becomes progressively louder, and the pressure in the airway may be as much as 100 cm of water less than the atmosphere when the airway closes off completely. Falling SaO_2 and increasing PCO_2 cause increasing ventilatory drive and effort, and the final attempt to breathe may be accompanied by strong contraction of other muscles, which can throw the sufferer to the floor or lead to injury of the bed partner—by the time a doctor's opinion is sought, the couple is seldom sleeping together.

The effects of obstructive sleep apnea are often severe. Obviously, snoring and disturbed sleep, and excessive daytime sleepiness (hypersomnolence) may cause functional problems in the family and at work—or school, because children are not immune from the condition. Other effects have their basis in the physics of airway obstruction and closure and in the integrated physiology of cardiorespiratory function. The consequences in terms of physics relate to the progressive lowering of pressure in the chest, as the respiratory muscles struggle to overcome the obstruction; this means that the heart muscle has to generate an additional tension (equal to the negative pressure surrounding the heart) in order to continue to maintain an adequate blood supply to the brain and other essential organs. Blood pressure usually drops during apnea, but there is then an overshoot, with blood pressure rising greatly; the chain of events places a great strain on heart muscle, with bad results for anyone who also has coronary artery disease. Then there are the effects of severe falls in blood oxygen saturation, which include increases in heart rate and blood pressure and stimulation of stress hormones. Over a long time, the frequent episodes of increasing CO_2 and decreasing O_2 pressure lead to a depression of the normal breathing control mechanisms, adding a "central" component to the obstructive apnea. Chronic sufferers frequently have large hearts and retain fluid, leading to a diagnosis of heart failure. This is reason enough to investigate snorers experiencing fragmented sleep, but more importantly, to prevent other outcomes that are more common in those suffering from obstructive sleep apnea. These include heart attacks and stroke, both three times as common, and automobile accidents, where the rates are also much higher.

Treatment of obstructive sleep apnea is aimed at removing or reducing the obstruction in the upper airway; this may require surgery to remove tonsils or other sources of obstruction. Sometimes weight reduction is effective, though difficult to achieve in patients who are morbidly obese; because alcohol, smoking and drugs may predispose patients to apnea, it is helpful to wean them off these.

Colin Sullivan, an Australian whose career interest in sleep apnea began when working in Toronto with Eliot Phillipson, had the imaginative idea of using positive pressure at the mouth to prevent collapse of the upper airway. This may be achieved by a blower attached to a closely fitting mask over the nose and mouth. In 1980 he applied the method in a patient with severe obstructive sleep apnea, and observed reversal of the upper airway closure with a gratifying improvement in sleep quality. To his surprise, he found that the required pressure was easily found, thus allowing the "prescription" of pressure for an individual patient. Continuous positive airway pressure (CPAP) has revolutionized the management of obstructive sleep apnea. Before its introduction the only sure way to cure the condition was to surgically bypass the obstruction via a hole in the windpipe (tracheostomy). Long term follow-up studies demonstrated a dramatic improvement in the 5-year mortality, from about 10% to zero.

"CENTRAL" SLEEP-DISORDERED BREATHING

Central sleep apnea, in its pure form, is much rarer than the obstructive type; in such cases there is a reduction of airflow without any evidence of the diaphragm responding, and there is a loss of the normal respiratory rhythm control. As we've mentioned, there is some reduction in breathing during deep sleep, and this is normally of no consequence. However, there are a number of rare genetic disorders in which the automatic control of breathing is severely impaired, such as the condition known as "Ondine's curse" , described in Chapter 4. Sometimes central breathing depression may occur in patients with long-standing obstructive apnea, perhaps due to fatigue of the diaphragm or to the effects of severe lack of oxygen to the brain, an effect that also occurs at altitude.

Several family studies have shown that sleep apnea has a familial incidence. This might be expected from the familial incidence of obesity and of different facial structures. However, these other factors do not seem to explain the familial incidence entirely. A familial association between sleep apnea and the Sudden Infant Death Syndrome (SIDS) raises the possibility of a gene that controls sleep arousal, and aspects of breathing control also show familial clustering. Such findings have stimulated interest in the genetics of sleep apnea, but we are a long way from finding an apnea gene.

DISORDERED BREATHING DURING SLEEP COMPLICATING OTHER CONDITIONS

In the early 19th century, the eminent Irish physician John Cheyne described a patient in whom periodic breathing during sleep was prominent. In *The Dublin Hospital Reports* of 1818 he presented "A case of apoplexy, in which the fleshy part of the heart was converted into fat"; "the only peculiarity…was in the state of respiration…it would entirely cease for a quarter of a minute, then it would become perceptible, though very low, then by degrees it became heaving and quick, and then it would cease again". Almost 30 years later, in 1846, Cheyne's compatriot William Stokes reported in the *Dublin Quarterly Journal of Medical Science* that he had seen a patient with an identical phasic breathing, and ever since the pattern has been known as Cheyne-Stokes breathing. The diagnosis in Dr Stokes' patient was the same—"a case of weakened and probably fatty heart", and the clinical situations in which periodic breathing is prominent have been mainly associated with heart failure and poor circulation to the brain, but also in kidney and liver failure. Physiologists have always been intrigued by the condition because breathing is actually *increased* when assessed over several minutes—that is, the level of CO_2 in the blood is lower, rather than higher. A slowing of the circulation is thought to play a large role in its causation—depression of breathing leads to a rise in CO_2, but this takes time to reach the respiratory centre; the stimulus to breathing then reduces CO_2 but again lags in the signal lead to an overshoot, and the resulting low CO_2 inhibits breathing, leading to the abnormal cycling or "hunting" behaviour. However, it also seems clear that reductions in oxygen supply to the brain play an important role.

In the late 19th century the Italian altitude physiologist Angelo Mosso observed typical Cheyne-Stokes breathing at altitude, and in 1909 the famous Oxford physiologists John Scott Haldane and Claude Douglas noted that it was promptly abolished by administering oxygen. At altitudes of over 4000 m, where periodic breathing during sleep is common, arterial oxygen content in the awake state is only 80% of sea level values; during sleep O_2 saturation drops further to around 70%; interestingly there are also fluctuations in heart rate that have the same periodicity as breathing. Douglas and Haldane argued that the combination of low O_2 (a stimulus to breathing) and CO_2 (depressing breathing) led to instability of the brain stem central controller of breathing, and drew an engineering analogy—"It is evidently a phenomenon analogous to the hunting often produced by the governor of an engine; and what is remarkable is not that it should occur, but that its occurrence should be so unusual under normal conditions". This is unlikely to be the last word on this intriguing problem.

Sleep apnea may complicate other illnesses: Cheyne Stokes breathing occurs in patients with heart disease and strokes. Patients with chronic obstructive pulmonary disease (Chapter 19) and asthma may experience worsening of their breathing at night, because of the combined effects of compromised lung function and the changes occurring during sleep. Such patients can experience severe falls in oxygen saturation in arterial blood, which may be helped by CPAP.

Considering that we spend a third of our life sleeping, it remains a puzzling, if absolutely necessary state, and one that we seem unlikely to understand completely. We know that during sleep many brain functions become completely reorganized, including memory and mechanisms that coordinate and control the autonomic nervous system. What happens to the complex interactions between the brain and systems that regulate respiration and circulation, when they are faced with reductions in oxygen supply, remains something that will continue to intrigue the dwindling group of clinical physiologists for a long time to come.

CHAPTER 17

THE SINGING BREATH

"...after severally swelling a note, in which each manifested the power of the lungs, and tried to rival the other in brilliancy and force...while the audience eagerly awaited the event, that both seemed to be exhausted; and, in fact, the trumpeter, wholly spent gave it up...when Farinelli, with a smile...broke out in the same breath, with fresh vigour, and not only swelled and shook the note, but ran the most rapid and difficult divisions..."

Dr Charles Burney, recounting a duet between a trumpet and the castrato Farinelli in 1720.

The human voice has been described as the oldest and most sublime musical instrument. Yet another aspect of breathing whose origin has been lost in time, interest began to be shown in voice production once opera became an important form of entertainment in about the 16th century. A wonderfully detailed description of the larynx and its muscles appears in *De voci auditusque organis historia anatomica* of Giulio Casserio, published in 1601. Casserio was a student of Fabricius in Padua, and he succeeded him as professor of anatomy; the quality of his dissections and illustrations rival those of Vesalius, and in his use of copper plate engravings (Vesalius used woodcuts) he set a standard that was unsurpassed for a century. Casserio's work had been preceded by similar anatomical studies by Bartolomeo Eustachio, a contemporary of Vesalius but who worked in a clerical institution in Rome in the 1560s and 70s. Eustachio (eponymous discoverer of

the Eustachian tube, connecting the middle ear with the pharynx) did not publish his work, and it was not until the early 18th century that his engravings were rediscovered and published by the physician to Pope Clement XI, Lancisi. However, whilst the anatomy of the vocal organs had been well described in the 17th century, more than a century was to pass before there was any notion of how they functioned. Such understanding had to wait for instruments that allowed the vocal cords to be seen, advances in the physics of sound production, and modern concepts of lung function. It turned out that the singing voice was more than any musical instrument. The sound is produced by the vocal cords which are capable of changing their length and tension; the tube at the upper end of the windpipe (glottis) is also variable in volume and tension, and the driving pressure in the sub-glottal space is generated by the muscles of breathing. Finally there is resonance produced by various cavities in the body which are capable of adding huge richness to the sound.

THE ANATOMY AND PHYSIOLOGY OF THE UPPER AIRWAYS IN SINGING

By the 18th century, operas, oratorios and recitals had become very popular, and there was great interest in voice production. Because women were still excluded from church singing, it was the time of greatest popularity for the castrati. The combination of a mature lung capacity and immature vocal organ made for prodigious vocal gymnastics, typified by sustained high notes. The greatest of the castrati, Farinelli (Carlo Boschi) took London audiences by storm in 1734; it was said that the orchestra were so overcome by the brilliance of his singing.

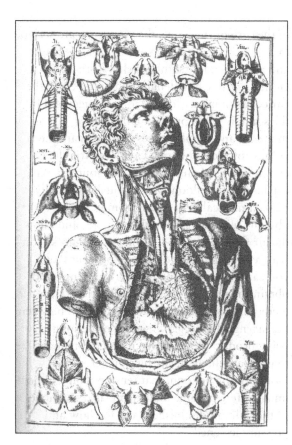

Figure 41 Casserio's 1601 dissection of the vocal organs.

His voice was described by Johann Quantz, flute teacher to Frederick the Great, as "a penetrating, full, rich, bright and well modulated soprano… His intonation was pure, his trill beautiful, his breath-control extraordinary, and his throat very agile". In terms of breathing capacity, it was said that he was capable of maintaining a high C for a full two minutes. The present day pulmonary physiologist (and singer) Don Proctor has calculated that this feat required a vital capacity of at least six litres, combined with the ability to constrain and control airflow to 50 ml/sec— extraordinary breath-control indeed! Farinelli spent two years in London, and then was lured to Spain by the Italian wife of Philip V, Elisabetta Farnese, who hoped that the singer might be able to lift the King from his deep depression. Although her wish was fulfilled, Farinelli spent the next decade singing the four arias that were the only ones the King wished to hear, every evening, thereby performing a miracle of complementary medicine.

The eighteenth and nineteenth centuries saw many singing teachers rise to eminence through many extraordinary techniques of vocal training, built more on experience than any theoretical knowledge of sound production. Then, in 1885, Manuel Garcia reported to the Royal Society that with an arrangement of mirrors he had been able to shine a light into the larynx and view the action of his own vocal cords—the birth of modern laryngoscopy. Garcia was said to be the ablest singing teacher of the century, and Professor of Singing at London's Royal Academy of Music. He described the wide adduction of the vocal cords during inspiration, and the action of the tiny muscles acting on two small angled cartilages (the arytenoids) attached to the rear part of the cords in order to bring them close and precisely together and generate the vibration that is the source of sound. The science of singing gradually grew, especially with the introduction of devices capable of measuring sound wave amplitude and frequency. The concept of resonance and resonant frequencies paved the way for theories of sound production. Sound is produced by expired air passing through the glottis, the space between the vocal cords or folds, forcing them apart, with their elasticity and the tension exerted by laryngeal muscles pulling them back, to set up vibration. Resonance is set up in the short tube above the vocal cords, and amplified by resonance in the vocal cavity. The frequency is determined by the mechanical characteristics of the cords and their tension; the muscles controlling tension govern the pitch. The vocal cavity acts as a tube whose volume can be varied to provide different resonances and sounds; X-rays of vocal cavity revealed that there were characteristic shapes associated with particular sounds. Early on it was found that the vowel sounds were each associated with a pair of peaks in their frequency ranges, or spectra, and in 1924 Sir Richard Paget succeeded in making models of the larynx in plasticine that when connected to an air source, produced the pure vowel sounds. More recently, sound production has been taken further by the work of scientists interested in voice production; the Australian astrophysicist Ian Johnston has provided an eminently readable book, *Measured Tones,*(1989), in which he provides a readable account of the physics of sound production by musical instruments. He recognizes the brilliant but simple studies of pendulums and vibrating strings made by Galileo Galilei provided the scientific foundation for this understanding. The revolutionary ideas for which Galileo was placed under lifetime house arrest by the Inquisition, impacted this and many other topics related to breathing. As for the physiology of singing, Donald F. Proctor, Professor of Otolaryngology at the Johns Hopkins School of Medicine, culminated a long and distinguished career with *Breathing, Speech and Song* (1980). Dr Proctor worked closely with Dr Jere Mead and Dr Arend Bouhuys in research that combined respiratory physiology and voice production, and forms the basis of current knowledge in the field.

The singing voice is a unique instrument, which makes the description of its physiology impossible, at least when it comes to finding suitable analogies. The sound is produced by a vibrating valve producing resonance in a cylinder; this suggests some similarity to a wind instrument, such as the clarinet. But the reed of a clarinet has fixed properties and its cylinder is of fixed length and volume (although both are effectively varied by the holes in the instrument);

in the case of the voice, the vibrations are set up in the vocal cords, which are of variable length and tension, and the tube is short—the *supra-glottal space*, whose length and volume may be varied. An analogy to the violin is suggested by the sounding box providing resonance, just as the vocal and nasal cavities do, but again the volume of the resonating cavity is variable. A commonly used analogy is to the sound making-capacity of a balloon, but no one has actually made a musical instrument from it, for fairly obvious reasons. If you fill a balloon and allow the air to escape whilst pulling on the neck, you will get a sound but it is soon apparent that you cannot produce precise enough tension to obtain the note you want—a reflection of the incredible coordination that is going on between the laryngeal muscles when a specific sound is being produced. Also, even if you did manage to generate the requisite tension across the mouth of the balloon, that tension would almost immediately become inadequate as the volume of the balloon diminished, and the flow and pressure lessened.

The most remarkable differences between the voice and mechanical instruments lie in the degree of flexibility in all aspects of voice production. The length, tension and shape of the vocal folds (or cords) are all independently variable; the driving pressure that initiates their vibration is infinitely variable; the length and volume of the supraglottic tube are variable; and the volume and shape of the resonating chambers which amplify the harmonic frequencies can also be varied. Finally the feedback nerve linkage between the heard sound and the muscles that generate it is uniquely capable of modulating all these functions within a split second. All of which brings us to the conclusion that we actually are a long way from "finally" understanding what is going on as we listen to the *liebestod* in Wagner's *Tristan und Isolde*.

We may reflect on the remarkable ability of professional singers to produce a given note just by thinking of it; there is no preceding tuning needed, such as with a violin. The ability rests on the remarkable biofeedback between the heard sound (perception) and the neural pattern in the brain cortex that provides the "central command" to the muscles of the larynx (vocal cords), supra-glottal space, pharynx and vocal cavity, and the muscles of breathing (air pump). Just by thinking of the sound to be produced, the singer is able to control the breath, contract the required small muscles of the larynx to open and tense the vocal cords, adjust the length of the supra-glottal space by dropping or lifting the Adam's apple, and modify the volume of the vocal cavity and mouth to obtain the resonance that determines the timbre of the voice. Each note represents the compound effect of the resonant chambers acting on the fundamental tone and overtones produced in the larynx, in order to amplify the specific harmonics required for the given sound. Broadly speaking, different vowel sounds are produced by variations in the volume of the supra-glottic air column, and consonants are formed by changing the shape of the mouth cavity and lips. How all this is unconsciously accomplished remains a mystery, but there is no doubt that training, by repeatedly linking the perceived sound to the brain's motor cortex, is required for its full development. The process is similar to the training that a piano player, or a tennis player for that matter, has to undergo to achieve high performance.

THE LUNGS AND THORAX IN SINGING

As the sound is generated in the larynx, the energy required to produce a note of a given loudness depends on the pressure difference across the vocal folds, and thus on the *sub-glottic pressure*. As we saw when considering the

factors that influence breathing capacity, most of us can generate a very large pressure in the lungs (at least 100 cm H_2O) if we take a deep breath, close the glottis and strain to breathe out; the pressure is much larger than is used to produce a loud, high note (about 40 cm H_2O). The sub-glottic pressure is a function of the inward recoil of the lungs and chest wall, and the expiratory, mainly abdominal, muscles. The recoil pressure depends on how deep the preceding inspiration has been, and possibly how heavy the chest wall is—there may be a reason for the bulk of the chest in the traditional Wagnerian performer, helping to generate loud and long-sustained notes. However, more important than power, is the ability to control it.

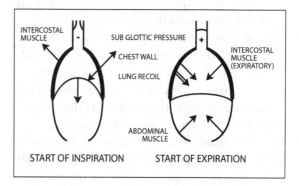

Figure 42 The factors contributing to sub-glottic pressure during singing.

Both the subglottic pressure and the airflow through the larynx during singing are controlled by the respiratory muscles. Much is made of the importance of diaphragmatic (as opposed to abdominal) breathing, but I suspect there is confusion about the differences between the two, and their effect on voice production. Let's be quite clear then, that the diaphragm is the inspiratory muscle, and the abdominals are the main expiratory muscles; to obtain the greatest inspiration the diaphragm has to be fully contracted and the abdominals relaxed. The reason you cannot run and sing at the

183

same time (other than in a chant "in step")
is that the abdominals also have to stabilize
the trunk to allow the legs to work effectively.
The intercostal muscles help in both phases of
breathing, although the way they act to control
the flow of air and the sub-glottic pressure is not
obvious at first sight.

Don Proctor, Harvard laryngologist, respiratory
physiologist and singer, has used his multiple
talents to research what goes on physiologically
during singing; in his book is a picture of
an antique harpsichord inscribed with the
motivating observation *sine scientia ars nihil
est*. Whilst accepting that *vice versa* is equally
as valid, Proctor and his colleagues Jere Mead
and Arend Bouhuys have applied state-of-the-art
scientia to illuminate the *ars* of singing. They
measured air flow and volume (by sitting in a
box called a body plethysmograph), partitioned
volume into chest and abdomen components
(through sensors applied to the skin), measuring
pressure in the chest (by swallowing thin tubes
with small balloons at the end), recording
electrical signals from respiratory muscles, and
taking cine-radiographs of the vocal cavities. All
these observations provide relevant information
regarding the breathing components of
sound production. It may sound extremely
uncomfortable and not conducive to relaxed
singing, but the techniques are routinely used to
assess function in chest disorders.

Although sound is produced in expiration, let's
first review what happens in inspiration.
Normally, if we are not exerting ourselves, we
breathe in through the nose, but the air passage is
narrow and also "floppy", tending to narrow if
we want to inspire rapidly. Usually then, the
breath is taken in through the open mouth, which
is only a tenth as resistant as the nose. A full
inspiration (a vital capacity breath) may then be
taken in, in less than a second. Full expansion

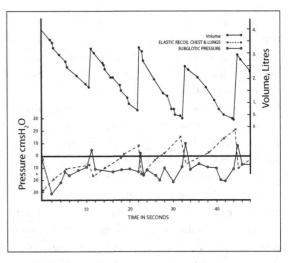

Figure 43 Don Proctor's recordings of the changes
in volume, elastic recoil pressure and sub-glottic
pressure during his singing of a Schubert song.

of the chest involves a full contraction of the
diaphragm, raising the ribs with the help of the
inspiratory intercostals and neck muscles, and
relaxation of abdominal muscles, allowing the
abdominal contents to descend and the abdominal
wall to protrude. Of course, a full inspiration may
not be needed, in which case it is better to limit
the abdominal movement than the chest
expansion. This is because sound production
requires pressure to be developed; recruiting the
elastic recoil of the lung and chest wall is the most
comfortable way to do this. If the chest is not
fully expanded, the subsequent expiration has to
be accomplished by contraction of the abdominal
muscles, and they have to do this against the
weight of the abdominal contents.

The role of the elastic recoil provided by the
lungs and chest wall cannot be overemphasized.
If you take a deep breath in and then relax,
three-quarters of the air is exhaled at a rate that
cannot be exceeded by forcibly breathing out.
Also the recoil pressure, and thus the maximum
achievable subglottic pressure, is not related to
the size of the lungs, which perhaps explains why

184

singers do not have larger lungs than their less vocal peers—although to achieve the sustained note of a Farinelli you do need large lungs.

Sound is produced during expiration, and if a long-sustained note is needed the flow through the larynx is constant. The larynx is partially closed in a precisely formed shape; as air passes through the cords tend to open, but also a negative pressure is generated just outside the cords—ie. on the mouth side rather than the lung side of the cords. This effect of a jet of air was first described by the eighteenth century physicist, Daniel Bernouilli. In everyday experience, the Bernouilli effect is what causes the shower curtain to annoyingly billow in on you; the jet of water produces a slight negative pressure to do this. The tiny fluctuations in positive and negative pressures across the vocal fold are what cause them to vibrate and generate the note. Although airflow is constant for a given note, it is the pressures that need to be kept constant throughout the production of the sound; this is not as easy as one might think. As I pointed out above, if you breathe in fully and then relax, most of the air will come out in less than a second; a brake has to be applied to control the flow initially. This braking effect during expiration is supplied by the <u>inspiratory</u> intercostal muscles; the abdominal muscles cannot provide it, and Proctor and his colleagues showed that the diaphragm behaves completely passively during expiration. Again, we have to consider the pressure available in the lungs to maintain a constant sound; at first there is too much pressure available, needing a brake to be applied; then as the note continues and lung volume falls, the elastic recoil is gradually lost, the inspiratory intercostals relax, and the abdominal muscles are more and more brought into action, together with the expiratory intercostals. Fine control of the abdominal muscles, during both inspiration and expiration is a *sine qua non* of the operatic singer, and is achieved through

repetitive training. During inspiration, abdominal contraction controls the position of the abdominal contents, indirectly the length of the diaphragm. If the abdominal contents are high, the diaphragm is long, and is able to lift the lower ribs and expand the chest effectively. During expiration abdominal mūscels help to control the reduction in chest volume, maximizing the effect of elastic recoil. Don Proctor observed that the inward movement of the abdomen during a sustained note comes with "a sense of absolutely effortless swelling or continuity of tone". The steady flow of air and constant subglottic pressure is now seen as an extremely complex, coordinated activity carried on by the brain, automatically if not unconsciously.

It has been shown that a given tone can be produced with a variety of expired flows and pressures, but in terms of comfort and efficiency only one combination is appropriate for a given singer. The combination is learnt, on the basis of the heard tone and the perceived effort required to produce it, and generally, it includes the lowest flow compatible with the pitch and intensity of the sound.

Having considered what is required for a sustained note, we may also observe what happens during shorter sung phrases. Within the lung's vital capacity (VC), most of the time is spent at around 50% VC, with variation from 20-80%; a full inspiration is required relatively rarely, but clearly this depends on what is being sung. Operating in this range of VC helps the singer to interrupt singing for the shortest possible time, in order to take a breath. Loud tones—requiring high pressures in the chest— are achieved with deeper breaths and greater abdominal muscle contraction, especially once the lung volume has fallen to below the point at which elastic recoil has disappeared (below functional residual capacity, FRC). From there to complete expiration (residual volume, RV) the expiratory muscles are working hard and adequate flow becomes impossible to achieve because of airway narrowing. Sometimes the view is expressed that "singers are taught to breathe in by bringing their bellies out"; the physiological studies of Proctor and Mead have shown that a strategy of "belly still" proceeding to "belly out" after adequate chest expansion has occurred, is more efficient.

My own singing is lamentably coarse; this description takes in both the quality of my voice and the fact that the only time it was regularly used was on coaches transporting the rugby team home, an environment singularly lacking any acoustical properties. The emphasis on the physiology of sound production may not appeal to more accomplished singers, but perhaps even to them some insight into the process may lead to greater comfort during their performances. However, it must be apparent to all that while we can dissect various aspects of great singing, we are a long way from understanding how great singers produce their sublime music.

186

CHAPTER 18

THE OFTEN DIRTY AIR WE BREATHE

"Some mines are so dry that they are entirely devoid of water and this dryness causeth the workmen even greater harm, for the dust, which is stirred and beaten by digging, penetrates into the windpipe and lungs and produces difficulty in breathing and the disease the Greeks call asthma. If the dust has corrosive qualities, it eats away the lungs and implants consumption in the body. In the Carpathian mines, women are found who have married seven husbands, all of whom this terrible consumption has carried away"

Georg Bauer (Georgius Agricola), De re metallicum 1556

'A young gentleman...was very obliging. ...and I asked him whether there was a great fire anywhere? For the streets were so full of dense brown smoke that scarcely anything was to be seen. "Oh dear no, miss," he said, "This is a London particular." I had never heard of such a thing. "A fog, miss," said the young gentleman. "Oh, indeed," said I.'

Charles Dickens, Bleak House, 1853

We all know that John Scott Haldane's "pure country air" (Chapter 8) is hard to find nowadays. Of course, it has never been found in cities, and over the centuries London was singled out as the city having the dirtiest air. Public complaints regarding London's dirty air began in the thirteenth century, and in 1661 John Evelyn addressed his pamphlet Fumifugium to Charles II; he considered the "evil" air as "epidemicall; indangering as well the Health of your Subjects, as it sullies the Glory of your Imperial Seat". Later, in 1854, Sir John Simon presented a report to the Court of the City of London in which he identified smoke from coal fires as the major culprit, observing that "we do not with impunity inhale day by day so much air which leaves a palpable sediment". The paintings of JMW Turner, Claude Monet and James McNeil Whistler, all three fascinated by the effects of sunlight filtered and scattered by fog on the Thames, graphically attest to the severity of the problem in the 19th and early 20th centuries.

One hundred years after Simon's report, on the night of December 8th 1952, I had to grope my way home after assisting the senior surgeon at St Mary's, Mr. Arthur Dickson Wright, in his operating list.[1] Once described as the "last of the truly general surgeons", whose list might contain operations as diverse as the removal of a cancer of the rectum to resection of the pituitary gland at the base of the brain, he liked to operate late at night when the theatre was unoccupied by any other surgeon. This left his long-suffering nursing staff waiting for hours in uncertainty, and his students having to find their way back to their digs well after the last bus and tube train. The way back to my rented flat in Sutherland Avenue led through

---

1 An unflattering picture of the private side of Mr Dickson Wright has been provided by his daughter Clarissa, who achieved fame as one of the two Fat Ladies in the TV series of that name. Titled Spilling the Beans her book recounts the dysfunctional and abusive family life, of which no one at St Mary's had the slightest inkling.

the back of Paddington rail station and over the Grand Union canal at "Little Venice". The struggle back on that night is forever etched in my memory; mouth covered with a wet handkerchief, I crept from street corner to street corner, barely making out the signs from a few inches distance. The intensity of the relief at finally making my way upstairs to the flat was matched only by the intensity of the black circle of soot left on the handkerchief where it had acted as a partial filter.

The week of December 6th to 13th 1952 saw three times as many deaths as usually occurred in London; although the excess of deaths was mainly due to respiratory illness (there was a 9-fold increase in deaths from bronchitis), deaths from heart conditions also were over twice as common. Whilst the deaths were mainly in older individuals with pre-existing chest problems, deaths in children and young adults were also three times the norm for the time of year; even some cows, brought into the city for an agricultural fair, fell victim to fatal respiratory illness. Although hardly a "wakeup call", it still took four years for the Clean Air Act of 1956 to be passed, imposing regulations regarding fuel use; probably the most effective regulation was one banning coal burning for domestic heating. The focus in these early measures was the reduction in smoke particles and sulphur dioxide—understandably, because at the time of the worst smog the concentration of both pollutants had increased four-fold.

LUNG DEFENCES

Given the innumerable gases and particles that commonly may occupy the air we breathe, it may even be surprising that serious problems are not more frequent. However, the respiratory system has a host of mechanisms helping to protect us from the necessarily intimate contact with our environment. First, there is the structure of the lungs with their branching system of progressively smaller airways, ensuring that larger and heavier particles settle out in the larger airways from where they may be readily coughed up. The walls of the bronchi contain little "goblet" cells that secrete a sticky mucus to capture particles, and a carpet of fine hairs (cilia) that beat in a rhythmic coordinated way to propel the mucus layer upwards. The final contributors to this Homeland Security are large macrophages that roam the alveoli and small airways, ready to gobble up any microscopic terrorists such as bacteria and viruses, and atmospheric particles. If anything nasty does manage to get through into the airway walls a secondary defensive wall is provided by lymph tissue and mucous glands that respond with an inflammatory train of events, with secretion of chemical messengers that are able to call on the immune system reserves of the rest of the body.

In spite of the defences, there is still a high incidence of asthma and chronic bronchitis. Children are especially prone to asthma, the incidence exceeding 20% in some countries, and there is the strong evidence that air pollution stunts the development of children's lung function. The harmful effects may be very subtle; for example, there is a complex interaction between different pollutants at concentrations that individually do not seem too dangerous, but which in combination may lead to lung damage.

Finally, we are constantly, and rightly, reminded of the deleterious effects on the earth's atmosphere, with damage to plant life, global warming and depletion of the ozone layer in the high atmosphere.

188

AIR POLLUTION, CAUSES AND EFFECTS

In the 50 years since the London disaster, there has been much research on air pollutants and their effects; more gases are now recognized as being toxic, and particles are graded according to size because fine particles, whilst they may not weigh much, reach farther into the lung than larger ones. Measurements can be confusing, at least in part because of the units that are used; particles can be weighed, and they are expressed in micrograms per cubic meter of air ($\mu g/m^3$); gas concentrations, because they are too small to be expressed in %, are measured in parts per million (ppm, equal to 0.0001%). Finally, the effects of various pollutants on the airways vary among individuals due to a variety of factors, some of which are not too clear. However, the effects are invariably greater in individuals subject to asthma, who develop airway narrowing (bronchoconstriction) and inflammation at lower exposure levels: their "airway reactivity" is greater than in non-asthmatics.

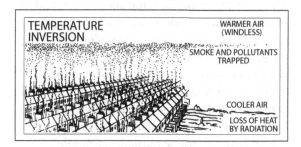

Figure 44 Factors contributing to inversions

Whether air pollution reaches dangerous levels or not in a given location is related to the extent of local emissions from industry and motor traffic, and geographic and meteorological conditions. Thus in the London disaster a cold air mass settled in the low lying Thames Valley, causing a greater need for domestic fuel burning (of sulphur-containing Welsh coal) but also trapping a stagnant air mass. Air may be trapped between a body of water and surrounding hills, as in Los Angeles and also my own city, Hamilton Ontario, lying between Lake Ontario and the Niagara Escarpment. Temperature inversions also contribute to the trapping of a dense cold air mass at ground level under a layer of warmer air a few hundred feet above; the effect is clearly seen on calm days as a dense brown haze that has a clear horizontal ceiling.[2] Ground level wind will tend to clear pollutants rapidly, but if the air is still the sun's heat does not penetrate the layer of pollutants, tending to perpetuate cooling at ground level.

THE SULPHUR DIOXIDE FAMILY

There have been several research approaches to the effects of pollutants, from carefully controlled experiments in animals and humans exposed to graded concentrations of individual pollutants, through long term studies of children

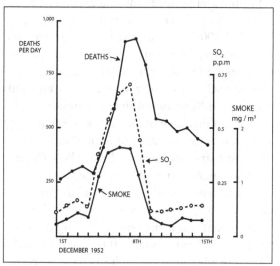

Figure 45 Particles, sulphur dioxide and excess deaths in London, December 1952

189

2   "Inversion" refers to the fact that the ground is usually warmer than the air high above, allowing smoke to rise and be cleared by wind.

living in areas with different levels of pollution, to the monitoring of hospital admissions with respiratory disorders such as asthma with later correlation to data obtained from the analysis of air samples.

If we first consider the chemical gases that may affect our health, most are oxides produced by combustion or the action of sunlight. The first to be recognized was sulphur dioxide (SO_2), mainly formed during the combustion of fossil fuels, such as coal, that contain sulphur as an impurity; for this reason SO_2 pollution mainly occurs in heavily industrialized areas. At least part of the reason the Clean Air Act worked was the availability of an alternative fuel—smokeless anthracite that conveniently could replace the "soft" coal. The data obtained during the London disaster showed a linear relationship between SO_2 concentration and daily death rate; on December 3rd the concentration was 0.15 ppm and deaths numbered around 260; by December 8th SO_2 concentration was 0.7 ppm and 800 deaths occurred. The observations were followed by research that measured lung function in individuals living in areas with differing SO_2 in the air. In 1965, Walter Holland and Donald Read, two British researchers who established the value of an epidemiological approach to the problems of air pollution, reported that workers in the British Post Office working in London, had more symptoms of chest problems (cough, sputum and dyspnea) and lower pulmonary function, compared to their compatriots living outside the city in areas where the SO_2 was about half that in London.[3] The large amount of research since the suggests that cities that are subject to an average annual concentration of greater than 0.04 ppm of

190

SO_2 show an increased incidence of chronic bronchitis. The effects of SO_2 are probably mediated by sulphurous acid (H_2SO_3, formed from the combination of SO_2 and water); as well, sulphuric acid (H_2SO_4) may be formed from SO_2, water, and Ozone (O_3). Droplets of sulphuric acid and ammonium sulphate contribute to atmospheric haze.

In many countries, reductions in the use of coal in industry and to generate energy for electricity have led to reductions in atmospheric SO_2; in Hamilton, the average yearly SO_2 level has fallen during the 40 years that I have lived there from over .03 ppm to less than .005 ppm. In Eastern European countries, on the other hand, industrial cities have seen the concentration rising progressively. Sulphuric acid is used in many industries; its production exceeds that of any other chemical.

CARBON MONOXIDE

Although we began thinking about air pollution in terms of sulphur dioxide, mainly because it was the main culprit in the London smogs, the greatest pollutant, in terms of tons emitted yearly to the atmosphere, is carbon monoxide (CO). The product of incomplete combustion of carbon compounds, most of the CO is produced by transportation. The main source in cities is slow moving, gasoline burning, automobiles; speeds above 50 km/hr lead to lower CO emission, and diesel engines emit much less than gasoline engines. A few decades ago high levels of CO were recorded on the streets of European cities; the record seems to be held by London, with levels in excess of 200 ppm.

We all know that carbon monoxide can be lethal; at the time coal-gas fired stoves were popular, "sticking your head in the oven" was a common way to commit suicide, and

---

3   They also showed a dramatic interaction between the worker's location and cigarette smoking: city dwellers smoked more than their rural counterparts.

malfunctioning propane stoves account for several accidental deaths every year. It was the great French physiologist Claude Bernard who, in the mid-19th century, fist discovered that carbon monoxide kills by taking the place of oxygen in the hemoglobin molecule, and death is secondary to oxygen lack. Not all the oxygen binding sites need to filled with CO, for oxygen carrying capacity to be seriously impaired; as little as 40% will do. It is reassuring that exposure to environmental CO nowadays is unlikely to cause carboxyhemoglobin to exceed 1%. "Personal" pollution by cigarette smoking, however, often causes carboxyhemoglobin levels in excess of 15%, probably contributing to atherosclerosis, the main cause of heart attacks and strokes..

NITROGEN OXIDES

Nitrogen oxides are emitted from motor vehicles and a number of chemical industries. Air being a mixture of 80% N_2 and 20% O_2, it is not surprising that some of the N_2 is oxidized in combustion engines to form nitrogen oxides (NO_x). Nitric oxide (NO) is formed first, further oxidation producing nitrogen dioxide (NO_2). As is the case with sulphur oxides, combination of nitrogen oxides with water yields nitrous acid (HNO_2) and nitric acid (HNO_3). Although the concentration of nitrogen oxides does not reach levels at which health effects are seen, with hydrocarbons from fossil fuels, they are the source of the "photochemical smog" that that plagues Los Angeles and many other cities, in which high concentrations of ozone are found.

OZONE

In 1952, AJ Hagen-Smit, a chemist in Los Angeles established that under the influence of solar energy an atom of oxygen is split off nitrogen dioxide (NO_2) to form ozone (O_3), a sort of oxide of oxygen which is highly reactive, and a member of the "free radicals" that are capable of cell damage. Ozone formed in this way is known as "ground-level" ozone to distinguish it from the ozone formed at great altitudes, again under the action of solar energy, but which acts as a protective layer that reduces the amount of ultraviolet light that reaches the earth's surface.

Ozone was discovered by Christian Friedrich Schönbein, a German chemist working at the University of Basel in the 1820s. He noticed a distinctive smell during experiments on electrolysis of water; he named the gas from the Greek word ozo (smell). He had taught German in England where he met Michael Faraday and attended a demonstration of electric sparking, during which the same pungent smell occurred. Later he recognized the smell during the oxidation of phosphorus which occurs in thunderstorms. Further investigation of the gas revealed it to be intensely corrosive. His work must have made an impression, because in 1865 WS Gilbert wrote one of his "Bab Ballads" on it, calling it "Policeman Ozone" and "the best disinfectant that's known, they've shown". Another line of this ballad stands out as prophetic—"And up in the clouds I'll be bound it is found"; I have no idea why he thought this. It was more than a century after Schönbein's discovery, at the time when Germany was developing its V2 "flying bomb", that ozone was detected in increasing concentrations at altitudes higher than 10,000 m. Postwar, ozone was recognized as causing deterioration in foam rubber in jet aircraft, and aircrew experienced cough and chest tightness that they correctly ascribed to it. Improvements in cabin pressure compressors have alleviated this problem.

Chemical reactions involving ozone take place rapidly, leading to great fluctuations in ground level ozone concentration over short periods of time; typically, during hot summer weather ozone concentration rises in the early afternoon and falls later in the day as the solar energy diminishes. For this reason, during "smog alerts" asthma patients are advised to stay indoors in the middle of the day.

Ozone that enters the lung in even small concentrations damages the delicate membranes that line small airways, leading to inflammation and increased reactivity of the smooth muscle in airways. Not surprisingly, the effects are more marked in asthmatic subjects. The changes in the lungs make it easier for bacteria to gain entry into the lungs to cause pneumonia, and make it more likely that other particles are retained in the lung to cause their own effects. In this way, smokers are at increased risk of lung cancer and chronic obstructive lung disease if they live in a polluted city such as Los Angeles. Striking pathological changes signifying inflammation in small airways have been found *post mortem* in people who have died in Los Angeles, compared to Miami, which experiences much lower ozone concentrations.

OTHER POLLUTANTS

Up to now, we have considered polluting gases— CO, SO_2, NO_2, and O_3. In addition, a variety of industrial and domestic processes, many coal-fired, and automobiles produce small particles of carbon, iron oxides, lead compounds and a great many other chemicals. Small particles in the atmosphere contribute to fog; larger particles tend to settle out, but small particles can remain suspended in air, and are also capable of penetrating deep into the lungs, where they remain as intensely black areas. Pathologists used to estimate the length of time someone had lived in London from the size of such areas *post mortem*. The first chapter of Charles Dickens' novel *Bleak House* is mainly taken up with a description of a densely foggy day in London, and the young gentleman terms it "a London particular", which seems to indicate that even in the mid-nineteenth century the makeup of London fog was appreciated. Nowadays, much is known about the physics of particles; the rate at which they settle out depends on their density, shape and volume, but to simplify their measurement, air is drawn through progressively finer filters, and the amount caught at each stage is weighed. Each filter is known to pass regular spherical particles of a given diameter, so the results are expressed "as if" the particles were perfect spheres of a given "aerodynamic" diameter. All particles are lumped into "particulate matter" (PM), which I think has a nice Dickensian ring to it; the diameter is expressed in micrometers (or microns, μm), and the amount in micrograms per cubic meter of air ($\mu g/m^3$). Particles that have an aerodynamic diameter of less than 10 μm (PM_{10}) remain suspended in still air, and have the potential to be breathed into the lungs and settle out in airways and alveoli; the smaller the size, the more likely are they to reach alveoli; particles having a diameter of less than 2.5 μm ($PM_{2.5}$) are the most likely to be retained in the lungs to cause damage. Increases in $PM_{2.5}$ are associated with increased incidence of hospital admissions for respiratory symptoms and reductions in the development of normal lung function in children.

COMBINATIONS OF POLLUTANTS

"Particles" doesn't seem very specific, but it has proved difficult to define their composition much farther. They may consist of relatively inert elemental carbon (from incomplete combustion of fossil fuels); be formed of metallic oxides of iron, mercury and lead; contain toxic organic compounds; or contain acids from the reaction of ozone with SO_2 or NO_2 (sulphuric and nitric acids). Although some of these could be potentially very dangerous, their incidence and impact tend to be close to their site of production, and generally their effects are reflected in the total airborne concentration. The exception to this generalization is the acidic particles, which are widely distributed and cause injury and inflammation related to the amount of acid deposited in the lungs.

The formation of acid particles by the reaction of ozone on oxides of sulphur and nitrogen, leads to dissociation between ozone and $PM_{2.5}$ concentrations during a period of smog formation that lasts for longer than a few days. The process may best be illustrated by what happened in Windsor, a Canadian city joined to Detroit by the busiest transborder bridge to the US, in June 2003. During four days when there was prolonged sunlight and very little wind, ozone concentrations rose in the middle of the day from .01 ppm to 0.08 on day 1 and to 0.11 on day 4; during the same time $PM_{2.5}$ increased progressively from 10 $\mu g/m^3$ on day 1 to 50 on day 4. The ozone produced each day for a few hours led to particles being formed that remained and accumulated from day-to-day, adding to the continuing burden from other sources, such as nitrogen oxides.

The linkage between different pollutants makes it difficult to assign damaging effects to each of the individual components. SO_2 and NO_2 both lead to the formation of acids (sulphuric and nitric acids) by combining with ozone; their effects may be combined into a single effect (acid vapour). Large studies that compare the effects of pollution in areas having different constituents suggest that each of the main components (SO_2, NO_2, ozone, acid vapour, and $PM_{2.5}$) contribute an effect independently of the others. For example, a recent study was carried out in 12 communities in California experiencing widely varied exposure to the different pollutant categories, to examine the part played by each in possibly harming children's lung development. Nearly 1800 children were recruited into the study at the age of 10, and followed for the succeeding 8 years. In 2004, Dr W James Gunderman and his colleagues reported that children exposed to NO_2, acid vapour and $PM_{2.5}$ showed deficits in tests of pulmonary function, which left them prone to impaired function by the time they reached adulthood; ozone did not show an independent effect. Children who lived in communities with the highest $PM_{2.5}$ (an annual average concentration of 30 $\mu g/m^3$) were five times as likely to show clinically significant decrements of function, as those in the lowest (5 $\mu g/m^3$). Slightly greater differences were observed between the communities experiencing highest and lowest concentrations of NO_2 (0.04 vs. 0.005 ppm) and acid vapour (0.012 vs. 0.003 ppm). As the greatest source of pollution in southern California is the internal combustion engine, rather than coal fired industry, elevated SO_2 was not observed in the study. These results, as well as providing ample evidence for the need to reduce automobile emissions, also provided possible targets for the needed "clean" air. Such targets are going to be very hard to meet if the progressive increase in auto vehicles continues; during the last three decades commercial transport has shifted from the railways to the roads, leading to a huge increase in diesel fuel use. However, at the same time there has be a surge in the development of cleaner engines, and the appearance of a few electricity-powered and hybrid cars, a hopeful sign.

In spite of evidence gathered over the past 50 years, linking particulates to effects on the development of lung function in children, the conclusions continue to be questioned (mainly by politicians and industry lobby groups) and ascribed to other variables in the surveyed populations—such as economic, racial, activity levels and stature differences for example. In 2006 the prestigious *New England Journal of Medicine* published the results of a study which contributed to our understanding of the mechanisms underlying the linkage. Professor Jonathan Grigg and his colleagues at the University of Leicester in the United Kingdom obtained cells from deep in the lungs of children by having them inhale a mist of a weak salt solution and collecting the mucus that they coughed up. The cells were macrophages, which engulf particles reaching the deep alveolar regions; the group identified the PM_{10} carbon particles under the microscope and calculated the area they occupied; the value obtained in an individual was then related both to lung function measures and to atmospheric PM_{10} found in the locality where they lived. The results in the 64 children aged 8-15 showed relationships between the pollution indices and macrophage particle area, and between the particle area and lung function decreases, with other confounders being excluded. An increase of 1.0 µg/m² in environmental PM_{10} was accompanied by a 0.1µm² increase in macrophage carbon. In turn, a 1.0µm² increase in macrophage carbon was accompanied by a 17% reduction in maximum airflow (FEV_1). The type of carbon found in macrophage cells was typical of the carbon particles emitted in diesel exhaust fumes, the main source of atmospheric pollution in this British city. The mopping up of particles by macrophages is the first step in a complex train of events that eventually leads to airway inflammation and obstruction to airflow into the lung.

There are many other linked factors that affect the quality of our air, especially locally, whether personally, as in cigarette smoking; in our place of work, as in second hand smoke; at home, where incomplete combustion of fuel for cooking may occur; and related to our work in certain industries, such as mining and welding. Other particles may lead to an allergic inflammation in airways, causing asthma, or in the air sacs (alveoli) to cause alveolitis. Their number is well into several hundred, and they range from the exotic to the downright disgusting. An eclectic selection might include the large (30 µm diameter) but light ragweed pollen that in North America is a major cause of asthma between late August and the first frost; the tiny (3 µm) spores of fungal thermophylic actinomycetes which thrive in mouldy hay and cause "farmer's lung"; the protein covered faeces of house dust mites, which live in their millions in our mattresses, and account for many cases of asthma in humid climates; avian protein shed from bird feathers, causing "bird fancier's lung"; fine cotton dust, causing byssinosis and "mill fever"; and the dust of many woods, from the lowly boxwood to the majestic Californian Redwood, that may cause asthma in woodworkers. Some particles may stick around for long periods, adding to the difficulty of making an association between exposure and symptoms. For example, when researchers investigated the high incidence of asthma in the remote tiny south Atlantic island of Tristan da Cunha they found a high incidence of allergy to cats, even though the last cat on the island had died 25 years previously.

The number of animal and plant products that may cause inflammation in the airways or alveoli provides a great challenge to respirologists who have to become amateur sleuths when tracking down causes for asthma and pneumonitis. All have experienced this difficulty, and our clinical experience is filled with examples, from the primary school teacher who was allergic to the class pet guinea pig to the young man who was sensitive to his the Eider down filling his grandmother's gift of a duvet.

Among the examples above are airborne particles and chemicals that may be encountered at work. The field of occupational lung disorders has expanded greatly in the last few decades.

OCCUPATIONAL LUNG DISORDERS

When it comes to identifying historically "the father" of a medical field, there is often a lively debate, but in the field of occupational lung disease there is only one indisputable holder of the title. Bernardino Ramazzini published *De morbus artificium* in 1700. Although this masterwork was published 150 years after Agricola's observations quoted at the start of this chapter, Ramazzini provided the first "modern" scholarly description of many occupational diseases. The first chapter, which lays out the general principles regarding the factors underlying the damaging effects of occupational exposures, also deals with diseases encountered in miners. He identified the importance of composition and concentration of particles in the air in producing lung damage, and made a number of suggestions to improve the conditions underground. Ever since, Ramazzini has been the starting point for any review of pneumoconiosis, the group of conditions associated with lung fibrosis due to inhaled silica. Silica is silicon dioxide, a component of quartz and the most abundant mineral in the rocks that form the earth's crust; the structure of silicate particles produced in mining and grinding rock is very variable, which to a large extent determines the severity of lung damage. The mineral with the worst reputation, and deservedly so, is asbestos. Exposure to asbestos particles may occur in the vicinity of mines and in occupations that use it, as well as in miners. These situations are associated with a fibrotic lung disease (asbestosis); malignant growths in the pleura covering the lung (mesothelioma); and lung cancer.

I saw my first patient with asbestosis at London's Hammersmith Hospital in 1960; only in his mid-thirties, he had noticed difficulty in breathing when he exercised and complained of a tight feeling in his chest when trying to take a deep breath or yawn. Unusually for patients in our clinic, he had never smoked but for eight years had worked as a grinder of asbestos in a factory that made brake linings, changing his job three years before I saw him. I asked him what the atmosphere had been like—a white dust made it hard to see across the factory floor and impregnated his clothes. He had been advised to wear a mask, but the discomfort of breathing through it in the heat of the workplace led to him not using it most of the time. His chest x-ray showed the fine lines of fibrosis in the lungs; his vital capacity was reduced to half of normal and the gas exchange capacity was only one third. Over the next three years I followed his progressive downward course, as his lung volume and gas exchange capacity halved again; he was never free of a feeling of suffocation that eventually could only be relieved by morphine.

The asbestos fibre is long, slim and light; it settles only slowly in the air, but when breathed it shoots down the airway like a mini-javelin, finally impacting in the deepest parts of the lung. It can work its way through to reach the internal pleura covering the lung to cause scarring (pleural plaques) and a malignant tumour—mesothelioma. In the lung substance an intense immune response is mounted by the body, which governs the intensity of the residual fibrosis. The needle like fibres are composed of silica and magnesium, with outer hydroxide ions that can damage lung cells; the cells attempt to take up the fibres but can only do this with short fibres. The asbestos becomes coated with a protein leading to typical "asbestos bodies" that can be identified in sputum. The inflammation in the lung eventually leads to scarring (fibrosis), and the alveoli become distorted and stiff, at which point they do not expand and their function is severely compromised.

Many particles in the air are capable of causing lung damage; their size, shape and weight determine where they settle in the lung and their chemical composition determines the type of inflammation. Additionally, the reaction varies amongst individuals in terms of the immune response. Some particles may be inert and a reaction to them only occurs if the person is sensitized to them. Asbestos is one of the worst, because its size and shape mean that it penetrates deep into the lung; its physical, chemical and electrical properties cause immediate damage, and the immune response leads to widespread fibrosis which is capable of causing death in a few years. Exposure to coal dust at one time could be very extensive, but once mining had become mechanical and less dependent on miners being at the coal face, the incidence of coal workers' pneumoconiosis has fallen. Particles of carbon settle out in the smaller airways but do not lead to severe inflammation; over many years of exposure emphysema and localized fibrosis occur. The reaction is more marked in miners working with coal that contains quartz because of its silica content.

Whatever the cause of widespread fibrosis in the lung, the effects are similar. The lung becomes stiff and the lung volume gradually shrinks. Breathing becomes difficult and increases are achieved mainly by rapid shallow breaths—breathlessness on exertion is the main complaint. In later stages of these conditions, most of which are progressive to a lesser or greater extent, the diffusion of oxygen into the alveoli and across into the blood becomes poor; any exertion leads to a fall in blood oxygen, multiplying the sense of dyspnea, and eventually preventing any activity.

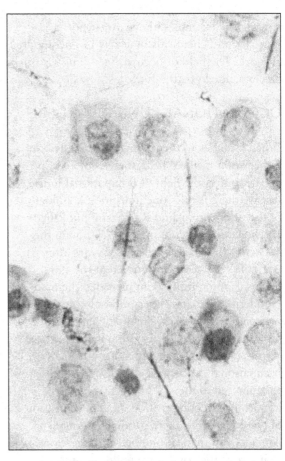

Figure 46 Needle-like fibres of asbestos surrounded by lung macrophages

Obviously all the lung conditions caused by dusts are capable of prevention, through control of exposure, but this is never as easy as it sounds. Again, asbestos is a case in point. Its name is taken from the Greek word for "inextinguishable", and its fire-resisting properties have been used since antiquity. A common early use was in the wicks of torches; Pliny, in 50 AD, observed that the makers of the lamps used by the vestal virgins protected themselves with masks. Its incorporation into industrial processes can be dated to 1878 when a mine was established in a small Québec township, named Asbestos, and followed by mines in Russia and South Africa. There is an astonishing number of applications for the fibrous mineral, but major users became the manufacturers of cement, floor tiling, insulation, brake and clutch linings and the plastics industry. Insulation of the engine rooms of naval vessels and submarines, generated many cases where the patients presented 5-10 years after World War II. Applications that with hindsight appear to have been inappropriate include its use as artificial snow in the movie industry; in gas mask filters; and in cigarette filter tips. The industrial production of asbestos world-wide reached 10,000 tons p.a. at the beginning of the 20th century, increased to 3 million tons in the late 1060s, and reached 5 million tons at the end of the century.

The first cases of asbestosis were described in workers employed in a Norwegian factory in 1906, and in the following year Hubert Montague Murray, in a report to the Commission on Compensation of Industrial Disease, described the typical effects of asbestosis in the sole survivor of a group of ten men employed at one asbestos textile factory. By the 1930s it was generally accepted that asbestos was extremely toxic to the lung, and legislation was brought in to limit exposure; how could it be then, that 30 years later workers were still being exposed to dense dust?

Well, the answer is that it has proved difficult to reduce asbestos exposure, in spite of the fact that legislation to reduce dust exposure were brought in as early as 1931 in the United Kingdom, with the Asbestos Industry Regulations. First, asbestos is an important, even life-saving, material that became part of thousands of products. Alternatives that fit its bill completely have not been discovered or invented; the closer synthetic fibres got to having similar properties, the more likely they

were to cause similar problems. Second, masks that effectively excluded the tiny fibres require such a fine filter that they cannot be worn comfortably; workers require hoods supplied with forced clean air—cumbersome to wear for heavy tasks; additionally, special clothing is needed to avoid dust being carried into the worker's home. Third, the monitoring of air quality presents problems in terms counting fibres caught on a membrane filter. The present American standard has been legislated at 0.2 fibres per cubic centimeter of air, counted under a light microscope at a magnification of 500 times. Before legislation, workers were routinely exposed to 20 fibres/cm^3, and even as high as 100/cm^3. Considering that 1 cm^3 is the volume contained by a teaspoon, such figures are staggering. Finally, as the only proven method to reduce exposure is filtration of the air, standards have to be met for the disposal of the filters.

Whilst we are thinking quantitatively about numbers of fibres, studies that have counted the number of fibres found in human lungs have been revealing. Electron microscopy allows even small fibres to be counted; in city dwellers, fewer than 100 fibres are found in a milligram of lung tissue; this still sounds a lot, but not when compared with the non-mining inhabitants of an asbestos producing town such as Thetford Mines in Québec, who have ten times this amount. Miners with asbestosis may have more than a million fibres/mg of lung.

Legislation has gone a long way in most countries to reduce the incidence of asbestos related diseases, and to protect and compensate workers. The difficulty in achieving industry standards is illustrated by one large US manufacturer moving its operations to Spain, where the standard was less stringent. However, the success of class action suits brought to the courts by workers has provided a stimulus to preventive action by most of the industry. Workers are monitored, and any asbestos related problem leads to removal from work, and compensation, where necessary. In addition to asbestosis, compensation for the malignant tumour of the pleura, mesothelioma, and lung cancer is usual practice.

THE LEGISLATIVE IMPERATIVE TO CLEAN UP THE AIR

Dr David Vincent Bates, the doyen of Canadian air pollution researchers, wrote eloquently of the need to combat the effects of environmental pollution; he pointed to successes in reducing the effects of asbestos and sulphur dioxide, to suggest that the imposition of standards and effective public policy decisions can lead to a brighter future for the lungs of generations to come.

Medical specialists like to feel that theirs is <u>the</u> specialty that is the most challenging, most rewarding and most likely to benefit mankind. Respirologists feel this way because the lung is assailed by hundreds of potentially harmful substances that manage to find their way into its functioning interior. This leads to lung problems being common, potentially serious and often difficult to diagnose and treat. It is also why many, exemplified by David Bates, passionately take up the cause of protecting our atmospheric environment.[4] They have acted as

experts testifying to governments and so helping to influence legislation to control pollution and reduce cigarette smoking. The first Clean Air Act in the United Kingdom was passed in 1956, after the Beaver Committee brought out its report in 1954; thus legislation to reduce open coal burning took four years to enact after the disastrous London smog of December 1952. The result was a dramatic reduction in smoke particles, and more modest reduction in atmospheric sulphur dioxide, during the succeeding ten years. In 1970, a committee of the Royal College of Physicians (stacked with eminent respiratory physicians) published a report, *Air Pollution and Health*, in which it was pointed out that reductions in pollution following the 1956 Clean Air Act had "happily" been associated with some declines in morbidity.

The legislation of standards for air pollutants has involved debate between the harmful effects on health, and the cost of the measures required to bring them about; cost in this sense has nothing to do with the cost of illness but the cost to the polluting industries or individuals (in the case of automobile emissions). The prime mover of the US Clean Air Act of 1970 was Senator Edward S Muskie; he clearly saw this tug-of-war and came down firmly on the side of health when he introduced the Act to the US Senate—"Our responsibility is to establish what the public interest requires to protect the health of persons. This may mean that people and industries will be asked to do what seems to be impossible at the present time." The Act proposed sweeping measures to achieve standards for the major pollutants, and led to major declines in emissions of nitrogen and sulphur dioxides and particulate matter. Amendments to the Act were legislated in 1990, and although lengthy and complex, the

198

---

4   Dr. Bates, in his book *A Citizen's Guide to Air Pollution* quotes the influential economist John Kenneth Galbraith—"In fact, no intellectual, no artist, no educator, no scientist, can allow himself the convenience of doubting his responsibility. For the goals that are now important there are no other saviors. In a scientifically exacting world scientists must assume responsibility for the consequences of science and technology...". David Vincent Bates worked at the University of British Columbia, becoming Dean of the UBC Medical School.

He died in 2006.

balance was seen by many observers to shift towards the cost. The improvements of the previous 20 years appear to have stalled, much to the dismay of health advocates. In 2003, the prominent respirologist David J Tollerud testified to a subcommittee of the US House of Representatives that "it is estimated that that 141 million Americans live in areas that expose them to unsafe levels of ozone and particulate matter. That means that half of America is breathing polluted air".

In Canada, National Ambient Air Quality Objectives were established in the mid-1970s as part of the Canadian Environmental Protection Act. They are a little schizophrenic in that whilst the objectives in most instances exceed the USA standards, they are guidelines and do not legislate specific action if they are not achieved. Nevertheless, there has been a steady improvement in air quality in most Canadian cities that suggests that this middle-of-the-road approach has some benefits. The most dramatic reduction has been seen in the pollutant most easy to control, that of SO_2 which originated mainly from the stacks of coal fired electrical generators. However, even here changes are slow—the several hundred coal fired generators in the American mid-west still contribute tons of SO_2 to pollution in Ontario and the Great Lakes states. There have been falls in NO_2, O_3, and PM_{10} resulting from the imposition of emission controls in the automotive industry. Against these successes must be set the results of recent research studies mentioned above that show deleterious effects on lung health in children from pollutant concentrations that are within the range of what used to be felt as "safe". It is inevitable that the targets will continue to set at lower and lower concentrations, paralleling technological advances.

Nowhere has the struggle between industry and the population's health been better demonstrated than in the development and enforcement of standards in the asbestos industry. The harmful effects of asbestos were recognized as early as the 1930s, became clinically important in the 1960s, and have continued to increase to this day. Standards have proved difficult to impose, beginning in 1968 with 12 fibres per ml of air (a staggering number for only a teaspoonful of air), but falling to 2 fibres in 1976 and 0.1 fibre in 1990. That standards are only a part of what is needed is illustrated by the unfortunate inhabitants of Libby, Montana, a small town close to a mine excavating tremolite, one of the more toxic forms of asbestos, for 30 years before it closed in 1990. Hundreds of people living in Libby, not only the miners themselves, have died and more than 400 are suffering the effects of asbestos exposure. Asbestos is a more-or-less unique problem because the industry is localized, and its control has been mainly brought about by legal suits brought against individual companies, some of which have been forced into bankruptcy. Other companies have cynically relocated to countries having more lax standards than North America, such as Spain.

The effects of catastrophic reductions in air quality have been appreciated for eons. Writing to Tacitus in 105 CE, Pliny the Younger describes how he found his father who, at the time of the Vesuvius eruption of 79AD, was the Admiral of the Roman Fleet anchored in the Bay of Naples—"Leaning on two servants, he brought himself upright and immediately collapsed again, I suppose because his breathing was affected by the dense fog that obstructed his airways that were of a weak nature, narrow and subject to inflammation". In recent decades, we have learnt much regarding fogs, airway obstruction, and inflammation; what is needed now is to put this knowledge to work

so that air quality is defended and the effects
of air pollution eliminated. As David Bates
pointed out, the interaction between science
and public policy is extremely complex, the
balance between industrial development and
health concerns often shifting in favor of
one or the other. What do we take from our
experience of the conflict? The successes that
have followed reductions in cigarette smoking
and the early pollution controls should give us
confidence that acting on the findings of first-
class epidemiological science will bring tangible
rewards in health and quality of life, within a
surprisingly short time.

CHAPTER 19

WHEEZY BREATHING

"...for though the asthmatic expire more easily than they can draw in breath, yet the expiration is very slow, and leisurely , and wheezing; and the asthmatic can neither cough, sneeze, spit or speak freely"

Sir John Floyer, Treatise of the Asthma, 1698

Sir John Floyer, like many physicians who to this day have followed him, to specialize in asthma, was a sufferer himself "under the tyranny of the asthma, at least, thirty years, and therefore think myself to be fully informed in the history of the disease." Selectively drawing on authors before him, and from his perceptive observations of his own symptoms and those of his patients, he identified asthma as a condition in its own right, due to "a contracture of the muscular fibres of the bronchi". Unlike a number of his successors he realized that asthma was not a trivial disease, not easy to cure, and sometimes fatal. One can make a good case to argue that 250 years was to pass before much advance occurred in our understanding or treatment of this common and disabling condition. However, since the 1950s there have been continuous and spectacular advances on both these fronts. Asthma is now seen as a complex disorder in which inflammation of the airways that can extend from the nose to the deepest parts of the lungs. The causative factors range from our genetic makeup to the particles present in the air we breathe. For the individual patient this is a "good news, bad news" situation. On the one hand we have many treatment options, but on the other, identifying which factors predominate in an individual

requires uncommon expertise and skill in physicians called on to treat asthmatics.

EARLY DESCRIPTIONS OF ASTHMA

For me, the most impressive work on the history of medicine is a tome published in 1849 for the Sydenham Society. In *The Genuine Works of Hippocrates*, Francis Adams, Surgeon, presents his translation from the Greek of all the material that to that time was considered directly attributable to "The Father of Medicine", and known as the Hippocratic Collection. The result is a book of almost 900 pages that encompass Hippocrates' experiences, with detailed case reports, evidence regarding disease causation, treatments, and aphorisms.[1] There are several references to asthma, as an episodic respiratory difficulty similar to and linked with epilepsy—a notion that lasted for centuries. Hippocrates noted that asthma occurred in children, could occur in several family members and was influenced by the weather.

To give credit where it is certainly due, the famous twelfth century Jewish physician Moses Maimonedes, had also written a book with the same title as Floyer's—*A Treatise on Asthma*. Hailing from Cordoba, Maimonedes travelled to Egypt at the time of the persecution of Jews in Spain, and became the personal physician to the Sultan Saladin. He achieved fame and fortune by treating the Sultan's son, who had

---

1   For example, the first reads—"Life is short, and the Art long; the occasion fleeting; experience fallacious; and judgement difficult. The physician must not only be prepared to do what is right himself , to make the patient the attendants and externals cooperate"

asthma. Maimonedes left a wealth of writings on philosophical topics, and was an advocate of "evidence based medicine"; he emphasized the spasmodic nature of asthma and the importance of hygiene, diet and exercise in its management.[2] In the sixteenth century, the Italian physician Girolamo Cardano also achieved lasting fame by treating a famous asthmatic; he was summoned to St Andrew's to help treat the Archbishop, John Hamilton. Among several useful measures was the order to remove the Archbishop's feather mattress; this has sometimes been taken as the first recognition of allergy causing asthma, although we may wonder whether he really felt the Archbishop was leading too soft a life style—the concept of allergic responses would not be recognized for several hundred years. Bernardo Ramazzini, the "Father of Occupational Medicine" similarly identified a specific inhaled agent as causing asthma in bakers in his book *De Morbis Artificum* (Diseases of Tradesmen, 1713), but again recognition of allergy to wheat grain and its associated moulds and insects would have to wait for the 20th century.

In the 19th century another asthmatic physician, Henry Hyde Salter, provided a description of symptoms that can scarcely be bettered. In *On Asthma: Its Pathology and Treatment* (1860), he identified many of the features that are now seen as characteristic of asthma—the variability during the day and during the year, the effect of cold air and exercise, and of genetic predisposition. He emphasized constriction of bronchial muscle in causing acute asthma, and considered bronchi to be "irritable"; one can

read into this the later concept of "bronchial hyperresponsiveness" or, more colloquially "twitchy airways". Likening acute attacks to epileptic fits, Salter postulated a nervous mechanism acting through the vagus nerve, which had recently been described as capable of constricting airways.

Sir William Osler was by all accounts the most widely and well read physician of the late 19th century, but on asthma he seems to fall short of his usual pre-eminence as a clinician. His *Principles and Practice of Medicine* (1892) is thought to have been the most successful medical textbook of all time; yet we read that "bronchial asthma is a neurotic affection" and "Death during the attack is unknown", both statements that were unlikely to promote aggressive therapeutic efforts on the part of his readers. However, he did recognize the association of hay fever with asthma, and some of their causes, including grass pollen and house dust. The stage was set for the next advance—recognition of the role of allergic responses.

ALLERGY AND ASTHMA

Charles Harrison Blackley was an asthmatic physician in Manchester, who in 1873 first demonstrated the clear association between pollens in the air and the symptoms of hay fever and asthma. He invented an air trap, fitted with a timed shutter, and containing a sticky glass slide; he placed the trap on the roof of his house and periodically removed the slide, using a microscope to identify and count the particles caught there. The graphs in his book *Experimental Researches on the causes and nature of Catarrhus Aestivus* amply demonstrated the huge variation in the daily number of grass pollens during the summer, and the relation between the pollen counts and his symptoms of hay fever and asthma. He went

2   One of his aphorisms—"He who puts his life in the hands of a physician skilled in his art but lacking scientific training is not unlike the mariner who puts his trust in good luck, relying on the sea winds which know no science to steer by."

several steps further by placing pollen in the corner of his eye, producing conjunctivitis, and finally scratching a minute amount of pollen into the skin, to produce a brisk reaction.

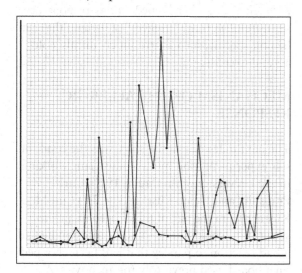

Figure 47 Charles Backley's graph of pollen counts over the course of several weeks. The original caption reads "Table of curves showing the number of pollen grains collected in each 24 hours on a surface of one square centimeter from May 28th to August 1st, 1866, the largest number, 880 being reached on June 28th."

Early in the 20th century, the Viennese paediatrician Clemens von Pirquet first used the term "allergy" (from the Greek word for "other") in putting forward the concept that reactions to foreign proteins, including pollens, involved antigen-antibody reactions that caused an abnormally sensitive state. With his colleague Bela Schick, von Pirquet was investigating diphtheria. As well as developing a skin test (the Schick test) for the diagnosis of diphtheria, they also observed serious reactions, including asthma, following administration of horse serum which at the time was used in an attempt to prevent the condition. To make the contrast to the beneficial, *prophylactic* effects (from the Greek word for guard), Charles Richet termed

the serious reactions to serum ("serum sickness") *anaphylactic* reactions ("ana" = not), in 1890. Anaphylactic reactions to allergens such as peanuts and shell fish remain potentially lethal in susceptible individuals. The severe reactions are due to a massive production of histamine.

To this day, skin tests are used in asthma patients to identify possible allergic "triggers", at least in part so that they may be avoided. The strategy was originated by a German dermatologist, Joseph Jodassohn, who in 1895 used patch tests to identify allergies in his patients with asthma. A small piece of lint was impregnated with dilute solutions of foods and other sensitizing agents and taped to the skin, and later observed for signs of inflammation. Nowadays, a drop of an allergen extract is placed on the skin and a tiny prick is made is made through it into the superficial layer of the skin, and the extent of any inflammation is measured to provide an index of the strength of the allergic reaction.

Although incompletely understood in the early 20th century, the immune or allergic response quickly caught on as an important factor in asthma, and by 1911 immunization to specific antigens was being used to treat patients. At the Inoculation Department at St Mary's Hospital, Leonard Noon and John Freeman conducted clinical trials of desensitization to grass pollens in patients with hay fever. The department head was Sir Almroth Wright, a larger than life scientific entrepreneur who offended the establishment by unashamedly approaching the pharmaceutical industry and notable individuals for money to support the department. A vigorous champion of vaccination, he once stated "The physician of the future will be an immunizer". With his support, Noon and Freeman made extracts of Timothy grass pollen, and placed drops of increasing concentration

203

"of the toxin" into the eye to obtain the lowest concentration that led to conjunctivitis, an index of allergy severity. Susceptible individuals might react to as little as 4 "units" (later known as Noon units); 1 unit represented the amount extracted from one millionth of a gram of Timothy grass pollen. Healthy controls showed no reaction to 20,000 units. They then injected very dilute concentrations into the skin of hay fever sufferers, regularly increasing the dose and monitoring the resistance by the eye test. Noon described the results obtained in 4 patients in a 1911 paper to *The Lancet*; resistance to the provoked inflammation increased in all, but not to normal. Freeman noted the danger of provoking a severe anaphylactic reaction if the concentration was increased too quickly. A paper by Freeman followed 3 months later, and was more encouraging; 20 patients were inoculated, and their comments recorded; there was one failure and two inconclusive results, but the remainder judged the treatment satisfactory.[3] Acceptance of the allergic theory may be judged by the fact that asthma and hay fever were to be found in the allergy sections of textbooks of the 1920s and 30s. However, clinical studies that followed Noon's and Freeman's papers suggested that only half of asthmatic patients reacted to known allergens, leading to the division of asthma into *intrinsic* (non-allergic) and *extrinsic* (allergic) types. Their work also emphasized the factors that are common to both asthma (in the lower airways) and hay fever (rhinitis, involving the nose and upper airway). Nowadays this is embodied in the concept of "one airway, one disease".

Since the time of Noon and Freeman, the number of substances known to cause allergic asthma has grown hugely, to include many plants, fungi and moulds; insects, fish, crustaceans and mammals; and many compounds encountered at work. Such allergens are nowadays thought of as "inciters" of a heightened airway response, to separate them from "triggers" of asthma that can be non-specific, such as irritant chemicals, cold air and exercise.

MECHANISM OF THE ALLERGIC RESPONSE

The next milestone in the story was the result of self-experimentation by two physicians working in the University of Breslau in 1920, Carl Prausnitz and Heinz Küstner. The 24 year-old Küstner from the age of 6 had been exquisitely sensitive to cooked fish—on one occasion he had a bad reaction to parsley that had been chopped on a board used previously for anchovies. A very small amount of fish extract when injected into the skin caused a large weal followed by a cough and wheezing, but when injected into his colleague no reaction occurred. The two then separated Küstner's serum and injected a small amount into Prausnitz's skin; 24 hours later, injection of the fish extract into the same area produced local inflammation. The experiment was repeated after treatment of the serum to show that the agent that transferred sensitivity from Küstner to Prausnitz was a protein, which became known as *reagin*. It was 1967, almost 50 years later, before the protein carrying the mediator of the acute allergic ("reaginic") reaction was placed in a subdivision of the globulins of plasma proteins (immunoglobulin E, or IgE), by two immunologists working at the Children's Asthma Research Institute and Hospital, in Denver, Colorado. Kimishige and Teruko Ishizaka used a combination of techniques to show that the "reaginic protein" could be obtained from blood taken from ragweed-sensitive subjects.

204

---

3   One was a Canadian who only had hay fever in August—thus probably sensitive to ragweed rather than grass; he was followed to June only!

In the late 1960s asthma was defined merely as "reversible airflow obstruction"; the links between the antigen (pollens, etc), the production of IgE, and the narrowing of bronchi remained conjectural. However, the stage was set for an explosion of research into the allergic inflammation of the bronchial walls. The cells taking part were identified, the ways in which cells are activated, attracted, multiplied and spread and the "mediators" that communicate between them, were all shown to be important. This information had to be integrated into what we knew about inflammation generally, both acutely as well as the chronic changes that occurred after years of recurrent asthma.

INFLAMMATION IN THE AIRWAYS

Modern ideas about inflammation began with the great German pathologist Rudolph Virchow; to the features of increased blood flow and seepage of plasma into affected tissues, he added accumulation of white blood cells.[4] In his book *Cellular Pathology*, published in 1858, he advanced many innovative ideas that drove research for decades, especially in the chemical components of cells. The introduction of cell staining with specific dyes for histology by Paul Ehrlich in 1888 was a notable advance, not least because he conceived the notion of a specific "receptor" on the cell surface to which the dye becomes attached. As different cells took up different dyes he made a conceptual leap in inferring that receptors for a variety of chemicals might be present on cell surfaces. He was responsible for the characterization of white

blood cells into types that remain accepted to this day. These included neutrophils (with non staining granules), eosinophils (granules taking up red eosin dye), basophils (taking up blue basic, alkaline, dye and similar to mast cells found in many tissues), and lymphocytes (small cells found also in lymph nodes). It took many years to determine the part played by cells in asthma, at least in part because few histological studies had been made in the condition. Thickening of the bronchial wall and an increase in the thickness of smooth muscle that circles the bronchi, together with accumulation of eosinophil cells, had been noted by William Osler, for example, but the first comprehensive study was not carried out until 1922, when Harry L Huber and Karl K Koessler, of the University of Chicago, submitted a paper to the *Archives in Internal Medicine*. Clearly, the Editor was impressed, for the published paper ran to 70 pages in length, and had many (expensive) colour figures. Although only 6 patients formed the basis for the study, careful measurements provided important information. The bronchial walls in asthmatics were twice as thick as in non-asthmatics, congested and inflamed, with large mucus-producing glands; bronchial smooth muscle was also twice as thick; these effects combined to make the airways very narrowed. The study thus provided evidence of both inflammation and smooth muscle growth; in addition, eosinophils were the dominant cells in both blood and tissues. As the eosinophil was recognized as the typical cell of allergic inflammation, the study was consistent with the emerging belief that asthma was an allergic disorder. However, two cases showed a predominance of neutrophils rather than eosinophils, indicating that other "non-allergic" mechanisms could also be important, including "intoxication with peptones or amines, bronchospastic poisons, which are formed by the action of micro-organisms on tissues."

205

---

4   Generally accredited as one of the fathers of modern medicine, Virchow also gained notoriety when he was challenged to a duel by Otto von Bismarck. However, the German Chancellor had second thoughts on being told that Virchow's chosen weapons were to be sausages laced with cholera bacteria.

During the past two decades we have learnt more about the cellular aspects of asthma due to the introduction of fiberoptic bronchoscopy. A flexible narrow tube is passed through the nose or mouth into the airways; fiberoptics enable small biopsies to be safely taken from the bronchial wall under direct vision. The biopsies are examined for cells that signify inflammation. Inflammatory cells can be washed out by broncho-alveolar lavage (BAL), and recently techniques have been devised to count the cells in specimens of sputum coughed up spontaneously or as the result of inhaling a mist of salt solution. In addition to confirming that eosinophilic and neutrophilic inflammation can cause asthma, the new information has added the concept of "airway remodelling"—long term structural changes in the bronchi—to the older concepts of airway inflammation and bronchial muscle contraction. The current view is that eosinophilic inflammation results from sensitization to environmental particles such as allergens (in seasonal asthma) and chemicals (in occupational asthma). Neutrophilic inflammation on the other hand, is more likely to be seen in infections by bacteria or viruses, and in chronic exposure to tobacco smoke and pollutants. Recurrent inflammation is thought to lead to remodelling, with thickened bronchial walls and large mucus glands, changes that are also common in chronic bronchitis.

In the last few years of the 20th century chest doctors were beginning to feel quite smug; the causes of asthma, especially in terms of allergic responses, were "understood", the means of assessing severity—with lung function and allergy skin testing—had been standardized, and treatment with inhaled steroids and bronchodilator drugs was generally successful. However, by the turn of the century the picture was becoming more complicated, and the complacency became seriously eroded. Mortality from asthma seemed to be steadily increasing in several countries, allergy did not appear to explain all the flare-ups that asthma sufferers were plagued by; the molecular, chemical mechanisms underlying bronchial inflammation were shown to be far more complex than we had thought; and the Human Genome Project was about to revolutionize concepts of asthma causation. One of the first facts that challenged previous concepts had to do with the role of viruses in causing asthma.

THE IMPORTANCE OF VIRAL INFECTION

The "common cold" is the bane of the British, who stoically put up with a week-long attack of annoying symptoms once a year; the experience often leads to a good-natured criticism of doctors and scientists in general who "can't even find the cause or cure for the common cold". However good-natured, the criticism is hardly justified. Since the end of World War II the British Medical Research Council has maintained a Common Cold Unit on Salisbury Plain in the South West of England. Volunteers were paid to spend time there taking part in experiments to study the spread of the illness, and its management. Along the way the research team established methods for the recovery and isolation of respiratory viruses, and they showed that several viruses, differing widely in their structure, could cause the symptoms; they included influenza, para-influenza, adenovirus and rhinovirus. The type of illness produced by the viruses to some extent could be related to the size of particles on which they were carried into the respiratory tract. Sniffed in on a coarse spray they caused nasal symptoms, whereas a fine aerosol deposited the virus deep in the respiratory tract to cause inflammation in very small airways (bronchiolitis).[5] The site of infection was also related to the temperature at which viruses replicate best; rhinoviruses thrive at a temperature of around 33°C, making the nose their preferred habitat; other viruses such as influenza multiply best at 37°C, found in the deeper regions of the lung, where they may cause pneumonia.

Viruses consist of genetic material (single stranded RNA or double stranded DNA) in a protein envelope, and they can only live and reproduce inside living cells. Viruses gain entry into the cell by binding to the cell wall, followed by transfer of the genetic strand, which then uses the cell's own RNA and DNA to replicate. The commonest portal of entry for viruses into the body is the respiratory tract, where they cause inflammation that varies in intensity from mild nasal mucus production to life-threatening pneumonia.

Wheezy bronchitis preceded by a cold is a common clinical condition in young children, and for many years this asthmatic condition was thought to be due to a viral infection; several studies showed that such infections were linked to asthma exacerbations. However, the crucial studies were a collaborative effort between Dr DAJ Tyrrell's team at the Common Cold Unit and Professor Stephen Holgate's asthma research group at the University of Southampton. Together they followed over 100 wheezy children aged 9-11 years during 13 months, monitoring symptoms and flow rates to quantify asthma, and collecting nasal secretions and a finger tip blood sample for evidence of viral infection. In their 1995 paper in the *British Medical Journal* they reported that viruses were isolated in a staggering

80-85% of asthma attacks, with the dominant viral group being the rhinoviruses. Since that time the association between asthma and viruses, especially rhinoviruses, has been confirmed in several studies, some of which seriously challenged clinical dogma.

In Canada, the most dramatic of the seasonal outbreaks of asthma occurs in early September, coinciding with increases in pollen counts from the hardy ragweed ptlant.[6] But it is also the time that the school year begins, bringing with it an increased incidence of colds. When Malcolm Sears and Neil Johnston surveyed schoolchildren in the Hamilton region they found that the incidence of virus infections, especially by the rhinovirus, closely paralleled symptomatic asthma. They also found that the increased incidence in school-age children was followed by increases in symptoms in younger children and adults. The strong association between asthma and virus isolation during this time of the year does not let ragweed off the hook; there is a tight link between asthma and positive inflammatory reactions to the ragweed antigen pricked into the skin. In addition to emphasizing that the cause of asthma involves the complex interaction of many factors, such research has opened up the possibility of adding specific anti-viral treatment to the drugs already available for the control of asthma exacerbations.

207

---

5   Bronchioles are the finest airways, narrower than bronchi; bronchitis is characterized by mucus production and a cough; bronchiolitis with difficulty in breathing and wheezing.

6   To someone visiting Canada from the UK, some differences in the flora are intriguing. For example, stinging nettles are not to be found, but their absence is more than made up for by poison ivy. Ragweed, is not found in Britain, but is widespread in North America. A flowering bush that can grow to well over a meter in height, in the late simmer it produces a large pollen grains in huge quantities to which many asthmatics are allergic.

FACTORS DETERMINING THE SEVERITY OF AIRWAY INFLAMMATION

The cellular events that that occur in asthma are the object of intense research, which means that the topic becomes more complex day-by-day. What has become clear is that the whole immune system is involved, thus taking the response well beyond the airways. Although initially the focus was on the eosinophil, now we know that many other cells (including lymphocytes, macrophages, neutrophils, mast cells, fibroblasts, and others) are involved; the key regulators of the immune response appear to be the T-lymphocytes.[7] Because of the number of cells and chemicals that are involved, most review articles on asthma contain illustrations that their authors presumably believe are helpful; however the reader is faced with so many arrows connecting cells, tissues and chemicals that he or she is left in a state of utter confusion. The story, as far as someone that is not directly involved in the research can understand it, is that an allergen, such as a pollen grain, lands on the delicate lining membrane (mucosa) of the airway, that may or may not have been damaged by viruses, pollutants (such as ozone) or tobacco smoke. Some allergens contain surface enzymes that allow them to penetrate the lining of the airway. The sensitizing protein of the allergen then meets, and is engulfed by, an octopus-like cell (antigen presenting cell) in the bronchial lining; when activated, this cell is able to attract lymphocytes from the bone marrow; at this stage it is likely that genetic factors influence the strength of this response. Genetic factors may also influence the way different lymphocytes develop. Thus, some lymphocytes produce chemicals (cytokines) that promote the allergic response, and others produce cytokines that inhibit the response; it's often termed an "orchestrated" process, but it is impossible to conceive an orchestra that might produce beautiful music in the face of interactions, positive and negative, between each and every one of the players. The number of new cytokines being discovered seems to increase every month and more than a hundred have been characterized. The interactions between cytokines and inflammatory cells determine whether sensitization to specific allergens, and therefore allergic disease, occurs in an individual. The lymphocytes grow locally where the allergen first settled, and the cytokines stimulate them to produce specific IgE antibodies, attract large mast cells and produce molecules on local blood vessels (adhesion molecules) that can attract eosinophils to the area. The IgE attaches to eosinophils and mast cells, so that when the antigen eventually comes into contact with them, they set in train the inflammatory process. Dr Ben Burrows and his colleagues at the University of Arizona in Tucson, showed that patients with higher levels of IgE in their blood had more severe asthma and rhinitis. The importance of IgE has also been shown by recent studies which have used a drug that blocks IgE formation (omalizimab); the drug prevents allergic inflammation and is effective in patients with asthma.

208

---

7   "T" is for "thymus-derived"; these lymphocytes act to coordinate the immune response, different groups of them having helper and suppressor effects on the growth and function of the B-lymphocytes (B for "bursa", a structure in birds where they were first identified); a final type of the T-cells ("killer" cells) has the capacity to eliminate "foreign" cells. It has also been shown that lymphocytes are derived from primitive cells in the bone marrow and later migrate to the thymus and lymphoid tissues, where they differentiate into their various types and develop their specific functions. B-cells mainly act to produce antibodies.

Probably the most dramatic event that occurs at the start of an asthma attack, is the emptying of the granules in mast cells and eosinophils. The granules consist of chemicals that cause the smooth muscle to contract (another reaction in which genetic factors are prominent), cause blood vessels to relax and become leaky, activate the mucus glands and stimulate local nerve endings. The main chemical in these reactions, and the first to be discovered, was histamine.

Histamine is one of many biologically active peptides, formed from amino acids. As well as forming the building blocks of proteins, peptides form hormones, enzymes and the chemicals that transmit nerve impulses. Together with adrenaline (epinephrine) and noradrenaline (norepinephrine), histamine strongly affects small blood vessels—they are said to be "vasoactive". The main figure in the discovery of histamine was Sir Henry Hallett Dale, who became the first Director of the British National Institute of Medical Research in 1914 and won the 1936 Nobel Prize, jointly with Otto Loewi, for work on the chemical transmission of nerve impulses.[8] Working with George Barger, Dale extracted a chemical from ergot (a fungus that grows on grain) that produced a strong contraction of cat uterus. A substance having a similar action had been isolated from the stomach, and they showed it had the same chemical structure as the ergot based substance; they named it histamine. Tiny amounts injected into the skin had a dramatic effect—a "wheal and flare" response like a nettle or insect sting. The flare is due to dilated skin capillaries and the wheal to the leakage of serum through the walls of capillaries. In a large dose it caused "histamine shock" with a large fall in blood pressure, similar to anaphylactic, and surgical, shock. In contrast to its effect on capillaries, which dilate, histamine causes the muscle of airways to constrict. When released from mast cells that have been activated by allergen reacting with IgE bound on the cell surface, histamine causes the airway inflammation and smooth muscle contraction that characterizes asthma attacks. Histamine release also occurs as the result of other "injuries"—such as cold air and virus infection, which explains the asthma attacks which sometimes occur in non-allergic individuals.

Dale exerted a huge influence on the future of mediator research, which revealed that histamine wasn't the only chemical to cause constriction of airway smooth muscle. Towards the end of World War I a brilliant young Australian physician visited his laboratory to learn more about the methods used there. Charles Halliley Kellaway had won the Military Cross whilst serving in Flanders and had been posted to London in an administrative position that gave him time to also embark on his research career. Dale was clearly impressed by him, and sponsored Kellaway for a prestigious Studentship, which allowed him to spend 1922-3 at the National Institute of Medical Research. Returning to Australia as the director of the Walter and Eliza Hall Institute in Melbourne, he was to play a major role in the development of medical research in Australia. Kellaway chose as his research focus the mechanisms whereby

---

8   Loewi famously had a dream—or, actually two dreams; he awoke after the first knowing that it had been important but unable to recollect any details. Luckily the dream occurred again and he was able to wake up, jot down the details and actually hurry to the laboratory and carry out the dreamt experiment. This was to perfuse two frog hearts connected in series so that the perfusate went from the first to the second; the vagus nerve to the first was stimulated, leading to a slowing in its rate, and soon after the second heart also slowed. Clearly a chemical had been liberated by vagal stinulation, later shown to be acetylcholine. This was the brilliant first demonstration of a chemical neurotransmitter.

snake venom acts. He found that tissue injury and the accompanying anaphylactic reaction was associated not only by histamine, but also a previously unknown chemical that had similar effects but was hundreds of times more potent, and slower but longer lasting in its action. The characterization of this chemical, 'slow reacting substance of anaphylaxis' (SRS-A) took many years, culminating in a landmark publication with his co-worker Everton Trethewie in 1940. The paper presented results obtained in a vast array of experiments which used Dale's approach of "bioassay", in which blood and tissue fluid was collected and processed, followed by its introduction into baths containing smooth muscle, such as guinea pig gut, and the strength of the resulting contraction was measured. The chemical structure of SRS-A did not follow until 40 years later, when improvement in biochemical methods allowed two post-graduate students to help their supervisors win the Nobel Prize. Priscilla Piper worked with John Robert Vane (another of Dale's protégés) on mediators of inflammation, and then with her colleagues at the Royal College of Surgeons in London, used the new methods in 1980 to "define unequivocally" SRS-A as a leukotriene. Work carried out by Pierre Borgeat, a Canadian graduate student working in the laboratory of Bengt Ingemar Samuelsson at the Karolinska Institute in Stockholm, had established the structure of this group of compounds as a combination of peptides and lipids. Vane and Samuelsson were jointly awarded the Nobel Prize in 1982, with Sune Karl Bergström. The identification of SRS-A as a member of the leukotrienes set the scene for one of the few novel treatments for asthma, the leukotriene antagonists.

Nervous factors have always been implicated in asthma, leading Osler, among others, to draw a parallel with epilepsy; the renowned 17th century Belgian physician Jean Baptiste van Helmont named asthma as "The falling sickness of the lungs". Asthmatic individuals were frequently labeled as "neurotic" and "hysteric", and many became chronically anxious, probably with good cause. In recent years such concepts have changed, as understanding of the autonomic nervous system, and its relation to stress and the immune system have increased. The lung and airways are plentifully supplied with nerve endings from the sympathetic and parasympathetic (or vagal) networks. Stimulation of these nerve endings leads to the release of chemicals, mainly acetylcholine and noradrenaline, that attach to a variety of receptors on specific cells, stimulating their function. In the lungs, sympathetic receptors (so called beta-adrenergic receptors) are in smooth muscle, and their activation leads to relaxation—bronchodilation. In contrast, stimulation of the vagal nerve endings leads to bronchoconstriction and also mucus gland stimulation. The widespread distribution of the autonomic nervous system to blood vessels and all body organs, and the central brain centres that partially control them means that there is scope for interaction between asthma and the function of many organ systems, such as, for example, the gut. There is scope also for asthma to be a manifestation of mind-body interaction, not only in provoking asthma by stress and anxiety, but also in its control through relaxation, meditation and controlled breathing.

Repeated asthma due to allergic, IgE mediated mechanisms probably account for at least some of the chronic changes in the wall of the airway ("remodelling") which can occur surprisingly rapidly and also early in life; the changes tend to lead to a gradual increase in the severity of the attacks due to the increasing number of inflammatory cells and thickness of smooth muscle, and a resistance to various forms of treatment.

The mechanisms involved at the tissue level have been the subject of successful research, which has led to improved treatment of asthmatic patients. In contrast to this research, which has employed techniques of increasing sophistication, has been the number of questions raised by epidemiological studies. Information regarding the prevalence, morbidity and mortality associated with asthma, has been obtained from simpler studies using questionnaires, skin testing and lung function (mainly spirometric measures of airflow, and the response to inhaled bronchoconstrictors— histamine and methacholine). In large part, such studies have raised questions regarding the effects of genetic factors versus environmental factors in asthma. For example, well standardized studies have shown that the incidence of asthma in the United Kingdom, Australia and New Zealand is about ten times that in Scandinavian countries. On a smaller scale, compared to children in cities, children who grow up close to farm animals are half as likely to develop asthma or hay fever. Early exposure to viruses, bacteria and fungi may protect people from the later development of asthma. These and other studies support the so-called "hygiene hypothesis" of asthma causation. Repeated studies have shown also that the incidence and mortality have been rising during the past twenty years, again most impressively in the UK, Australia and New Zealand.

The findings of large epidemiological studies have generated testable hypotheses regarding the relative importance of heredity versus environmental factors underlying the incidence of asthma. For example, is the high, and increasing, incidence in Australia due to the predominance of British people in the early immigrant population, or to the very high prevalence of dust mite faeces in domiciliary air and lack of ventilation, secondary to the adoption of air-conditioning? We wait for the relative power of heredity *vs.* environment to be quantified.

ASTHMA GENETICS

Heredity was emphasized as an important factor in asthma by Sir John Floyer in the 17th century and more recently, allergic disorders have been recognized as having a familial incidence. At least 50% of the offspring of parents with asthma will experience wheezing during childhood. Modern techniques of molecular biology, combined with greater understanding of the ways in which the various processes are controlled, have revealed that allergic inflammation and increased responsiveness of the bronchial muscle are separate genetic traits. Research carried out many years ago by Freddy Hargreave at McMaster University indicated that the severity of asthma was reflected in the combination of skin sensitivity to allergens and hyperresponsiveness to inhaled histamine, suggesting that the two processes were separate but combined to dominate the clinical expression. Both these features— allergic inflammation and bronchial muscle hyperresponsiveness are genetically determined. At least 30 genes have been identified as important in determining the occurrence of asthma and allergy, and genetic findings can predict the probability of poor lung function in childhood. Clearly, with the successes of the Human Genome Project, this sort of genetic information is set to increase greatly over the coming few years. A number of companies have invested millions of dollars and several years of research to find the genetic basis of asthma. One impressive study was carried out by the company Genome Therapeutics, who applied "positional cloning" techniques to 480 families containing at least two asthmatics, who were identified by the Southampton University group headed by Professor Stephen Holgate. Linkage studies showed that asthma families were statistically more likely than controls to have abnormalities (polymorphisms) in the amino acid sequence of a region of chromosome 20. The gene involved was named ADAM33, because it encoded an enzyme (A Disintegrin And Metalloprotease) found in smooth muscle cells. Subsequently, polymorphisms in this gene were shown to predict deterioration in lung function and impaired lung function in children.

A different approach to the genetics of asthma was taken by Dr Noë Zamel and his colleagues at the University of Toronto. A problem facing researchers who wish to find linkages between genes and clinical expression of various disorders, is that in a varied population there may be so many genes playing a significant role, that statistical relationships become impossible to find, unless huge numbers are studied. A solution is to study a population that is more uniform in its genetic background, and yet has a high incidence of asthma. One such population exists on the remote South Atlantic island of Tristan da Cunha, situated halfway between Cape Town and Buenos Aries.

Tristan da Cunha was only settled in the early 19th century, and records have documented additional settlers, so that intersecting family trees can be constructed for all 90 families of the total population of 301, present in 1993. Physicians from visiting ships had reported a high incidence of asthma, and when the entire population had to be evacuated to the United Kingdom in 1961 due to the eruption of the island's volcano, two physicians at the Brompton Hospital, Ken Citron and Jack Pepys found an incidence of asthma symptoms in half the evacuees. Zamel and his colleagues, with the island's doctor, Dr Peter Sandell, constructed a genealogy—everyone on the island was a cousin of everyone else; performed allergy skin tests—half showed positive responses; and recorded symptoms and lung function tests—57%

showed some evidence of asthma.[9] Blood samples were taken and DNA from white blood cells was examined with radioactive probes, to identify segregation of gene markers that matched to features of asthma. This painstaking research revealed two genes that appeared to confer susceptibility to asthma, located on chromosome 11, and subsequent studies have confirmed the finding in larger, more varied, populations.

Canada has seen a great increase in the number of immigrants from many parts of the world. Comparisons between asthma sufferers from different ethnic backgrounds provide some indication of the relative importance of genetics and environment in causing the condition. Chinese children have a lower prevalence rate than in age matched Canadian children; the rate is lowest in children born and raised in China, intermediate in those who had migrated to Canada, and highest in those born in Canada. The findings suggest interaction between genetic and environmental factors.

The recent research into the genetics of asthma has shown that asthma is a complex "polygenic" disorder, in which the effects of many, perhaps hundreds of genes interact to confer susceptibility to allergic reactions and a heightened response of bronchial smooth muscle. Given a genetic predisposition, there are also interactions with environmental factors such as allergens, viruses and pollutants. Not only have we learnt much about the causes of asthma, the new information has sparked new approaches to prevention and treatment.

---

9   Including allergy to cat dander, even though cats had been eliminated from the island 20 years previously—many of those who were sensitive to cat had never seen one! Which just goes to show how persistent dust can be.

TREATMENT OF ASTHMA

When we come to consider the treatment of asthma, the actions of various drugs are best understood against the background of the processes involved, but in many cases their usefulness was discovered long before their action was understood. We now have a large armamentarium, with drugs that are effective in controlling bronchial smooth muscle contraction, inflammation of the airway wall, the allergic response, and the production of inflammatory mediators (cytokines). We can say that now, but to begin with treatments were used without any real understanding of the way in which they worked.

One consequence of this fact is that whereas drug treatment for asthma used to be based on concepts of bronchial spasm, their action is now interpreted in terms of their effects on inflammatory cells, nerve endings, smooth muscle and mucus glands.

Atropine, and parasympathetic inhibitors. In common with many present-day drugs, drugs for asthma have their origin in plant products. Probably the first plant to be used was the hardy annual *Datura stramonium* (Jimson weed, thorn apple), in India, perhaps as long as 5000 years ago. In the 17th century henbane and belladonna were found to have similar effects in the relief of wheezing. These plants yield atropine and related compounds that inhibit the release of acetylcholine from vagal (parasympathetic) nerve endings; atropine reduces airway constriction (though not dramatically) and also mucus production. Initially the leaves, roots and stalks were burnt and the smoke inhaled by the patient—an early form of inhalation therapy, and in the 19th century, cigarettes containing the powdered plant were popular, especially those that also contained opium or cannabis. In the

1950s atropine methonitrate was found to be effective in cigarettes and later as an aerosol. Finally, a new atropine derivative, ipratropium bromide, was developed in the 1970s; this is effective as an aerosol and has fewer side effects than the previous atropine preparations. Because more potent drugs have been developed for asthma, ipratropium is reserved nowadays for patients with a lot of mucus, being a useful agent for chronic bronchitis.

Adrenaline, and sympathomimetic drugs. The use of the tea plant, the *Camellia* species, also began in antiquity in India and China, and was particularly popular in Ancient Greece where it was known as "the divine leaf". The other stimulant drink with its origins in the ancient past, coffee, also became very popular throughout the Western World. The drinking of coffee for asthma was promoted by Sir John Floyer in the 18th century and especially Henry Hyde Salter in the mid 19th, and the active constituent, theophylline, was identified in the 1880s and shortly after synthesized. The drug was effective when taken by mouth, but when a soluble derivative, aminophylline, was developed, it became a popular drug to administer intravenously in acute attacks. In the 1950s it became the most important drug available for life-threatening asthma; however, its dramatic life saving effect was short-lived and often accompanied by distressing side-effects of extreme anxiety, restlessness, vomiting and even fits. Theophyllines are classed chemically as *methyl xanthines*; they relax bronchial smooth muscle and reduce inflammation, although the actual mechanism remains a matter of debate. Their clinical use also remains debatable; although much less widely used than in the 1950s to 80s, they may still play a role when taken by mouth by patients with chronic severe asthma.

Among "adrenergics" or "sympathomimetics"—drugs that increase the effects of the sympathetic nervous system—the first to be used was ephedrine, obtained by the Chinese some 5000 years ago from the evergreen plant known as Ma Huang (*Ephedra sinica*). Extracts from the green branches of the plant are present in many traditional Chinese remedies, and the dried branches of the plant can be chewed. The active drug was isolated and named in the late 1880s, but it was not until 1924 that its properties became well known. KK Chen and Carl Frederic Schmidt, from the Peking Union Medical College suggested that in addition to its cardiovascular effects, ephedrine may dilate bronchi, arguing from its structural similarity to adrenaline.

In 1895, George Oliver and Edward Sharpey-Shäfer, of London's University College, found that an injection of adrenal gland extract resulted in large increases in blood pressure, and only 3 years later John Jacob Abel, of Johns Hopkins University isolated the active principle, adrenaline. Adrenaline was first used to treat severe asthma in 1903, when Jesse M Bullowa and David M Kaplan from the Montefiore Home for Chronic Invalids in New York, gave subcutaneous injections of the drug to three patients experiencing severe symptoms, which resolved a few minutes after. With intravenous aminophylline, subcutaneous or intravenous adrenaline became standard treatment for severe bouts of asthma, and patients who were known to be subject to sudden severe attacks were taught to give themselves subcutaneous injections. With the introduction of aerosol treatment in the 1960s, injected adrenaline and aminophylline became less used, although self-administered adrenaline (Epi-pen) remains first aid treatment of severe allergic reactions, for example to peanuts and insect stings.

Chemically, adrenaline is an amine which when injected mimics activation of the sympathetic nervous system, producing increases in heart rate and blood pressure—it is one of a number of "sympathomimetic amines". Henry Dale previously mentioned in connection with the discovery of histamine, investigated the mechanism underlying the sympathomimetic effects of adrenaline on muscle. With brilliant intuition he called it the "receptive mechanism for adrenaline", thus, as early as 1906, he conceived the idea of receptors on cell walls that allowed proteins to act as messengers and activate a variety of processes. In 1946, Raymond Ahlquist, at the University of Georgia, recognized that the effects of different sympathomimetic amines varied. For example, some increased heart rate, but produced very little constriction of the pupil, whilst in others the reverse was the case. He proposed that there were two main types of receptor—the *alpha* receptor was responsible for blood vessel constriction, pupil dilation and intestine relaxation, and the *beta* receptor was responsible for dilation of blood vessels and bronchial airways and stimulation of heart muscle. In 1967 the concept was expanded by AM Lands and his colleagues at the Sterling-Winthrop Research Institute in Rochester, New York. By comparing the activity of different beta-stimulants in terms of their effects on the heart, bronchi and blood pressure, they proposed two types of β-receptor—β_1, having a large effect on the heart, and β_2, which have a large bronchodilator effect. Needless to say, there are now other types of β-agonists, but the β_1/β_2 classification remains the one in general use. Finally, when we consider treatment, drugs may stimulate (an "agonist" effect), or inhibit (a blocker or "lytic" effect).

From a physiological point of view, new synthetic drugs were developed, beginning with isoprenaline and later becoming more selective—to obtain good bronchodilation with fewer effects on the heart—the "selective beta two (β_2) adrenergic receptor agonists". The most popular of such drugs was salbutamol—the "blue puffer" was a fixture in the pockets and purses of asthmatics throughout the 1960s to 1990s. Longer acting β_2-agonists such as salmeterol and formoterol were introduced in the last decade of the century. However, by that time a broader range of management options were available, leading to less reliance on β_2-agonist inhalers as the sole treatment for asthma. In part this was because there had been a conceptual shift from asthma being due to broncho-constriction, to the pathological features of airway inflammation.

Corticosteroid drugs. The beginnings of an approach to treating asthma as an inflammatory disease occurred in 1932, when cortisone was first used in its treatment by AH Fineman, of the Sydenham Hospital in New York. He gave extracts of the adrenal gland to four patients, because he considered that several features of asthma, including weakness, loss of appetite, low blood pressure, and low blood sugar were consistent with failure of adrenal function—they were "present in Addison's Disease, except in a more marked degree". The patients were given an extract of animal adrenal glands by injection for up to 4 months; one patient improved greatly, one slightly, one not at all, and one got worse. We might judge this result to be disappointing, but the editor of the *Journal of Allergy* thought them worth publishing, and Dr Fineman concluded they "warrant its further trial in a larger series of patients". The active principle in the adrenal gland, cortisone, was isolated and synthesized by Edward Calvin Kendall at the Mayo Clinic in the late 1940s; in 1948 there was enough to enable his clinical colleague Philip Showater Hench to treat some patients with rheumatoid arthritis. So miraculous

were the results that within a year of their publication Hench and Kendall were awarded the 1950 Nobel Prize. Also, within a few months, John E Bordley and his colleagues at Johns Hopkins, reported the successful treatment of five patients with severe asthma, and in the following year (1949) the same group reported a placebo controlled study of 23 patients; in addition to a dramatic clinical effect in 17 patients they also noted that cortisone inhibited allergic skin reactions and the blood eosinophil count. The early results were followed by large scale controlled trials sponsored by the British Medical Research Council, in both chronic asthma and acute life-threatening asthma (so-called "status asthmaticus"). The results, published in 1956, were more impressive in the acute condition, possibly related to the small dose and short duration of cortisone treatment in the chronic group.

In a similar way to the development of β_2-againsts given by metered-dose canister, steroids were synthesized that could be given by inhalation, to avoid the unpleasant and potentially lethal effects of cortisone given by mouth. Early in the era of steroid therapy, its dramatic effects on eczema and other skin disorders were the stimulus for the search for topical (locally acting) steroid preparations; first used in skin ointments, some were again miraculously effective in low concentration, and it was a small step to use them in a powder or solution given by inhalation as a puffer. Hydrocortisone, triamcinolone, and later betamethasone, beclomethasone, budesonide and fluticasone were shown to be powerful inhibitors of asthmatic bronchial inflammation, and thus much more effective in achieving long-term benefit than β_2-agonists. In the last decade, inhaled steroids have become "first line" treatment, with β_2-againsts being relegated to "relievers" of symptomatic wheezing. Along with the development of the drugs has come improvement in their administration—the optimal inhalation method, use of spacers to achieve an effective particle size, and changes in the propellant which generates pressure in the canister.

Cromoglycate. Steroids inhibit bronchial inflammation by binding receptors on the surface of cells; cell activation and recruitment of cells via cytokines is also prevented. Other drugs having some of these properties have been developed, and they also are effective in asthma. The first to be discovered was sodium cromoglycate, which is chemically similar to khellin, a drug obtained from the seed of a Eastern Mediterranean plant, of the same family as parsley and carrots, that had been used to treat chest problems since ancient times. The discovery was made by Roger Altounyan, a physician and asthma sufferer who worked for Fison's, a large British fertilizer manufacturer which with this drug intended to make a major foray into the pharmaceutical field. Altounyan was the main subject in the search for a khellin-like compound that might be effective in asthma. With each compound, he tested its ability to prevent asthma, which he provoked using inhalations of histamine and pollen extracts to which he was sensitive. Over ten years many compounds were tested, until in 1967 cromoglycate was found to have a useful protective effect. Inhaled as a powder from an ingenious "spinhaler" that Altounyan invented, it proved especially valuable in childhood allergic asthma and athletes with exercise-induced asthma.[10] In some ways this was a lucky find, because the succeeding two decades of intensive work led to only one other similar drug, nedocromyl. Both drugs acted on

the mast cell, preventing release of histamine and others mediators of inflammation; however, compared to more recent agents, they were only effective in limited situations, and they have been discontinued.

Leukotrienes receptor antagonists. Recently drugs have been developed that inhibit the inflammatory response by acting on leukotriene receptors. Leukotrienes are potent bronchoconstrictors that are formed in activated mast cells and eosinophils; they attach to receptors on airway smooth muscle. Receptor antagonists block this linkage and thus prevent bronchoconstriction. Montelukast and pranlukast are two drugs that have undergone large trials, and are now used for their bronchoprotective effect in resistant asthma.

Inhibitors of the allergic response. Finally, drugs that target the immune system by reducing the production of immunoglobulin E antibody are being investigated.

In spite of the recent increase in asthma, often called "an epidemic", and increases in deaths from asthma, most experts now feel that all asthma symptoms are capable of being controlled. However, this implies that asthma sufferers can be recognized, assessed, provided appropriate treatment and educated in aspects of their own management. In the face of increasing mortality from the condition, the obverse of the coin is that many patients do not recognize or choose to ignore symptoms, are inadequately assessed, poorly treated and not educated. Why, may be hard to understand because the measures involved in recognition, assessment, treatment and education are well understood, and neither complex nor costly.

Drugs administered by inhalation. Anyone who has had asthma for a few years will tell you that

---

10 As a former Spitfire pilot, he brought his aeronautic expertise to invent a small device in which powder contained in a capsule was dispersed by a tiny propeller.

inhalers are a growth industry. Since they arrived on the scene some forty years ago, we have learnt much about them—what influences their effectiveness, and the variety of medications and delivery systems has increased dramatically.

Inhalation treatment for asthma is probably as old as the medical profession itself. As soon as some plant extracts were thought to be useful it became clear that they worked best when inhaled rather than taken by mouth. Infusions were made and the steam inhaled, or the plant was vaporized on a hot brick, or even smoked in a pipe. Many of these ancient inhaled remedies remained unchanged for centuries, and were recommended still within living memory. Inhaled steam from a witch hazel extract and menthol cigarettes were common remedies; indeed tobacco cigarettes were first used for medical purposes before they became popular. Inhalers became popular for the treatment of asthma in 18th and 19th centuries, and devices became increasingly sophisticated.

The use of inhaled adrenergics, steroids and other agents has already been mentioned, but to give credit where it is due, one of the first to use this route of administration was a London general practitioner. Dr Peter Camps was a GP who also practiced surgery at the Teddington Cottage Hospital in West London. In 1929 he wrote *A note on the inhalation treatment of asthma* which was published in the *Guy's Hospital Reports* in which he honestly credits three of his patients who, "tired of my efforts, sought relief by a treatment …advertised in the lay press, and having obtained it reported the good news to me in the right spirit. (Our failures seldom come back to us)". Inhalation of adrenaline vaporized with oxygen promptly aborted acute asthma, and prevented nocturnal asthma when taken at bed-time. Camps also used atomized ephedrine, but he found it

less effective than adrenaline. In his paper, he set out some ideas for research into aerosol treatment; he identified four aspects—physical, physiological, pathological and psychological. All four aspects would be intensively researched in the succeeding fifty years. The brief allusion to psychology in Dr Camps' paper may be seen as the fore-runner of two features in modern asthma research and treatment— irst, the absolute necessity of controlled trials to reduce bias and suggestion in the response to treatment; and second, the need for a "holistic" approach to asthma management, in which patient education plays a strong role.

From the physical stand-point, different methods were developed to generate the most effective size of particle and dosage; radioactive aerosols were used to demonstrate that only a small proportion was retained in the lungs, most of the rest being swallowed. In the mid-1950s small pressurized canisters and valves were devised, which allowed an accurately metered dose to be delivered; even small children found them easy to use.

Once it became possible to measure particle size, it became clear that this was an important determinant of the therapeutic effect; like the bears' porridge in the children's tale the particles may be too small, too large or just right. Very small particles may remain suspended and be exhaled without dropping on the airways. Large particles tend to impact on the throat and mouth, and are then swallowed. Particles having an "aerodynamic" diameter of around 5 μm are most likely to be deposited in the bronchi, to exert maximum effect. Many of the early aerosols were very variable in size and density, but engineers were able to devise valves and jets that made the dose delivered to the airways more predictable. However, some problems remain, due to differences in the way the inhalers are used by patients, some of whom require a lot of education in their use.

Dr Camps used an oxygen cylinder to power his nebulizer, but this method could only be used in hospital. Later, a hand-held bulb became very popular, but a major breakthrough in 1955, was the invention by Philip Maschberg of a valve to deliver a known amount of medication from a small canister—the pressurized metered dose inhaler (pMDI). The pressure was provided by Freon, volatile chloro-fluoro-carbon (CFC). This type of inhaler was convenient and effective in delivering a succession of increasingly sophisticated drugs, both beta-agonists and steroids. In 1996, after the acceptance of the Montreal Protocol, CFCs were replaced by hydro-fluoro-alkanes (HFC), which are less damaging to the ozone layer. The pMDI is often used with an attached chamber, a little smaller than a beer can; the method has proved useful for two reasons; first, large particles settle out before the patient inhales; and second, less "hand-breath" coordination is required. Many patients have difficulty in actuating the device whilst breathing in slowly and fully.

Dry powder inhalers (DPI) began life in the 1930s; the powder was placed in a rubber bulb and puffed out through a mesh to keep large particles from being inhaled. Dr Altounyan's Spinhaler was popular in the 1960-70s, and later devices use plastic bubbles containing a measured dose, which the patient can inhale from a multi-dose disk.

We now have a myriad of inhalers, marketed by many pharmaceutical companies, and the choice between them is often difficult. The market is in billions a year, world-wide.

SPIROMETRY, THE ESSENTIAL ASSESSMENT TECHNIQUE

One of the keys to asthma management is the measurement of airflow. Although recognized and implemented by Henry Hyde Salter in the mid-19th century, it took more than a hundred years before spirometry became routine. Humphry Davy designed a spirometer in 1800 and John Hutchinson used a modification to measure lung volumes in a large series of healthy subjects, and showed the clinical value of the measurements in a variety of conditions in 1846. Twenty years later, Salter reinvented the instrument and a recording device, to produce a "spirograph" with which he assessed patients with asthma. In spite of these early suggestions regarding its clinical importance, it was not until the 1950s that spirometry caught on, with the introduction of the "timed vital capacity". Vital capacity (VC) refers to the total volume that someone can breathe out following a full inspiration, which was the main measure that Hutchinson made. The recording obtained with a spirometer allows the amount expired to be measured with respect to the duration of expiration (seconds). This was a key advance because it measured the rate of flow of air from the lung, the main physiological disturbance associated with airway obstruction. Given this fact and the relative ease with which spirometry is performed, it seems strange that nearly 100 years was to elapse before it became a routine clinical technique.

Robert Tiffeneau was a Parisian pharmacologist, who searched for a way to measure changes in the airways due to adrenaline and other agents. In 1947, with his colleague A Pinelli, he described the "capacité pulmonaire utilisable à l'effort" (CUPE). The measurement was proposed to measure the breathing capacity for exercise, in which a breathing frequency of 30 breaths/min is reached. This allows inspiration and expiration to take 1 sec each; Tiffeneau thus measured the volume expired in 1 sec. Although there was a delay in the acceptance of this Gallic index to be accepted, or even noticed, by the English-speaking respiratory fraternity, the volume expired in the first second of a forced expiration (FEV_1) became the principal tool in the diagnosis and assessment of severity and for following progress. The vital capacity (VC) is also measured; the ratio of FEV_1 to VC, normally greater than 80%, is another index of airflow slowing. The extent to which the FEV_1 is reduced reflects the severity of airflow limitation, and indicates the level of treatment required; the improvement that follows an inhalation of β_2-agonist shows the degree of "reversibility". Tiffeneau also suggested that when the FEV_1 is relatively normal, its repeated measurement following inhalation of brochoconstrictor agents. The inhalation of graded doses of histamine or methacholine is now used routinely to measure bronchial hyperresponsiveness.

Today, spirometry is cheap, and simple to perform ("even a doctor can do it!"), and so has become the yardstick on which management depends. The first line of treatment is provided by inhaled corticosteroids (because the initiator of asthma is airway inflammation); the dose is increased until symptoms have cleared and the FEV_1 is normal. The dose may then be reduced to find the lowest dose that maintains this function. This "optimal" dose is maintained for at least a year, even if the patient is symptom free, because this improves the long term outlook. Inhalers of β_2-agonists are used for rapid relief of wheezing, but the lowest use possible is the main aim. Other anti-inflammatory agents and bronchodilators are added where needed. Treatment is accompanied by a programme of education that allows patients to understand and control their condition.

ASTHMA MORTALITY

Our improved understanding of the causes of asthma, and the advances in treatment, has without question improved the quality of life in asthma sufferers. However, the incidence of death remains much higher than in the general population, and in many regions gradually increased through the 1980s and 90s. This has been ascribed to increases in air pollution, second-hand smoke, allergies, reduction of exposure to allergens in early life, among other factors, but the reasons remain elusive.

The rising mortality rate became especially apparent in New Zealand, where mortality in the age range 5-35 years quadrupled between the mid-1960s and mid-1980s. Dr Malcolm Sears then began a single-minded and lengthy crusade to combat the trend, which began during a trial of a new medication. Patients in the trial first had to stop their usual β_2-agonist inhaler and then take the new medication or a placebo. Several patients improved dramatically, and Sears guessed they were taking the active drug; to his astonishment, he later found that these patients were in the placebo group. The notion that β_2-agonists taken regularly several times during the day might lead to a worsening of asthma, led to a formal study of the question. At the time a short-acting β_2-agonist, fenoterol, was a popular bronchodilator and usually taken up to four times a day; in the study, this regime was compared to a placebo inhaler over a period of six months. Again, the investigators were surprised to find that asthma control was better with placebo treatment and worsened on fenoterol. They were very surprised because fenoterol had proved very effective when given acutely to asthmatics. Clearly over the long haul the drug was harmful, and the findings provided another example that the two processes of bronchial muscle contraction and inflammation were, at least in part, separate processes. Long term fenoterol made the airway inflammation worse. A parallel study showed a link between fenoterol and mortality: an increase in fenoterol use of one canister per month was associated with a threefold increase in mortality. The New Zealand Department of health withdrew fenoterol from use in 1990, and by 1992 mortality had fallen to almost a quarter of its previous high level; hospital admissions for asthma were also dramatically reduced. Because similar findings were reported with other short-acting β_2-agonists, ever since, patients have been taught to avoid regular or frequent use of their β_2-agonist, and instead to increase inhaled corticosteroid. These changes in prescribing habits were initially criticized by the pharmaceutical industry, but as the baby was not thrown out with the bathwater and short-acting β_2-agonists remain valuable "rescue" drugs the guidelines for their use became universally accepted.

The increases in mortality rates from asthma occurred at the same time as our increased understanding in the causes and treatment of the condition, and raised questions regarding asthma management. Why the increases progressed during the last two decades of the 20th century remains a matter of some debate; probably the asthma was under-diagnosed and its severity underestimated; treatment may have been inadequate and inconsistent; there may have been delays in applying research findings into routine clinical practice. There remains the fear that maybe, asthma is becoming more severe and more prevalent, due to environmental and host factors. However, mortality rates appear to reach a plateau in the late 1990s, giving rise to the hope that a corner has been turned. Recently, results were published of a 10-year study of deaths from asthma in Swedes aged less than 35; the incidence of death showed

a two-thirds decrease between 1994 and 2003. The study provided some clues regarding risk factors for death—under-treatment being top of the list; food allergy was implicated in 1/3, and exposure to animal dander in 1/5. It seems clear that better characterization of allergic factors and more aggressive treatment of asthma symptoms should improve the outcome of asthma patients.

MODERN MANAGEMENT OF ASTHMA

Asthma is a common condition with an appreciable morbidity and mortality. However, much is now known about the factors contributing to its cause and we have a range of effective drugs which have been studied in large, well controlled, randomized trials. Thus, it might be reasonably assumed that its management is simple and widely effective, but prospective long term follow-up investigations have revealed that many asthmatic patients are poorly controlled. Most chest physicians have encountered preventable deaths, such as the tragic occurrence of children who have died in their sleep. Clinical trials have shown that education of patients and their families is one key to good control. Other important factors include adequate initial assessment of severity, identifying causative agents, and measuring lung function. Inhaled corticosteroids to control bronchial inflammation are now considered first-line drugs, and inhaled β_2-agonists are used to control wheezing. Optimal inhalation technique has to be taught and reinforced during follow-up of progress. Guidelines for treatment have been developed, validated and published: there seems to be little excuse for the poor control revealed by long-term case control studies.

The story of asthma illustrates the evolution of medical science from observation and empirical application of simple practical treatments,

through an understanding of the physiological
and structural changes in asthma, to reach
the modern era, where treatment is guided
by measurement of airflow and the extent of
inflammation, and is evidence-based. The future
holds many challenges, not least in the area
of environmental air quality, but also with the
promise that eventually we will understand
what makes some of us (up to 20%) genetically
susceptible to developing airway inflammation
and over-reactive bronchial muscle.

CHAPTER 20

BREATHING SMOKE, AND ITS CONSEQUENCES

"A custome lothsome to the eye, hatefull to the nose, harmfull to the braine, dangerous to the lungs, and in the blacke stinking fume thereof neerest resembling the horrible Stigian smoake of the pit that is bottomlesse."

King James the First, 1604

In his "Counterblaste to tobacco" James I of England, Jamie the Saxt (sixth) to the Scots, got it right. However, his diatribe against tobacco smoking—"this filthy custome"—is not counted amongst his main legacies; more durable were the flag (the Union Jack) and the translation of the Bible authorized by him. Tobacco importers into the United Kingdom, from Sir John Hawkins and Sir Walter Raleigh 50 years before, continued to thrive in spite of the royal pronouncement. Cigarette consumption steadily rose through succeeding centuries. Closely paralleling this increase was an increase in two conditions that affected breathing—obstructive lung disorders and lung cancer. Millions have died from these conditions, and continue to do so: they are the focus of the present chapter. A question that lurks behind the story is—why did it take so long to recognize the association between them and smoking, and to do something about it?

PREVALENCE OF CIGARETTE SMOKING

The Aztecs, who had smoked tobacco for more than 1500 years, used hollow reeds in which to pack the leaf; in the first major change in the habit, a manufacturing process to produce cigarettes was devised in the 1870s. This had the double effect of increasing consumption and the concentration of toxic chemicals inhaled by smokers. Skilful advertising, that went as far as trumpeting "smoking is good for you", and a variety of social factors led to a steady increase in the smoking population, reaching its zenith in the Second World War, when Allied troops were issued free cigarettes cheaply made and with a high tar content. By the 1950s, 70% of British men were smoking regularly and women were smoking in increasing numbers.

In the USA the prevalence of cigarette smoking was small in 1900, but the *per capita* consumption in the USA increased ten-fold between 1900 and 1920 to reach about 700 cigarettes per annum per head of the population. The distribution of free cigarettes to the armed services led to sharp increases between 1915-20 and 1940-45, and overall *per capita* consumption in North America reached 3,500 in 1950, peaking at 4,300 in 1963. Data on smoking habits first appeared in a survey by the *Milwaukee Journal*; in 1935, 62% of males in the area were regular smokers, compared to 17% of females; by 1960 there was little further increase in males, to 70%, but the prevalence of adult female smokers had dramatically increased to 50%. Thereafter, a number of surveys showed a steady decline in cigarette consumption; in 1980 approximately 30% of both adult females and males smoked regularly. These historical figures contribute to the rates at which lung cancer mortality increased, both in the general population and in males versus females. The fact that smoking reached its peak in the mid-1960s implies that lung cancer rates will be highest in people that are now aged

60-80, but should then gradually decline. This appears to be happening.

Of course, such smoking statistics can never tell the whole story, because of large differences between individuals in smoking habits, including number of cigarettes smoked per day, the type of cigarette smoked (filter *vs.* plain, tar and nicotine content, depth of inhalation, etc). Habits, either individually chosen or promoted by cigarette manufacturers in their advertizing, have changed over the years. Surveys have shown that daily consumption in men has always been higher than women, that more men inhale deeply and also smoke cigarettes with higher tar and nicotine content. Also, women have used filter-tip cigarettes in greater numbers than men; a survey in 1964 showed 79% of adult women smokers and 54% of men used filter-tips. Unfortunately, filters have only a small effect on cancer-causing particles.

The average age that adults begin smoking has also changed; in the 1930s the average age at which women began to smoke was 35, but this has now dropped to 16, similar to men. Indeed the prevalence of smoking among teen-aged women now exceeds that of men.

INCIDENCE OF LUNG CANCER, AND THE LINK TO SMOKING

Before the 1920s, lung cancer was rare. However, over the subsequent two decades, an increasing incidence was noted, but put down to improved diagnosis and related factors. Incidence and mortality increased rapidly. An age effect was noted, with 60 year-olds being roughly 100 times more likely to be diagnosed than 40 year-olds, together with a gender effect—men being approximately 7 times more likely than women. In the 1960s, incidence in men peaked and began to fall, whereas in

women the incidence continued to increase; by 1983 the ratio of males to females had fallen to less than 3. In retrospect, it is easy to see that these trends followed trends in smoking habits, with a lag between the two of 20-30 years.

It was not until the 1950s that epidemiologists began to equate increases in mortality from a number of respiratory and cardiovascular disorders to increases in cigarette consumption.

Probably the most famous research on smoking was that begun by Richard Doll and Austin Bradford Hill in the early 1950s: 40,000 British doctors were surveyed on their smoking habits and followed for the ensuing 50 years.[1] The initial study revealed that risk of lung cancer increased with increases in amount smoked, by as much as 30 times, in those smoking in excess of 40 cigarettes daily.

The Royal College of Physicians of London, in what was probably its first real foray into the field of public health, commissioned a report on the health aspects of smoking. When published in 1962, it began a revolution in smoking habits; its major conclusion was that smoking was "the" cause of lung cancer, and also contributed to respiratory and cardiovascular ill health. The study of Doll and Hill in doctors, as well as providing mortality statistics, was able to follow the effects of stopping smoking; as the results appeared, the doctors rapidly appreciated they were being killed as well as their patients;

223

---

1 Doll and Bradford Hill were knighted for their ground-breaking work on links between tobacco and disease; Doll was nominated several times for the Nobel Prize, but was unsuccessful, perhaps due to the perception that epidemiology was less of a science than the technological advances in medical science of the latter half of the century. In terms of benefit to mankind, however, there can be no doubt regarding the value of his work.

between 1951 and 1964, over 50% of those in the study stopped smoking and the medical profession became a powerful force, both in education and in agitating for preventive action. After 15 years of stopping smoking, the death rate from lung cancer had fallen almost into the non-smokers' range. Politicians were slower to act: tax revenue from tobacco was vast, and of course the tobacco industry vigorously fought the findings.[2]

The second Royal College Report in 1971 lamented the inaction of the government, and dwelt at length on all the measures that might be taken, because tobacco sales had continued to rise. In most countries it took some time for action to be taken, in spite of the well publicized huge cost of smoking-related disease; however, advertising bans and educational programmes eventually brought changes. The prevalence of smoking in the adult male UK population fell from 55% to 33% between 1970 and 1990; in females there was a fall from 42% to 30% during the same period. By contrast, in populous "emerging" countries, such as India and China, consumption is increasing in parallel with affluence; in China cigarette sales increased from 500 billion in 1978 to 1,700 billion in 1992. The cigarette manufacturers opposed legislation, but it soon became clear, and eventually public, that they had known the health risks for many years. The manufacturers, now multinational conglomerates, persisted in denying the health effects, and even began to target advertising towards children and enhancing the nicotine content of cigarettes, to hasten the addictive process. However, in 1997 the Ligett Group, makers of Chesterfield cigarettes once advertised to "Cause no ills", finally admitted that smoking was addictive and a major cause of heart and

lung diseases and reached a monetary settlement with twenty-seven US States. In spite of all the anti-smoking initiatives, it is an uncomfortable fact that tobacco company profits have increased by more than 4-fold in the first decade of this century. Several Canadian Provinces are in the process of suing tobacco companies for health costs of smoking-related diseases.

EFFECT OF AMOUNT SMOKED

All large prospective studies have shown that lung cancer incidence and mortality increase with increasing duration and number of cigarettes smoked. This is impressively shown by data obtained in a study of US veterans. This led to the concept of "pack-years" of smoking, in which average cigarette usage in packs of cigarettes per day is multiplied by the total duration in years. Whilst this index is used extensively in clinical assessment, it seldom appears in epidemiological studies, mainly because of the unreliability in subjects' recall of their past cigarette usage. Most prospective surveys have used current smoking at enrolment as the index of smoking intensity, and in the best studies the smoking habits were documented regularly at follow-up. We do not have the information to quantify the difference in risk between, say, smokers with a 50 or 100 pack-year history, nor whether a 50 pack-year made up of 1 pack smoked for 50 years is equivalent to 2 packs smoked for 25 years. Recent studies have shown that for a given pack-years value, lower intensity smokers (<20/day) have a higher risk ratio than higher intensity smokers (>20/day). Duration is more important than intensity. The finding is consistent with experimental carcinogen studies in animals.

Another factor that, to this day, is insufficiently appreciated, was also revealed by the US veterans study is the age at which smoking

---

2 At its peak, the tax on cigarettes equaled the cost of the National Health Service.

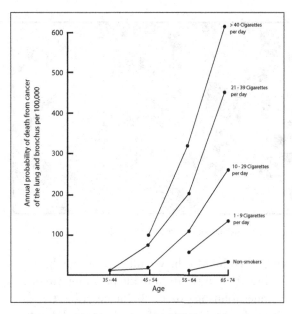

Figure 48 Death rates (per 100,000) for males, categorized by number of cigarettes smoked per day.

commenced. There is a steadily increase in cancer death rates as the age of starting drops below 25 years; smokers who began before the age of 15, had a 3-4 times higher death rate at age 60 than those who began at 25 or over. Recently, this finding has been supported by animal experiments in which age influences the effects of carcinogens on DNA damage.

The effect of quitting smoking could be studied in Doll and Hill's study of British doctors; the incidence of lung cancer fell 5 years after quitting, but never reached the rate in life-long non-smokers. Fifteen years after stopping the rate had dropped from 16 times to twice the rate of non-smokers.

Finally, surveys showed that less than 2% of lung cancer deaths occur in lifelong non-smokers; however, women non-smokers have a much higher relative risk than their male counterparts.

COMPOSITION OF CIGARETTE SMOKE

More than 4,000 chemicals have been identified in cigarette smoke, and most of them are toxic. They range from simple gases to complex particles. Of the gases, carbon monoxide dominates, but nitrogen oxides, ammonia and even hydrogen cyanide are present in measurable amounts. The smoke also contains particles, which in addition to nicotine include phenol, aniline and several benzene compounds. Gases have the potential to be absorbed from the lung in relation to their solubility; carbon monoxide binds to hemoglobin in blood, displacing oxygen by as much as 15% in heavy smokers, who thereby suffer equivalent effects to someone who is anemic to the same extent. Gases and particles that settle out on the walls of the bronchi and alveoli to cause a variety of effects—inflammation, mucus secretion and interference with the tiny hair-like cilia that help to move particles and mucus back up the airways to be cleared. Particles, such as nicotine, may be dissolved and rapidly absorbed; the pharmacological effects of nicotine on the brain are felt within 10 seconds.

SMOKING AND CHRONIC OBSTRUCTIVE PULMONARY DISEASE (COPD)

Chronic bronchitis and emphysema are collectively known as chronic obstructive pulmonary disease (COPD); the dominant cause for both is cigarette smoking.

Habitual cigarette smoking makes the smoker 12 times more likely to develop chronic bronchitis and emphysema than the life-time non-smoker, just as they are 13 times more likely to develop (and die from) lung cancer.[3]

225

---

3   The risk of other serious conditions, such as stroke, heart attack and cancer are all increased by 2-3 times.

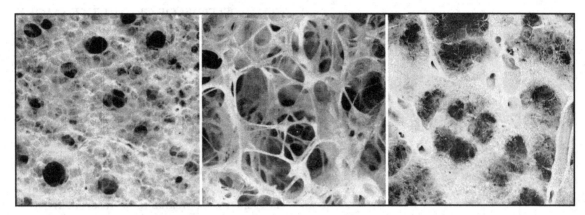

Figure 49 Normal lung (left) contrasted with emphysema, panacinar (middle) and centrilobular (right)

The main diagnostic criterion for the diagnosis of COPD and asthma is a reduction of airflow in the lung. By far the most robust measurement is the FEV_1, the volume of air exhaled during the first second of a forced expiration. This spirometry volume is compared to standards in the population, which take into account age, gender and stature. Most (over 95%) of the healthy population have an FEV_1 that is at least 80% of the predicted (standardized) value. The measurement is used to assess severity, disability, and the response to treatment; thus, it has become a mandatory measure in anyone with chronic or recurrent cough and wheezy breathing, and shortness of breath due to any cause. Also it is simple enough to be used in prevalence studies. For example, it was used in studies of children of smoking parents show evidence of poor lung development compared to their non-exposed peers.

EMPHYSEMA

The term "emphysema" is derived from the Greek word for "blown up" or "inflated", and was first used for collections of air in tissues; later it came to be applied to the generalized over-distension of the alveoli. The first clear description of pulmonary emphysema was published by Matthew Baillie in 1807, which included an illustration made post mortem of Dr Samuel Johnson's lung.[4] Baillie describes the distended lungs and air "cells", which did not collapse when the chest was opened at post mortem; he recognized the destructive nature of the condition, in which "the accumulation may break down two or three contiguous cells into one, and thereby form a cell of very large size". However, it is generally conceded that a modern understanding of emphysematous changes in the lung and how they affected function dates from the work of René Théophile-Hyacinthe Laënnec, inventor of the stethoscope and author of *A Treatise on the Diseases of the Chest.*[5] The

4   Dr Johnson was a heavy smoker, but apparently was quite guilty about it; his biographer, James Boswell quotes him as saying "to be sure, it is a shocking thing, blowing smoke out of our mouths into other people's mouths, eyes, and noses, and having the same thing done to us".

5   There are several translations of the title "De l'Auscultation Médiate ou Traité du Diagnostic et des Malaries des Poumons et du Coeur", first published in 1819. The full title of the translation by Dr John Forbes in 1821was "A Treatise on the Diseases of the Chest, in which they are described according to their anatomical characters, and their Diagnosis established on a new

English translation by John Forbes, published in 1821 is dedicated to Matthew Baillie, and Laënnec gives full credit to him, quoting at length from his descriptions of the pathology; however, he rightly avers that "the disease is very little known, and has not hitherto been correctly described"; that it is "by no means infrequent"; and that it is "in some sort merely an *exaggeration* of the natural condition", that is of the aging process. By combining the information gained in life through the stethoscope with the examination of lungs post mortem, Laënnec made a quantum leap—"In emphysema the air makes its escape from the air cells much slower than in the healthy state of the organ. This seems to indicate either more difficult communication between air contained in the air cells and that of the bronchi or else diminished elasticity of the air cells themselves. Perhaps both these causes conspire to produce the effect in question". Laënnec recognized that emphysema often coexisted with a variable degree of airway narrowing due to chronic bronchitis, but its essence was that of alveolar enlargement with destruction of alveolar walls. The concept of tissue destruction is crucial to the modern definition of emphysema; the implications were recognized in 1840 by the London pathologist Thomas Hodgkin who wrote that it was "more correctly considered as an instance of atrophy, since the total weight of the lung is evidently reduced, and the vascularity of the texture, and the absolute extent of the surface exposed to the inspired air, are diminished". It would be more than one hundred years before this pathological description would be improved by Jethro

Gough, and the reduction in lung elasticity would be measured by David Bates, both in 1952. Gough devised a simple method in which thin slices of the whole lung could be mounted on paper to enable measurements of the size of alveoli and bronchi, Emphysema was characterized by large air spaces, either affecting all alveoli in a segment of lung ("panacinar" or "panlobular") or mainly the central regions next to the small bronchi ("centriacinar"or "centrilobular")—the type associated with chronic bronchitis. Gough worked in Cardiff; many of his studies were on the lungs of Welsh coalminers; huge amounts of coal dust were deposited in their lungs, concentrated in the central parts of the lung lobule, leading to an appearance of large black holes scattered through the lung, and surrounded by relatively normal looking alveoli. The destruction was located in the parts of the lung where the relatively large coal particles had settled out.

The question, what causes emphysema? was much debated through the 19th century; the recognition that wheezing, or slowed expiration, associated with increases in lung size was an invariable feature of emphysema, suggested that alveoli enlarged and their walls eventually destroyed through the action of mechanical factors. The analogy was drawn to an elastic band which, with constant stretching and aging, gradually loses its elasticity and eventually breaks. This simplistic theory had to be thrown out after two Swedish physicians reported their findings in *The Scandinavian Journal of Clinical and Laboratory Medicine* in 1963.

Carl-Bertil Laurell and Sten Eriksson worked in the medical biochemistry department in Malmö; they were interested in one of the protein groups found in blood plasma, alpha-1-globulin. They embarked on a large study to investigate the variation in its concentration, and by chance

---

principle of Acoustick Instruments", which might be considered nowadays as a bit over the top, but when the book is read, fully justified. Laënnec was born in Quimper, Brittany, spent most of his career in Paris and died in Quimper from tuberculosis at the age of 45.

found very low levels in two emphysema patients in the local respiratory disease hospital. It was already known that this fraction of the proteins in blood was a potent inhibitor of the digestive enzyme trypsin which breaks down dietary protein—a "proteinase". Another example of a chance finding leading a prepared mind to a previously unrecognized discovery, Laurell realized that increased tissue protein breakdown in the lung might be an important cause of emphysema.[6] They found that severe deficiency of "alpha$_1$-antitrypsin" (α_1AT) had a familial incidence. Eriksson went on to study the families for his doctoral thesis; he found that 80% of males and 50% of females in families with severe α_1AT deficiency developed emphysema, most in their 40s, younger than usual patients. The work unlocked a door to a host of studies into the genetics, geographical distribution and biological effects of α_1AT deficiency, and to experimental emphysema produced by introducing proteinases into the airways of animals. Thus, the main hypothesis that resulted from this research was that emphysema results from the action of proteinases produced by activated leukocytes, on the elastic fibres of the alveolar walls. The elastases are liberated as only one group of many enzymes and cytokines produced during the process of inflammation, and normally they are rapidly inactivated so that their main effect is limited. In susceptible individuals, represented at the most extreme end of the spectrum by people who lack α_1AT, elastic tissue is lost, leading to breakdown of alveolar walls and

228

expanded air spaces. The stimuli that lead to leukocyte activation include cigarette smoke and air pollutants; there is a close relationship between extent of emphysema and smoking history, and the geographical distribution of emphysema follows that of air pollution. The condition also is traditionally linked to the other smoking related lung disorder chronic bronchitis.

CHRONIC BRONCHITIS

Laënnec noted thickening of bronchial walls and narrowing of the bronchial lumen in association with emphysema; he termed the condition chronic pulmonary catarrh, and identified several types according to the type of mucus that patients coughed up. An early, but perceptive, description of the effects of chronic bronchitis was that of Charles Badham who wrote *Observations on the inflammatory Affections of the Membrane of the Bronchi* in 1808. Dedicating his book to his most illustrious

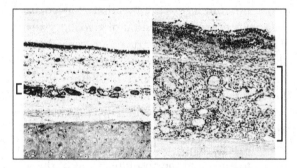

Figure 50 Cross section of bronchial wall showing thickness of mucous gland layer in normal bronchus (left) contrasted to chronic bronchitis (right)

patient, His Royal Highness the Duke of Sussex, he then provided a description of the "inflammatory affection of the part of the mucous membrane which lines the bronchial tubes", which could lead to "death... occasioned by the mechanical obstruction which ensues or by the interruption of the reciprocal operations of

---

6   Laurell's research led to the recognition of the essential function of a whole family of protease inhibitors that control the breakdown of protein as part of complex biochemical processes, such as blood clotting. Later it was shown that the deficiency of α_1AT was due to abnormal folding of the molecule during its formation in the liver, leading to new concepts of genetically mediated diseases.

the air and blood upon each other". In modern terms, Badham recognized that chronic bronchial inflammation and mucus production disturbed the normal distribution of air and blood to the alveoli where gas exchange took place. Soon after, in 1844, the term "chronic bronchitis" was used by William Stokes as a diagnostic label for patients who had a chronic productive cough for which no other cause was apparent, but over the next hundred years the diagnosis remained controversial because no clear pathological changes had been shown. In North America many authorities denied its separate existence; a standard textbook of the 1960s stated that it never existed alone, but was always due to other lung problems, or heart disease.

In 1932 the young Howard Florey, who later went on to win the Nobel Prize, jointly with Fleming and Chain, for the discovery and synthesis of penicillin, identified the problem as over-production of mucus, showing the enlargement of the mucous glands in the bronchial wall and overgrowth of mucus producing "goblet" cells in the lining. However, the definitive description had to wait until Lynne McArthur Reid, working at the Brompton Hospital in London in the late 1950s, showed how mucous gland enlargement caused airway narrowing and was associated with chronic inflammation of the bronchial wall. The work led to the "Reid Index"—the proportion of the bronchial wall taken up by mucus glands—that described the severity of bronchial wall inflammation. Normally about 25%, it may exceed 75% in severe chronic bronchitis (Figure 50).

The upshot of research during the 1950s and 60s was that two separate processes could be identified that were both triggered by cigarette smoking and air pollution—one in the alveoli and the other in bronchi. In the

alveoli, the effects appeared to be mediated by the liberation of enzymes, proteinases, which caused alveolar enlargement and destruction; and in the bronchi, inflammatory changes led to enlarged mucous glands and thickening of bronchial walls. Not surprisingly, as Laënnec had found, the two frequently coexisted; frequently, but not always. Patients were found who had died after many years of wheeze, productive cough and shortness of breath, whose lungs showed widespread bronchitis but no trace of emphysema. At the other end of the "spectrum" were patients—typified by those with α_1AT deficiency—with severe emphysema but without any bronchitis. Both chronic bronchitis and emphysema are characterized by the slowing of airflow into and (especially) out of the lungs; in the former, airway narrowing is the major problem, and in the latter a loss of alveolar structure means that the small airways are not supported and the lung does not retract effectively on breathing out, leading to mainly expiratory airflow slowing.

In 1961 it was my great good fortune to be appointed registrar to Dr CM Fletcher at the Royal Postgraduate Medical School at the Hammersmith Hospital in London. Charles Montague Fletcher was the son of Sir Walter Morley Fletcher, the first secretary of the British Medical Research Council; at Cambridge he won a rowing blue on his way to becoming a physician. As a young physician in Oxford, he was the first to administer penicillin to a human patient, a policeman with an invasive carbuncle: the staphylococcal skin infection responded, but because the production of penicillin from *penicillium* mould was so slow, and in spite of the extraction of the antibiotic from the patient's urine, he subsequently died. At the early age of 31 Fletcher was appointed director of a new unit in South Wales, set up to research into coal workers' pneumoconiosis, a lung disease caused by inhalation of coal dust. By applying several new techniques of measurement, he showed that changes in the chest X-ray were related to the extent of dust exposure and smoking, and how risks could be minimized. For this work he was awarded one of the highest civil honors, the CBE (Commander of the British Empire). Health education was one of his passions and for many years he presented the BBC TV series *Your Life in their Hands*, much to the consternation of the medical establishment, represented by the British Medical Journal, which ran a series of vitriolic editorials against letting the public onto the medical profession's private turf; 20 years later the BMJ apologized and acknowledged the value of his work. His work on the importance of cigarette smoking in causing chronic bronchitis had already been recognized by his appointment as secretary of the Royal College of Physicians Reports—*Smoking and Health* —published in 1962 and 1971. To learn more about factors that influence the development of airway obstruction, Fletcher and his colleagues, Dr Cicely Tinker and Richard Peto, recruited 900 Post Office workers and followed them for a decade, documenting symptoms and breathing capacity. As is the case in asthma, limitation of airflow was found to be best assessed by the FEV_1—the volume of air expired in the first second of a forced expiration. The study showed that the amount of sputum produced, and reductions in FEV_1, were both related to the amount smoked, but independently. The decline in FEV_1 in some of the workers could be as much as 4 times as fast their compatriots, suggesting that the degree of airway inflammation and lung destruction caused by smoking depends in part on genetically determined cell factors in the individual. In the 1960s there was a thirty-to-one difference in mortality from chronic bronchitis between the United States and Britain; it became known as the "British Disease", and appeared to

contrast with the incidence of emphysema, which appeared to be more common in the US. The opportunity to compare the incidence

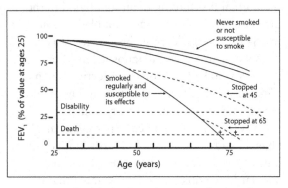

Figure 51 Charles Fletcher's diagram to illustrate the effects of smoking on the decline in FEV , and the effect of quitting smoking

of the two conditions was afforded by Dr Benjamin Burrows, of the University of Chicago, who suggested that patients attending his "Emphysema Clinic" be compared with those attending our "Bronchitis Clinic" at the Hammersmith Hospital. Fifty patients were studied in each clinic and followed for five years. In brief, there were no major differences between the patients in London and Chicago; Londoners coughed a little more, which we put down to greater exposure to air pollution, most of them having lived through the notorious smog years. As the study continued a proportion died and we were given the opportunity to examine the lungs and measure the degree of emphysema and bronchitis; it then became possible to identify the features that distinguished patients with bronchitis and little or no emphysema, from those with mainly emphysema. The differences were intriguing.

Typically, patients with bronchitis and severe airway obstruction were overweight, placid individuals with a bull neck and florid features; their lungs were normal in size and elasticity,

230

but their blood oxygen levels were low and carbon dioxide high—this was due to areas in the lower part of the lungs that were poorly ventilated, and to a reduced responsiveness of breathing to CO_2. The low oxygen makes them into "high altitude residents at sea level", their blood hemoglobin rising to similar levels as people living high in the Andes; low oxygen also constricts the small blood vessels in the lung causing the pressure to rise in the pulmonary artery. In time they develop features of "heart failure" (known medically as "cor pulmonale "), with swollen legs and large heart, due partly to the rise in pressure and partly to water retention by the kidneys. Tony Dornhorst, Professor of Medicine at St Thomas's Hospital, had described them as being "blue and bloated", which was later turned into the less elegant appellation "blue bloaters". In our Chicago-London comparison study we termed them "Type B".

The contrast between the type B patient and those who had severe emphysema ("Type A") could not have been more marked; such patients were skinny to the point of emaciation, intensely short of breath and agitated. Their lungs were voluminous and inelastic, but blood oxygen and CO_2 were usually normal at rest; however, when they exercised blood oxygen fell and their dyspnea was especially distressing. Fluid retention was rare and the heart not enlarged. In Dornhorst's words they were "pink and puffing"—later they were called the "pink puffers". Not surprisingly, many patients had features of both emphysema and chronic bronchitis ("Type X")—38 of the 100 in our study, compared with 27 characterized as type A, and 35 as type B.

The explanation of the striking differences between the "typical" clinical pictures we termed Type A and type B still eludes us; why should severe emphysema be associated with a pink and puffing, emaciated individual, and the blue and bloated, overweight bronchitic be found to have little or no emphysema? Perhaps the obese smoker necessarily breathes shallowly, leading to the deposition of particles in large airways, rather than alveoli, and the full picture develops from there. Perhaps the mechanisms that lead to alveolar destruction, with poor inactivation of proteinase enzymes, are also linked to other metabolic responses that control body weight. This is just another instance of disturbances of breathing spilling their effects into other body systems that include especially the autonomic nerves, immune reactions, heart and circulation, and the brain.

Because the two conditions of emphysema and chronic bronchitis frequently coexisted, and both showed severe airway obstruction, the term *chronic obstructive pulmonary disease* (COPD) was adopted in the 1970s, and has now replaced "chronic bronchitis and emphysema" as the main diagnostic term. The term may also include patients with long-standing asthma, who have airway inflammation and narrowing; the inflammation differs from chronic bronchitis in the cell types involved, and the airway obstruction is more variable, but the clinical picture may overlap chronic bronchitis. The definitions used to classify individuals as having emphysema, bronchitis and asthma are not mutually exclusive—frequently a patient will meet the criteria for all three.

The term COPD is also justified by the fact that treatment is determined by the effects, rather than the underlying cause. Two large multicentre controlled trials showed that long term oxygen treatment is beneficial in patients whose blood oxygen saturation is reduced—increasing their life expectancy by 5-6 years. The use of inhaled steroids and bronchodilators is indicated in patients who respond to them with an increase in FEV_1. Surgery to reduce lung volume and thereby increase elasticity, or even lung transplantation, is used in highly selected chronically disabled patients. Replacement of α_1-antitrypsin is expensive and as yet unproven. The treatment options are not large, placing importance on general measures to improve outlook and quality of life; smoking cessation and physical rehabilitation are mainstays of the clinical approach.

Patients with COPD become very disabled, mainly but not only because of shortness of breath. For a long time the severity of shortness of breath puzzled many physicians because it seemed out of proportion to the degree of airway obstruction, but a systematic approach to the problem, in which the symptom was measured during exercise, and various components identified, went far to solving the enigma. The sensation arises in the muscles of breathing and is appreciated as a sense of effort. As with any other muscle, the sense of effort depends on the one hand on the force being exerted, and on the other, on it and the capacity to meet those demands. In patients with COPD the effort expended in breathing is intense because the demands are increased and the breathing capacity reduced; the combination leads to an intensity of breathlessness during exertion that may be as much as ten times as high as that normally experienced. Because of the structural changes in the lung, its efficiency is poor and an increase in breathing is required to clear carbon dioxide; blood oxygen pressure falls, giving rise to an additional stimulus to breathe more. Increases in the resistance to airflow mean that greater pressures are required to move air, and loss of the lung's elasticity lead to overexpansion of the lung; breathing requires much more effort if the lungs are already expanded. Muscles generate their power most effectively when they start

232

contracting from a normal resting length; however, the overexpansion of the chest means that breathing muscles are already shortened before they begin contracting. Finally, the breathing muscles gradually weaken with age; to produce any pressure requires more effort. As we observed more and more patients, we began to realize that many of them were not limited by the sense of effort in breathing, but by a sense of fatigue in their leg muscles. All their muscles were weak, presumably the result of years of relative inactivity: those patients who had maintained their fitness were much less disabled than their unfit compatriots. Weaker patients obtained great benefit from a muscle strengthening programme, which has now become an important measure in our efforts to keep patients active and independent.

We end this chapter as we began it—with smoking. In his study of Post Office workers, Charles Fletcher, besides showing that the more cigarettes smoked the faster lung function declined, demonstrated the benefits of smoking cessation in slowing or halting further decline. The prevalence of smoking in most Western nations is declining and air quality has improved since the smog-days in 1950s London. The incidence of chronic bronchitis is falling, but COPD remains a major health problem—the fourth ranking cause of death in the US and costing its economy an estimated $30 billion each year. In less well developed countries the use of wood and animal dung for heating and cooking in poorly ventilated dwellings, together with increasing prevalence of smoking is inevitably causing an increase in COPD world-wide. One can hear the echo of Jamie the Saxt ringing down over five hundred years—"I told ye so". However, the clear benefits of stopping smoking provide a great incentive to increase our efforts to reduce the scourge of tobacco. As the last line of the second Royal College Report, written by Charles Fletcher, put it—"The goal is the preservation of the lives and health of thousands of smokers who would otherwise continue to become ill and die before their time".

In Canada now, the prevalence of smoking has fallen from over 50% a few decades ago to 19%, as a result of vigorous anti-smoking campaigns.[7] However, there remain groups of individuals in whom progress in smoking prevention is slow—in the young, in aboriginals, in women, in people already showing symptoms of COPD. A particular concern is the prevention of smoking in the young, who are at special risk; 50% of smoking teenagers will continue to smoke for at least 20 years, doubling their risk of premature death. Charles Fletcher—chest physician, researcher, brilliant public speaker and educator—used to become despondent when reviewing the results of education programs aimed at teenagers. Thirty years later, this group continues to pose a great challenge, in spite of advances in our understanding of the teenage brain; new approaches and fresh effort are needed before we can claim success in achieving our goal of eradicating the preventable diseases caused by smoking. Of these diseases COPD has smoking as its only cause, allowing us to hope that we might eradicate a condition that is responsible for a huge economic and human burden.

7   In 2008, Health Canada set out its Tobacco Control Strategy, with the main aim of reducing the prevalence further, to 12% by 2011.

CHAPTER 21

INFECTED BREATHS "Captain of the men of death"

"...(I have been seen by) the three most famous doctors on the island. One sniffed at what I spat up, the second tapped where I spat it from, the third poked about and listened how I spat it. One said I had died, the second that I am dying and the third that I shall die"

Frédéric Chopin, 1847.

The unfortunate Chopin was suffering from tuberculosis, and writing to a friend from the island of Majorca; he had gone there with his companion, the novelist George Sand, hoping to benefit from some good weather by the sea. The weather was poor and Chopin worsened—the third doctor was correct in his prognosis, and he died at the age of 39. Living in the mid-nineteenth century, he was in good company for many of the Romantics—poets, writers, musicians—fell victim to the disease. In 1815 Thomas Young estimated that it caused premature death in as many as one in four; in the US urban population the peak mortality rate reached 400 per 100,000. Whilst we remember the rich and famous who died young from the disease, tuberculosis was predominantly a disease of the poor and under-nourished. Improvements in housing and nutrition were followed by a reduction in mortality, before the discovery of antibiotics; in Great Britain the mortality by 1950 was only a tenth of what it had been 100 years before. After 1950, with the introduction of anti-tuberculous drugs , the decline accelerated about four-fold to reach its lowest incidence at the beginning of the 1980s; in England the notification rate reached 8.6 per 100,000, and mortality was less than 1 per 100,000. More recently there has been an increase related to HIV infection and AIDS, and to immigration, especially from the Indian sub-continent.

Tuberculosis is only one, though admittedly seen by most of us as the most lethal, of many infective agents that can wreak havoc in the lungs and eventually cause death. Their number contains viruses, bacteria, fungi, and parasites, and their effects range from colonization without serious sequelae to widespread pneumonia, where both lungs can become virtually airless, full of fluid and the products of inflammation. The effects of infection in the respiratory tract is often described as a battle between the virulence of the invading organism and the strength of the defences presented locally in the lungs and generally by the body's immune system. Although this "model" of respiratory infection has a number of shortcomings, it provides a good starting point for discussion. The combination often defines the characteristic effects of a given organism. For example, the organism *pseudomonas pyocyaneous* seldom causes a problem unless defence mechanisms lead to accumulation of mucus, as in cystic fibrosis; *haemophilus influenzae* causes the recurrent flare-ups of chronic bronchitis; and *legionella* is the cause of severe pneumonia (Legionnaires' Disease) in small epidemics of middle aged and elderly individuals, often with a chronic disease such as diabetes. The same interplay between the characteristics of the organism and the state of an individual's defence mechanisms, will determine outcome.

There are a number attributes which influence an invader's capacity to damage the lungs.

234

These include its size—the smaller, the deeper the penetration into the lungs; its ability to penetrate into the cells of bronchi and alveoli; the presence of a coat that makes it difficult for the lungs' scavenger cells (macrophages) to engulf and neutralize it; the ability to reproduce rapidly; and its capacity to damage cells of the lung and immune system through the production of toxins or incorporation into cell's genetic code. Set against these aggressive properties are the respiratory system's defence mechanisms. These include the tiny hairs (cilia) on the cells lining the airways; the mucus produced by bronchial (goblet) cells and mucous glands in the bronchial walls; the cough reflex. To these may be added the body's immune system, consisting of locally produced macrophages, and white blood cells—neutrophils and lymphocytes. After bacteria and viruses have been taken up—phagocytosed—by cells, the cells produce enzymes capable of destroying infective agents; they then die and the molecular debris can then be removed from the airways in mucus by ciliary action, and coughing. Molecules that get through the alveolar walls, and into the delicate structures that form the lung's framework, are removed by lymphatics, fine tubes that can absorb large molecules and transport them to central lymph nodes, which act as garbage cans for the lungs. Of course, the immune system is complex and has many mechanisms for dealing with invaders; however, it is highly sensitive to aspects of general health—for example the state of nutrition, and the age of the individual. Many respiratory infections, whether viral or bacterial, are only lethal at the extremes of life.

A number of conditions are associated with inadequate lung defences, making the affected individuals particularly prone to infections. Some are genetically determined, as in the ciliary dyskinesia syndrome in which the cilia

do not function, and in cystic fibrosis, in which very viscid mucus is produced that cannot be cleared. Other situations are caused by acquired factors; cigarette smoke paralyzes the cilia, and virus infections can have the same effect, allowing bacteria to secondarily invade the lung. Conditions in which the body's immune system is compromised are particularly prone to lung infection; again, such conditions rarely may be congenital, and more commonly are acquired—as in the Acquired Immunodeficiency Syndrome (AIDS), in the malnourished and in people with debilitating disease, such as cancer or diabetes.

In the case of tuberculosis, the disease runs a two phase course in the lungs. The first, which often occurs in children and is usually termed the primary form, is characterized by a vigorous local response in the lung. There is a small focus of infection to which macrophages are attracted , followed by T-lymphocytes from the immune system; the reaction in the lung is often overshadowed by enlargement of the lymph nodes at the root of the lung, and it is soon followed by a positive Mantoux skin test. The secondary form consists of a more chronic inflammation in the lung: lung tissue is destroyed and replaced by cavities and scarring (fibrosis).

I can recall seeing my first patient with severe pulmonary tuberculosis in 1958, as clearly as if it was yesterday. An Army sergeant-major was referred to the British military hospital where I was the medical specialist. He was waiting for me in the entrance to the hospital, standing rigidly to attention and clutching a blood-stained handkerchief in one hand and a chest X-ray in the other. I could see that the X-ray was grossly abnormal, and when I looked at it on a viewing screen I saw evidence of tuberculosis in both lungs. On the left side a huge cavity had ruptured into the pleural space, which contained air and blood

235

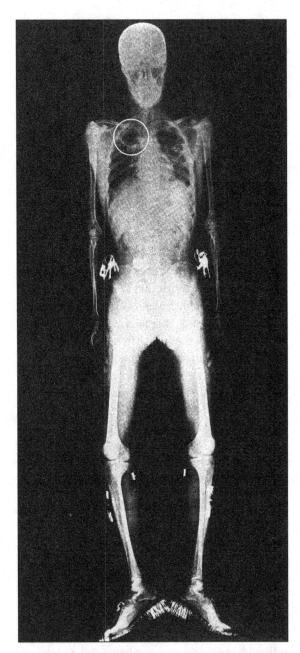

Figure 52 Röntgen's first radiograph of a man. In the upper region of the right lung (on the left of the picture) there is a large tuberculous cavity, seen as a white circle (circled in white).

(a "hematopneumothorax"). During the next few days we found that his wife showed a large

cavity in the lung and two of their four children, together with three of their schoolmates, had the primary form of the disease. Fortunately, they all responded well to treatment, but they remain to me a stark reminder of how infective the mycobacterium can be.

There are several reasons for choosing tuberculosis as an example of a serious lung infection, chief among them being its recognition since ancient times and the availability of epidemiological data since the early 1800s. Also, the tubercle bacillus, *Mycobacterium tuberculosus,* was the first organism to be recognized as the cause of a disease, by Robert Koch in 1882. Before Koch, Laennec had provided superb descriptions of both the clinical and pathological findings in *A Treatise on the Diseases of the Chest*, written in 1819, 5 years before he himself succumbed to the disease. Until the discovery of X-rays by Wilhelm Conrad Röntgen, Laennec's stethoscope was the tool in the clinical assessment of tuberculosis, but it was many decades before it was widely used. The same may be said of X-rays; although Röntgen's first picture of a man, taken in 1895, shows clear evidence of (apparently undiagnosed) advanced tuberculosis, more notice was taken of the keys hanging from the man's belt (he was clothed) than of the cavity in his lungs. Even in 1918, delegates to an international lung disease meeting were told that shadows on the chest X-ray were not likely to be significant if they were not accompanied by other clinical signs. Röntgen was the first recipient of the Nobel Prize for Physics in 1901.

Louis Pasteur had shown that micro-organisms were capable of fermentation, but at the time that Robert Koch presented his paper to the Berlin Physiological Society on May 22, 1882, tuberculosis was considered a familial disease, and there was great resistance to the acceptance

236

of his findings. The controversy was grounded in two different views of disease causation—the "cell theory" *versus* the "germ theory". Many eminent pathologists, chief among whom was Rudolph Virchow, believed that disease was due to a disorder of cell function, and sustained by cell division passing on the characteristics to "daughter" cells. Arguing against the cell theory was Pasteur, whose research into micro-organisms, suggested that germs were capable of invading the body to produce disease. Laennec, on the basis of close clinical observation of tuberculosis, was a strong supporter of this concept.

To counter the resistance that he expected to his observations, Koch brought with him to the 1882 meeting a laboratory demonstration of the organism. Koch's intuition did not fail him in this fear: Professor Virchow stormed out of the meeting in disgust. It seems quite likely that, at least in part, Virchow's anger was due to professional snobbery. Only six years before his dramatic presentation in Berlin, Koch was a lowly general practitioner, and a nonentity in the scientific world. He wrote to Professor Cohn in Breslau to tell him of his systematic research into the bacillus that caused anthrax, and presented his findings to a critical academic audience who were astonished at the quality of his work. Nine years after the Berlin meeting the great Canadian physician William Osler, in his *Principles and Practice of Medicine*, called it "one of the most masterly demonstrations of modern medicine" and expressed his opinion that in spite of great interest and intense research over the intervening years "the innumerable workers at the subject have not, as far as I know, added a solitary essential fact to those presented by Koch". More than a demonstration of the staining and culture characteristics of the tubercle bacillus, Koch was able to rout the opposition by providing scientific proof of the cause of an infection,

by testing the evidence against four criteria, which ever since have been known as "Koch's Postulates". Thus an organism, first, had to be capable of being isolated in every case of the disease; second, it had to be cultured and grown in pure form; third, the pure culture had to produce the disease when inoculated into laboratory animals, such as the guinea pig; and fourth, the organism had to be retrievable from the inoculated diseased animal and recultured. In this way, through innumerable studies of thousands of cases, Koch had proved the cause of tuberculosis to be the *Mycobacterium tuberculosis*. Koch's Postulates have stood the test of time; indeed, they have been adapted to establish cause and effect for other conditions, such as the link between smoking and lung cancer. In this respect his work had an impact that was similar to Darwin's *On the Origin of Species*; the theory of natural selection was seized by others to underpin their theories in other fields—such as Karl Marx who saw it "as a basis in natural science for the historic class struggle". Koch was later appointed to the department of health in the district, and applied himself to the problem of tuberculosis control. He was awarded the Nobel Prize in 1905.

Koch was desperate to improve the treatment of tuberculosis: following Jenner's success in immunization for smallpox, he developed an extract of a protein derived from cultures of the mycobacterium—tuberculin—that was given by injection. His faith in this regime was misplaced: it was no cure, and indeed caused a severe flare up in tuberculous skin lesions. The Viennese paediatrician who first used the term "allergy", Clemens von Pirquet, suggested that a local reaction to the injection of tuberculin into the skin might prove to be valuable in the diagnosis. The French physician Charles Mantoux took up the idea and modified it into a clinically usable procedure, ever since known as the Mantoux test. Apart from some technical improvements this simple skin test has remained the most widely used indicator of exposure to tuberculosis. Even his idea of vaccination treatment was to bear fruit many years later, when BCG inoculation was introduced. BCG stands for *Bacille Calmette-Guérin*, after Albert Calmette, a bacteriologist, and his assistant Camille Guérin, a veterinarian, who worked in the Institut Pasteur in Lille during the first two decades of the 20th century. They noted that repeated sub-culturing of the bovine tuberculosis bacillus eventually led to a non-virulent live bacillus, that prevented the development of disease in research animals. Although first used in human subjects in 1922, there was resistance to its use until after World War II. Then, BCG vaccination of 8 million babies was successful in preventing the expected post-war epidemic of tuberculosis. Now BCG is offered to individuals who do not react to the Mantoux skin test—they have not been previously infected with the bacillus—and especially if they are likely to be in contact with it (health care workers, etc). It has been estimated that BCG is 80% effective.

238

The work of Robert Koch provided techniques in the diagnosis of tuberculosis that remained unchanged well into the second half of the 20th century—not only the stains used to identify the organism in sputum and methods to culture it in the laboratory, but also the diagnostic inoculation of material into guinea pigs, and the Mantoux skin test, all remained as important clinical tools. It is only very recently that molecular techniques have been developed to provide more rapid results than can be obtained with these "tried and true" clinical methods.

Whilst mortality steadily declined in the first half of the 20th century, this was due to improvements in public health measures. In the 1920-40s a number of treatments were

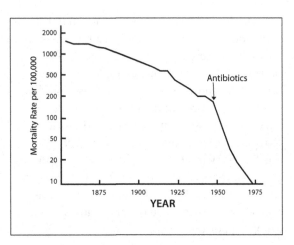

Figure 53 Standardized death rates (per 100,000) in England and Wales; the scale is not linear—there was a fall from 1600 to 200 between 1850 and 1950, when streptomycin began to be widely used, with a further fall to 10 by 1975

advocated, but none proved effective. Bed rest and interventions to rest the affected parts of the lungs seemed to be the tuberculous patient's only hope. Those who could afford it went to an alpine sanatorium; the great German novelist Thomas Mann wrote about his experiences in Davos in the 1920s in *The Magic Mountain*. Interestingly, there was a vogue for vitamin treatment—such as vitamin D, which went along with alpine sun exposure. One of the B vitamins, nicotinamide was also used; although by itself it was ineffective, several drugs were later developed from it, including the highly effective isoniazid and ethionamide. However, a revolution in treatment was ushered in by Alexander Fleming's discovery of a mould that had antibacterial properties. Whilst penicillin was found to be ineffective against the tubercle bacillus, streptomycin saved the day.

Albert Schatz, a graduate student at Rutgers University with the soil microbiologist Selman A Waksman, detected streptomycin in a culture of actinobacteria in 1943, and in 1944 Waxman showed that it was active against the tubercle bacillus. In the same year, two researchers at the Mayo Clinic, William H Feldman and H Corwin Hinshaw, infected guinea pigs with a virulent human strain of *M. tuberculosis*; streptomycin reduced the infection and was well tolerated, although their supply of the drug ran out before the study was completed. Then in a remarkable move Waksman persuaded Georg Merck, the owner of the pharmaceutical company that bears his name, to produce streptomycin in industrial quantities. Not only did Merck take on this multi-million dollar endeavour, but also he returned the patent to Rutgers, thus ensuring that research could continue. The first patients to be treated with streptomycin in 1945 were reported as showing a dramatic response, and the antibiotic was hailed as a wonder drug. At this point there occurred one of the defining moments in medicine, ushering in the era of the randomized controlled trial (RCT), laying the seeds of the later "evidence-based medicine". The first trial was conducted by the British Medical Research Council (MRC), which directed trials that became progressively more sophisticated over the succeeding 40 years. In the first, 104 patients with pulmonary tuberculosis were divided into two groups; 54 were treated with streptomycin and 50 were treated with bed rest alone. The trial showed improved mortality (4 died in the streptomycin and 14 in the control group), and better clearing of the bacilli in sputum (8 vs. 2) over the six months of treatment, but the mortality after five years was similar in the two groups (53% vs. 64%, respectively), because of the development of resistance to the drug.

At the same time that streptomycin was being developed, the Danish chemist Jörgen Lehmann working at Sweden's Göteborg University and its hospital, the Sahlgrenska Sjukhuset, synthesized a derivative of aspirin, para-amino salicylic acid (PAS), which interfered with the growth of the tubercle bacillus. The second MRC trial was begun in the same year as the disappointing long-term results of the first were published, in 1948. In this (second) landmark trial patients were randomized to receive streptomycin alone, PAS alone, or the two drugs in combination. After 6 months the results clearly showed that the combination worked best, the addition of PAS reducing the development of resistance to streptomycin, from 80% to 12%. Since that time combinations of drugs have been standard practice. In 1952 isoniazid was added to the regime after studies that showed it was very effective and safe; when all three drugs were taken for a year the number of permanent cures increased dramatically. Isoniazid was a major breakthrough, and had the welcome side effect of making patients happy; later, it was recognized as the first monoamine oxidase inhibitor—a class of drugs that proved effective in depressive disorders. However, this regime was expensive and it proved difficult to get patients to take it continuously for the full year. One reason was the large amount of PAS required; it came in capsules the size of four quarters piled up, and gastric side effects were frequent; it proved particularly difficult for children to take. During the 1960s to 80s, these problems were systematically tackled by one RCT after another under the direction of the MRC. The Tuberculosis Chemotherapy Centre was established in Madras in 1956, and trials were based in Hong Kong, Singapore, and East Africa, as well as Europe and America; new drugs were tested, different durations of treatment were compared and home based treatment compared to sanatorium care. At each step the design of the studies established solid evidence of each successive improvement in treatment. Among new drugs, ethambutol replaced PAS, and rifampin and pyrazinamide were developed in the 1950s, but no new agents have been introduced in the past 30 years. Home based treatment was as effective as in the sanatorium and relatives were no more likely to develop TB; direct observation of treatment was shown to be invaluable, leading to regimens that did not require drugs to be taken every day. The most successful strategies included an initial two month intensive 4-drug regime, followed by six months of a 2-drug combination. This regime is one of the standard approaches used to the present day; rifampin, streptomycin, isoniazid and pyrazinamide are given for two months, followed by rifampin and isoniazid for a further 4 months.

So successful were these trials that John Bunyan's "captain of all these men of death", the disease that had been the leading infectious cause of death for over a thousand years, was itself considered to be at death's door by the mid-1980s; indeed the MRC research units were all closed in 1986, ending a remarkable 40 years of continuous success. Many people, with the benefit of hindsight, criticized the closure of the research clinics, because at about the time of their closure it became clear that tuberculosis and HIV infection were very happy bed-fellows. Especially in the poorer countries of Africa the AIDS epidemic was accompanied by the resurrection of tuberculosis; as this coincided with the loss of the clinics and experienced medical and nursing staff, the infection became especially problematic. AIDS devastates the immune system, leading to aggressive forms of tubercular disease, and often drug reactions make it difficult for the AIDS victim to tolerate the usual drug combinations. Furthermore, resistance to the main drugs has become common, leading to failed treatment and relapses. To add a final level of difficulty, the antiviral therapy used for AIDS may interact with the main antibiotics. Although the problem is worst in Africa, tuberculosis is edging its way

back up the infectious disease leader board, even in rich countries of the developed world. There is renewed interest in the development of a preventive vaccine and antibiotics that are effective in a shorter time than the established drugs, and that cost less.

The battle seemed to have been won, but now there are new challenges; we have to hope they can be met with the same combination of imagination, intuition and science that was so successful in the past.

CHAPTER 22

BREATHING MACHINES

"To revive the animal...make an opening in the trachea... insert a tube of reed or cane...and blow into it...with a slight breath in the living animal, the lung will swell to its full extent and the heart becomes strong"

Andreas Vesalius, De Humanis Corpora Fabrica, 1543.

This book has been about the importance of breathing, for many reasons, but primarily to enable the supply of oxygen to all our cells, remove carbon dioxide and ensure homeostasis of our internal environment. If breathing is inadequate, blood oxygen falls, carbon dioxide increases and our internal environment becomes acid. Broadly speaking, there are two main causes of inadequate breathing. First, breathing may be just too difficult because our lungs are too damaged, our airways too narrowed, our breathing muscles too weak. And second, the mechanisms that control breathing may be impaired. Moran Campbell, with his usual flair for pithy descriptions, characterized the first as "can't breathe" and the second as "won't breathe". Of course, although there are pure examples of each, the combination ("I can't and I won't breathe") is common. In both situations it may be important to sustain breathing with the help of a machine.

The idea of sustaining breathing to maintain life had its origin deep in antiquity. In Egyptian mythology, the goddess Isis breathed into the mouth of Osiris to revive him. Galen, in spite of his weird theories of breathing, used a bellows to maintain ventilation of animals. Vesalius, though better known for his anatomical masterpiece, also conducted animal vivisections, opening the thorax to observe the actions of the heart and lungs, and provided the above directions to keep the animal alive when spontaneous breathing was impossible. As respiratory function became better understood, especially in the 20th century, artificial support of ventilation was seen to be a vital measure and a succession of methods was devised. All employed a machine to generate sufficient pressure to drive air into the lungs. The pressure applied was either negative, applied outside the chest, or positive applied in the airway. For both methods, it proved much easier to ventilate normal lungs (won't breathe or can't breathe because of respiratory muscle weakness) than lungs and airways that were stiff and narrowed. It's probably not surprising that the first widespread use of ventilators was for respiratory muscle weakness.

POLIO AND THE IRON LUNG

At school in the UK in the mid-1940s, each summer we went through a recurring terror—that we might contract poliomyelitis. In a large school everyone knew of someone afflicted, and even who had died, with the disease. A common theory, whether true or not I still am uncertain, was that a common site of its spread was the public swimming pool, leading parents to prohibit its use. If several cases occurred, the local pool was closed. In the US, outbreaks became particularly severe in the early part of the 20th century, with up to 50,000 deaths in a bad year. The deaths were nearly all related to paralysis of the muscles of breathing; in "mild" cases the intercostal muscles might be affected, but in "bulbar" polio the diaphragm became paralyzed and the mortality was close to 100%, with the child dying only a few hours after the first symptom of difficulty in breathing. The necessity of maintaining breathing was realized but established methods of resuscitation, manual chest compression and inflation with a bag and mask, could not be kept up for longer than a few hours. In 1928, Charles F McKhann, a young Assistant Professor at the Boston Children's Hospital, became aware of the work of Philip Drinker, an engineer working at the School of Public Health at Harvard, and asked for his help in managing a severe case of polio.

Drinker had been appointed to a commission at the Rockefeller Institute, formed to research new methods of resuscitation. His brother Cecil was a professor of physiology at Harvard, working on the control of breathing, and Philip went along to watch some experiments. Breathing was measured in cats by placing them in a box (a plethysmograph), with the head protruding through a hole and sealed around the neck, by recording changes in the volume of air in the box. Drinker placed a paralyzed cat into the box and found that breathing was readily maintained by means of a pump attached to an opening in the box; it proved easy to ventilate the cat for hours at a time. The notion that the method might be effectively applied to paralyzed humans was rapidly turned into reality by a local tinsmith, who built an adult-sized cylinder into which someone could be slid on a garage mechanic's "creeper". The hatch at the head of the cylinder contained a hole for the head, and a close-fitting rubber collar provided a seal. The pressure in the tank was varied by two vacuum cleaners made by the Electric Blower Company in Boston, one to exert negative pressure for inspiration and the other positive pressure for expiration. Later, the positive pressure blower was found to be unimportant as the lungs'

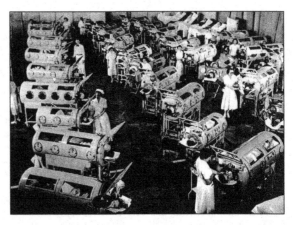

Figure 54 Tank ventilators being used in a US hospital at the height of the polio epidemic

own elasticity was sufficient to ensure adequate expiration. Drinker and his colleagues tried it out, and found that breathing was easily sustained—too easily if one was not careful. In the first trial, Drinker was ventilated for 15 minutes, and then worried the others by not breathing for 4 minutes. Hyperventilation had led to the blowing off of CO_2 and consequent respiratory inhibition.

In 1928, a clinical trial of Drinker's iron lung was proposed by Dr McKhann when one of his patients, an eight-year-old girl with polio, developed difficulty in breathing. The machine was brought into her room so that the child could be reassured and not scared by the noise of the vacuum pumps. The next morning she was blue from lack of oxygen and comatose; she was placed in the respirator and "In a few minutes, her normal color had returned and she tried to talk". She was treated intermittently over the next few days, but died from an extensive pneumonia five days later. The response to the single case report was dramatic; several medical engineering firms undertook to produce the Drinker respirator in Europe as well as the US, where within a few years every hospital had at least one of the machines. The demand for them often outstripped their supply, especially in some epidemics—such as that in the Eastern US in 1931, when "there were many accounts of several patients arriving at the same time at hospitals that had only one iron lung". In the early 1950s, large children's hospitals gave up whole wings to accommodate up to 50 of the machines; Drinker even developed one capable of accommodating two patients at a time.

The Drinker iron lung is an example of a medical treatment that, in spite of an evident need, was delayed for an unbelievably long time, but that after publication of a single case report (an "n of one" study to use the jargon of present-day evidence based medicine), so caught the imagination of the profession, that within a very short time it became standard treatment. But the principle of ventilating someone in a box by applying negative pressure around the chest, had been known for almost a century.

John Dalziel was the first to propose that patients with respiratory depression might be ventilated in this way. Dalziel, a physician in rural Scotland, presented his ideas in the *Journal of the British Association for the Advancement of Science* of 1832, describing an air-tight box in which the patient sat with his head protruding from the top; negative pressure was applied by bellows, and two windows allowed the movements of the chest to be watched. The first, and apparently only, record of its use appeared in 1840, when Dr Robert Lewins, from Leith—on the coast near Edinburgh—reported in *The Edinburgh Medical and Surgical Journal* that he had used the device in an unsuccessful attempt to resuscitate a drowned seaman; although the man was not brought back to life, onlookers were convinced of its success by the evident respiratory movements that were produced. Dr

Lewins himself was no less enthusiastic—"By elevating the piston of a large syringe which communicates with the interior…a partial void is created, to fill up which, the air from the atmosphere rushes into the lungs from the trachea". Then, in 1876, a young French physician, Joseph Woillez, described a cylinder that was virtually identical to the iron lungs manufactured fifty years later; however, the pump had to be powered by hand, thus limiting its use to acute resuscitation in mine disasters. The development of thoracic surgery gave another impetus to artificial respiration; the great Prussian surgeon Ernst Ferdinand Sauerbruch, Professor of Surgery at the University of Marburg, early in his career (1904) devised an operating chamber that was kept at a negative pressure—again, the head of the patient was kept outside—thus allowing the chest to be opened without the lungs collapsing. He also devised a positive pressure cabinet in which the patient breathed compressed air to prevent lung collapse while the chest was opened.

Respiratory physiology can only be understood quantitatively in terms of physics and engineering; of pressures acting on structures that have the properties of volume, resistance, elastance and inertia, to generate airflow and gaseous exchange sufficient to meet the demands of metabolism. To engineers the concepts are straightforward, almost trivial. This may account for the number of engineers who came to the rescue of their less knowledgeable clinical confreres by designing and manufacturing ventilators of ever-increasing sophistication. Perhaps the first modern engineer to become involved in ventilator design was Bernard Dräger, whose company Drägerwerk AG were renowned for their mine rescue apparatus. In 1907 they introduced the Dräger "Pulmotor" for resuscitation; the apparatus used cylinders of oxygen to generate sufficient positive pressure to inflate the lungs, and slight negative pressure to help deflation; a gramophone motor was used to cycle between inspiration and expiration. It was widely adopted and used by the Royal Humane Society, Police and Firefighters, but was never fully accepted by physicians; a prominent US respiratory physiologist, Yale's Yandell Henderson, sealed its fate by proclaiming that it was "a step backwards towards the death of thousands". The fear was that the pressure delivered to the lungs would cause rupture of the airways or alveoli, an example of a situation where an "evidence-based" approach would have upheld Dräger's engineering intuition. After Philip Drinker, another engineer, had demonstrated his "Iron Lung" in Europe in 1938, several firms, including Drägerwerk, began to manufacture tank respirators. In the late 1950s we used a Dräger iron lung in the British Military Hospital where I was working in Germany; beautifully designed and made, it incorporated a dome that could be bolted onto the head end of the tank; positive pressure applied around the head allowed the lower part of the tank to be opened for nursing.

"CUIRASS" VENTILATORS

Another promising approach was designed in the 1880s by the Viennese physician Ignez Hauke; his "Pneumatischer Panzer" consisted of a shaped container of sheet metal that could be strapped to the front of the chest—like the cuirass worn by Roman troops. The application of negative pressure to the space between the cuirass and chest wall with a hand driven pump achieved adequate ventilation, but only in patients who were relatively easy to ventilate, because it proved difficult to maintain an air-tight seal. Later he produced a tank ventilator that was to all intents identical to that of Woillez. Even the great Canadian inventor, Alexander Graham Bell, made a cuirass ventilator when

visiting England in 1882; the device was a hinged shell that could be strapped on the chest, negative pressure being applied with a bellows. Bell showed it to a "gentleman connected with University College in London" who promised to do some experiments with it, but that was the last that he saw of it. It was not until the 1930s that cuirass ventilators were commercially produced and powered by electrical pumps; they have been used, on and off, since then to provide some help to patients who need ventilatory assistance, but because they are cumbersome, uncomfortable and not very effective, one seldom sees them being used today.

POSITIVE PRESSURE VENTILATION

All the above techniques employed negative pressure around the chest to expand the lungs, and because of the need for a chamber or cuirass, limited access to the patient inside. Also, if there was difficulty in achieving ventilation, either because the airways were narrow or the lungs stiff, the pressures required became too large. The problem included the difficulty in maintaining an airtight seal around the neck. But the alternative—application of a positive pressure inside the airway—had been used since biblical times to resuscitate infants through mouth-to-mouth respiration.

In 1667 Robert Hooke used a bellows tied to the trachea to keep an experimental dog alive for several hours. John Hunter, described as "one of the three greatest surgeons (with Paré and Lister) of all time" used a double-chambered bellows in his surgical experiments in 1755, and suggested that the technique could be used to resuscitate drowned persons. The suggestion was taken up notably by the Royal Humane Society, but in the face of criticism—that excessive pressure might cause rupture of the lung—the use of bellows fell into disfavor until the late 19th century. Then the advent of inhalation anaesthesia saw several methods developed that used a pump to inflate the lungs through a mask or a tube inserted through the larynx. The rebirth of Hunter's method appears to have followed the successful resuscitation in a case of poisoning, in 1887, when Dr George Edward Fell, a Buffalo, NY, physician used a hand operated bellows and mask. A Cleveland, Ohio, paediatrician, Joseph O'Dwyer, who had a large experience in treating diphtheria, modified Fell's method by intubating the trachea through the larynx, and using a foot operated pump to generate pressure; this became known in 1888 as the Fell-O'Dwyer apparatus. Rudolph Matas, an innovative New Orleans anaesthetist, further increased the scope of the method by incorporating a laryngoscope to aid in the placement of the tube, and it became a standard method in chest surgery. Why another half century would have to pass before the principle was used to sustain breathing in the face of respiratory muscle paralysis, remains a puzzle. Was the communication and cooperation between anaesthetists and physicians so bad that the application didn't occur to them? Or was it a subtle turf war, the physicians distrusting their colleagues to manage any clinical condition outside the operating room? Whatever the reasons, everything changed in 1952.

In mid-summer of 1952, Copenhagen was hit by a particularly virulent outbreak of poliomyelitis. The situation was described in a brief preliminary report to *The Lancet* by Dr Henry Cai Alexander Lassen, Chief Physician to the Blegdan isolation hospital in Copenhagen, on January 3rd, 1953.

Between July and December of 1952, 2722 patients were admitted to the Blegdan Hospital with acute poliomyelitis; 866 were paralyzed and in 316 the respiratory muscles were affected; as many as 50 patients were admitted in one day, and up to ten of them had respiratory weakness. During the early weeks a crisis developed; previously the hospital had experienced an average of only 8 patients a year who had required ventilation, and there were only 6 ventilators available, one tank and five cuirasses. Of the first 31 patients with respiratory paralysis, 27 or almost 90% died. The clinicians were distraught, but also puzzled by this outcome, as the patients were well oxygenated, and appeared to be suffering from "a mysterious alkalosis"—a very elevated blood bicarbonate level. However, when the hospital's senior anaesthetist, Bjørn Ibsen, was consulted on August 27th, he immediately realized that the elevated bicarbonate was in fact due to the retention of carbon dioxide.[1] Analysis of the blood for its acidity (pH) showed an acidosis, thus proving him right. He suggested artificial ventilation via tracheostomy, a tube being inserted into the trachea through an incision in the neck just below the larynx, and ventilation accomplished by manually compressing a rubber bag connected to a cylinder of 50% oxygen. The patient breathed in and out of the bag, and carbon dioxide was removed by a canister of soda-lime between the two. This method was duly carried out on one of the patients, a desperately ill twelve-year-old girl, on July 28th; the next day the blood bicarbonate and pH were normal, and the patient was comfortable. In spite of what appeared to be an impossible logistic task, the method was adopted for all the subsequent patients with respiratory muscle involvement. Manual ventilation was achieved by students, working eight hour shifts, 24 hours

245

---

1   The reaction can be represented as follows— $CO_2 + H_2O \rightarrow H_2CO_3 \rightarrow HCO_3^- + H^+$, where H_2CO_3 is carbonic acid and HCO_3^- is bicarbonate; hydrogen ions (H^+) are generated—this is not an alkalosis, but a respiratory acidosis.

a day. Some patients required the support for as long as three months; 1400 students took part, and by the end of the outbreak mortality had fallen to around 25%. More than fifty years later, this story remains one of the most dramatic in the history of medicine, a testament to ingenuity and leadership of Dr Lassen and his colleagues. Furthermore, the legacy of their pioneering work has been huge.

The experience gained in treating bulbar polio and the evident successes of the iron lung in the 1930s and 40s, and of positive pressure ventilation in the 1950s, provided a needed stimulus for new approaches to prevention of polio and treatment of acute respiratory failure. In the 1930s President Roosevelt, who had been left crippled as a child by polio, boosted fund-raising (the "March of Dimes") for paediatric treatment and rehabilitation. The Danish experience of the early 1950s led to the concept of "Intensive Care Units" staffed by specialists; to innovation in powered artificial positive pressure ventilators; and to improvements in blood gas analysis, that enabled the CO_2 and O_2 pressures in arterial blood to be measured accurately. Within a decade giant strides had been made in all three areas, and after two decades a further impact was made by the application of early computers to clinical problems.

As surgery developed in the early 20th century, anaesthetists devised machines of increasing sophistication for maintaining respiration under anaesthesia. Gas and oxygen was delivered to the lungs via endotracheal tubes by positive pressure, generated through foot pumps or from gas cylinders. Electrical pumps came in the 1930s, and ingenious magnetic and spring loaded valves, actuated by changes in pressure, controlled the flow and phase of breathing (inspiration/expiration). Indeed, the valves provided ways in which control of the ventilator could be made completely automatic and eventually electronically "servo-controlled".
By the 1950s, different types of "intermittent" positive pressure ventilation (IPPV) were available; positive pressure was used to inflate the lungs and the recoil of the lungs and thorax produced expiration. The ventilators were set to generate a prescribed flow or pressure; the former produced sufficient pressure to achieve the given flow however difficult the lungs were to fill, and the latter merely produced the set pressure, and ventilation was controlled by varying the timing of inspiration. A further improvement was achieved by incorporating a pressure sensor that recognized the instant of a patient's own beginning inspiratory effort, causing the ventilator to cut in and carry most of the burden of breathing. Nowadays ventilators have all the bells and whistles one could possibly want; the effectiveness of ventilation is monitored, leaks in the tubing detected, and various patterns of breathing can be readily achieved. For example, a patient may be allowed to breathe on their own, and the ventilator helps to achieve adequate ventilation when necessary (mandatory ventilation). One of the problems of artificial ventilation is that a constant depth of breathing may lead to parts of the lung being poorly expanded; this is countered by building in regular deep breaths (sighs) into the pattern. Patients with lung problems that predispose to the closure of small airways can be treated with positive pressure during expiration to prevent this from occurring; this strategy—positive end-expiratory pressure or PEEP—may dramatically improve oxygen uptake by preventing some parts of the lung from collapsing during expiration. Finally, where there is obstruction in the upper airway, as in obstructive sleep apnea, constant positive airway pressure (CPAP) applied through a nasal mask can prevent airway collapse and thus completely remedy the problem.

With all the improvements in ventilators came improvements in other aspects of patient management. One early problem that occurred in patients being ventilated for long periods via an endotracheal tube was damage to the trachea that could lead to scarring and narrowing. Such patients were left with difficulty in inhalation, accompanied by an audible screech or "stridor", as uncomfortable for the listener as the actual sufferer. This nasty complication was lessened by the use of endotracheal tubes having longer cuffs that self inflated to a much lower pressure than the older tubes.

My early experiences in the use of ventilators, gained in the 1950s, were difficult, and extremely time consuming; the iron lung was placed in a medical ward, often an isolation unit. Often, the nursing staff were not expert in their use, because the ventilators were not constantly in use, and the monitoring systems that control pressure and airflow were primitive compared to modern machines. Today, ventilators are almost exclusively found in intensive care units, and the staff is well-trained and experienced. The large number of ventilators that are currently available, and their variable specifications and performance characteristics, may make for difficulties in when choosing one for a local need. However, it is generally agreed that "the type of ventilator used …is of less importance than the experience of the person using it"—a quote from a book co-authored by Moran Campbell, who also famously stated that "the problem with some intensive care specialists is that they're more intense than careful". In the mid-1960s Campbell was approached to prepare a report for the British Medical Association, regarding the development of specialized ICUs in Britain. Although reluctant to take on the task, because the Hammersmith Hospital in which he worked had not set one up, he chaired the committee which in short order produced its

report. It proved relatively easy to recommend specifications for such units, but there were serious concerns regarding their cost, in the face of little evidence that patient outcome was significantly improved. In Campbell's view the most important issues had to do with intangibles, such as responsibility; that is, who takes care of the patient? A key function is communication—between physicians and staff, and between staff and relatives and patients. However sophisticated the machines, they can never replace humans in such essential functions.

NOTES, ACKNOWLEDGEMENTS AND BIBLIOGRAPHY.

Chapter 1.

The quotation from Hippocrates is taken from *The Genuine works of Hippocrates* by Francis Adams, first published in 1849, but reprinted in 1985 for the Classics of Medicine series published by Gryphon Editions, Ltd.

The first four chapters of the book deal with different aspects of the structure and function of the lungs. There have been many erudite reviews of the history of respiratory physiology, and of medicine as a whole, and I have drawn extensively on them. Charles Singer's books remain probably the most readable accounts, even though they date back to the 1920s, attesting to his long and influential career- *A Short History of Anatomy and Physiology from Galen to Harvey* (1925), republished by Dover, 1956; *A Short History of Scientific Ideas to 1900*(Oxford U.P., 1959); and *A Short History of Medicine* (Oxford U.P., 1928). All are profusely illustrated and, in common with several later authors the diagrams portraying Galen's views are modified from those in his first book. He seems to have been the first to try diagrammatically to explain the logic behind the linkage of concepts of life forces. His diagram (Fig.1) linked the four Grecian "essences" (or "elements")- water, air, fire and earth- to their properties- hot, dry, wet, cold- and to four "humours"- blood, phlegm, back bile and yellow bile. Later authors added bodily systems- heart, liver, spleen and brain- to the scheme, but looking at the concepts from our 21st century vantage point the logic disappears, or at least does not make much sense. Jacalyn Duffin, for example, transposed 'yellow bile" and "blood" in the diagram, presumably to reconcile some of these problems. Writing in 1999 in her book *History of Medicine (A Scandalously Short Introduction)*, she shows sympathy with the Greeks, by posing the question cited on page 5.

John F. Perkins, Jr, contributed an exceptionally fine introductory chapter (*Historical development of respiratory physiology*) to Section 3 of the Handbook of Physiology published in 1964 by the American Physiological Society. John West edited *Respiratory Physiology* for the People and Ideas series also published by American Physiological Society (1996), which contains chapters by many of the leading researchers of the second half of the 20th century. The subject matter of another book in this series- *Circulation of the Blood*, edited by Alfred P. Fishman and Dickinson W. Richards- overlaps and expands on several aspects of respiratory physiology, although it was published some 30 years before, in 1964. One of the most readable and beautifully illustrated accounts of the history of respiratory physiology is by Poul Astrup and John W. Severinghaus- *The History of Blood Gases, Acids and Bases* (Munksgaard, 1986). A feature of all four books is the portraits of all the prominent men in the history of this topic, allowing me to omit them in the present book.

A series of articles titled *The Thorax in History* by RK French of the Wellcome Unit for the History of Medicine at the University of Cambridge was published in volume 33 (1978) of *Thorax*.

Before classic papers were accessible electronically, Julius H. Comroe, Jr, , collected many into the two volumes of *Pulmonary and Respiratory Physiology* in the series Benchmark Papers in Human Physiology (1976). A similar task was undertaken, though less completely, by John F. Fulton in his *Selected Readings in the History of Physiology* (1930).

I was fortunate to have access to the historical collection of the Royal College of Physicians of London, with the help of the Archivist, and was able to study the works of Boyle, Harvey, Hooke, Lower, Mayow, Malpighi, Priestley, Servetus, Vesalius and Willis, and had permission to photograph the illustrations in this chapter. A number of these works have been reprinted in The Classics of Medicine Library, including Servetus (with a translation by CD O'Malley, 1953) and Harvey (translated by Geoffrey Keynes, 1928).

Harvey's life and achievements are chronicled in Gweneth Whitteridge's book *William Harvey and the Circulation of the Blood* (Macdonald, 1971). *The Curious Life of Robert Hooke* by Lisa Jardine is an entertaining account of his life and of the beginnings of the Royal Society (Perennial, Harper-Collins, 2003).

Figure 1 is based on Charles Singer's diagram of the ancient scheme of inter-related elements, humours and qualities described by Hippocrates, from *A Short History of Medicine*, published by Oxford University Press, 1928. Figure 2 is from the same source. Figure 3 is form Malpighi's *de Pulmonibus* (1663) and figure 4 from Mayow's *Tractatus duo quorum prior agit de respiratione* (1668) both Royal College of Physicians ©. Figure 5 is in the public domain and may be accessed through Wikipedia. Figure 6 is from Humphry Davy's *Researches, Chemical and Philosophical* (1800) ©.

In the history of the discovery of oxygen, the Phlogiston Theory (page 15) is difficult to understand, as it implicates a negative attribute (phlogiston). Priestley's experiment with mercury (Hg), which he heated with a burning-glass to produce mercuric oxide may be expressed using modern notation, as follows— $2Hg + O_2$ (in air) $\rightarrow 2HgO$. Then when he took mercuric oxide and subjected it to extreme heat, a gas was produced, which was "much better than air", allowing a flame to burn brighter and for longer. He had collected oxygen- $2HgO \rightarrow 2Hg + O_2$. So dominant was the Phlogiston Theory that Priestley was unable to make the logical leap and infer that he had produced a gas that was present in air, and that in pure form sustained combustion.

Chapter 2.

The early developments in metabolic biochemistry are described in the beautifully illustrated *Discovering Enzymes* by David Dressler and Huntington Potter (Scientific American Library, 1991). Here also will be found an absorbing account of the arguments between Pasteur and Liebig. Astrup and Severinghaus in their above-mentioned book devote a chapter to Lavoisier, and his *Elements of Chemistry* is available in the series *Great Books of the Western World* published by the Encyclopaedia Britannica.

An up-to-date and readable account of metabolic biochemistry is provided by Eric Newsholme and Tony Leech in their *Functional Biochemistry in Health and Disease* (Wiley-Blackwell, 2009).

The biochemistry of muscle contraction is meticulously referenced in Dorothy M Needham's massive work *Machina Carnis* (Cambridge University Press, 1977).

The importance of Chevreul in recognizing fat as an important metabolic fuel was emphasized by Caroline Pond in her book *The Fats of Life* (Cambridge University Press, 1998).

An engaging account of Hans Krebs' life and the discovery of the Citric Acid Cycle (including the letter from the Editor of *Nature* declining publication of the paper presenting its first description) appears in his *Reminiscences and Reflections* (Oxford U.P., 1981).

Chapter 3.

The daVinci quotation is from *Selections from the Notebooks of Leonardo da Vinci*, edited by Irma A. Richter (Oxford University Press, 1952).

Leonardo's anatomical drawing (Figure 8) is #1228lr in the Queen's collection in the Royal Library in Windsor Castle.

Figure 9 is from Malpighi's *de Pulmonibus* (1663) ©.

My copy of Gray's *Anatomy* is the facsimile edition of 1858, published in *The Classics of Medicine Library* (Gryphon Editions, 1981).

Ewald Weibel has provided an authoritative account of the history of lung structure in Chapter 1 of *Respiratory Physiology. People and Ideas*, edited by John West (1996); the left hand portion of Figure 10 is from this source. Also Weibel's *The Pathway for Oxygen* provides a brilliant introduction to the marriage of structure and function in the lung, and to comparative physiology. The right hand portion of Figure 10 is reprinted by permission of the publisher from *The Pathway for Oxygen: Structure and Function in the Mammalian Respiratory System* by Ewald R. Weibel, p. 273, Cambridge, Mass: Harvard University Press, Copyright © by the President and Fellows of Harvard College. Figure 12 is also based on a figure from his book (p. 236). Weibel and Gil's demonstration by electron microscopy of the alveolar surfactant lining layer is described and illustrated (Figure 13) in their chapter of *Bioengineering Aspects of the Lung*, also edited by John West (Dekker, New York, 1977).

Fritz Rohrer's studies are published in *Pflügers Archiv gesammte Physiologie* vol. 162 (1915), pp225-200, and vol. 164 (1916), pp295-302.

Benoit Mandelbrot's book *The Fractal Geometry of Nature* (WH Freeman Co., 1977) provided the background to fractal geometry applied to the bronchial tree, and figure 11.

Chapter 4.

Thomas Willis' *The London Practice of Physick* is available in facsimile in *The Classics of Medicine Library* (Gryphon Editions, 1992). Early work on the measurement of blood gases is described in John F. Perkins chapter *Historical development of respiratory physiology)* in Section 3 of the Handbook of Physiology(American Physiological Society,1964) and Astrup and Severinghaus- *The History of Blood Gases, Acids and Bases*.

Figure 14 of Nathan Zuntz appears in several historical accounts, and was taken from one of Marsh Tenney's annual reports of the Puritan-Bennett Foundation.

The classic description of the oxygen dissociation curve by Bohr, Hasselbalch and Krogh is in *Skand Arch Physiol* 16: 402-412, 1904, from which Figure 15 is taken ©.

In 1961 a meeting was held in Oxford to commemorate the centenary of J.S. Haldane's birth, and attended by most of the respiratory physiologists of the day. The Proceedings were published as a book- *The Regulation of Human Respiration*- edited by Dan Cunningham and Bryan Lloyd (Blackwell, 1961), and contain notable contributions by many experts. There is also an account of

Haldane's life and work, by his college and successor C.G. Douglas, and a complete bibliography. Details of his life also appear in a book by his son, J.B.S. Haldane (*What is Life?* Lindsay Drummond, 1949). The second edition of *Respiration* by J.S. Haldane and J.B. Priestley was published in 1935, the year of Haldane's death.

Figure 16 is from the paper by Christiansen, Douglas and Haldane in the Journal of Physiology (vol. 48: 244-271, 1914).

A delightful account of the life and work of August and Marie Krogh is provided by their daughter Bodil Schmidt-Nielsen in the *Journal of Applied Physiology* (vol. 57: 293-303, 1984); this paper provides references to their major contributions to respiratory physiology.

The papers by R.L. Riley and his colleagues, presenting the concepts of ventilation perfusion relationships were published in the *Journal of Applied Physiology*, vol. 1: 825-847, 1949, vol. 4:77-101, and 102-120, 1951. Hermann Rahn's analysis was virtually contemporaneous and published with Arthur Otis in the same journal, vol. 1:717-724, 1949; he also published "A concept of mean alveolar air and the ventilation-blood flow relationships during pulmonary gas exchange" in the *American Journal of Physiology* vol. 158:21-30, 1949. These papers occupied me for long periods in the 1960s as I worked to complete my thesis for the degree of M.D. at the University of London (1964). The thesis described the blood gas changes during exercise in health and in patients with COPD, in terms of changes in dead space and venous admixture. The material was also published as two papers in *Clinical Science* (vol. 31: 19-29 and 39-50, 1966).

Chapter 5.

The three quotations that begin the chapter are from classic texts on integrative physiology, each in its own way describing the interconnectedness between systems. Claude Bernard's book is available in facsimile in the Classics of Medicine Library. Joseph Barcroft's 1934 text is a "must read" for physiologists, and has also been published in facsimile (Hafner, 1972). And Lawrence Henderson's *Fitness of the Environment* (1913, reprinted by Beacon Press in 1958) is an amazing book, when one takes into account that it is almost a century since it was written. Chapters on water and its properties, the oceans, carbonic acid and the elements of most importance to life, are well worth reading again.

The approach I have taken to neutrality control, or hydrogen ion homeostasis owes everything to Peter Stewart. When he published his book *How to Understand Acid-Base* (Elsevier North Holland, 1981) it became something of a *cause célèbre*; discussion at physiology meetings dealing with acid-base was likely to become heated, even a shouting match, much to the entertainment of the onlookers who were not directly involved. The problem was that Peter went back to classical physicochemical relationships that Lawrence Henderson would certainly have endorsed, and then applied modern computer techniques to solve equations that previously were too complex. This showed that that approaches developed in the previous 50 years, requiring empirical concepts that too often were arcane, or depended on circular arguments, were no longer required. To his followers, his approach may logical sense and clarified the mechanisms that acted to change, or respond to, hydrogen ion concentration. To his detractors, such as the UCLA Professor Daniel Atkinson, adoption of Stewart's approach "would seriously undermine attempts at rational understanding of pH homeostasis" . An impression of the vitriolic exchanges may be gauged by Atkinson's assertion that "The number of women wearing green hats does not depend on the number of men present, or on the number of bare-headed women any more than [H^+] depends on the strong ion difference". More recent discussion has been less heated, and Stewart's "strong ion difference approach" is increasingly accepted as the most rational way to understand acid-base interactions. His followers now have a web site where a new edition of Stewart's book may be accessed (www.acidbase.org).

I attempted to provide a simplified description of Stewart's approach in the second edition of my book *Blood Gases and Acid-Base Physiology* (Thieme, 1987).

Chapter 6.

The Hutchinson quotation, and Figure 22, are taken from his lengthy paper in the Transactions of the Medico-Chirurgical Society of London (vol. 29 of 1946) ©,of which there are extracts reprinted in Julius Comroe's Pulmonary and Respiratory Physiology (Part 2; Dowden, Huntington and Ross, Inc., 1976).

The quotation of Fenn is from his paper in the American Journal of Medicine (vol. 10, 77-90, 1951). This article, 60 years after it was written, remains the single readable description of the mechanics of breathing. The quotation was also used by Moran Campbell in his Foreword to the two part multi-authored *The Thorax*, edited by Charis Roussos and Peter Macklem (Marcel Dekker, Inc., 1985), which remains the most authoritative text on the topic. Figure 21 is adapted from figure 1 in Dennis Osmond's chapter in Part A of this work.

I was able to view the works of Vesalius, Fludd and Mayow (from which figures 18, 19 1nd 20 are taken) ©.

John Clements chapter in *Respiratory Physiology: People and Ideas* in addition to recounting the history of surface-active forces in the lung also provides an account of the recognition by the Rochester group that von Neergard's work on the mechanics of breathing that preceded their own studies by 25 years, and the possible reasons for such a delay.

Fritz Rohrer's publications are to be found in *Pflügers Archiv* (vol. 162: 225-299:1915; and vol. 164, 295-402: 1916), but there is a translation of large portions in Comroe's Pulmonary and Respiratory Physiology (Part 2; Dowden, Huntington and Ross, Inc., 1976). Jere Mead's appreciation of Rohrer's work appears in his review of 1961 in *Physiological Reviews* (vol. 11, 281-330) and his chapter in *Respiratory Physiology: People and Ideas.*

Norman Staub provided an appreciation of Charles Macklin's life and work in a paper which had the appropriate dedication "A prophet is not without honour save in his own country" (*Canadian Respiratory Journal*, 1: 199-207, 1994).

Hutchinson provided the first description of lung volumes in health and disease, and it is interesting to reflect that his studies remained the most comprehensive for over a century. The first real breakthrough towards the use of spirometry in daily clinical practice did not occur until Robert Tiffeneau recognized that the rate of airflow was at least as important as the size of the lungs, in determining breathing capacity. His 1947 paper (in *Paris Med.* vol. 37, 624-678) described the FEV_1 measurement, but it took another decade before the English-speaking world took any notice, after Brian Gandevia and Philip Hugh-Jones suggested that the FEV_1 as a fraction of the vital capacity (FEV_1/VC) provided a reliable index of airflow limitation (in the *Thorax*, vol. 12:290-293' 1957) . Tiffeneau was also the first to describe the methacholine provocation test, nowadays a standard method for assessing airway reactivity. J.-C. Yernault (*European Respiratory Journal, vol.* 17:2704-2710, 1997) provides more details.

Chapter 7.

I make no apology for quoting Wallace Fenn at several points in the book. As well as being an awe inspiring figure in the respiratory physiology of the 1950's and 60's he was able to advance concepts that were elegant and deceptively simple. The quotation at the start of the chapter is taken from his Introductory Remarks at a symposium on The Regulation of Respiration, held at the New York Academy of Sciences in 1960 (*Annals of the New York Academy of Sciences* vol. 104: 415-417, 1960).

Beginning this chapter with Elliott Phillipson's studies in awake animals in whom carbon dioxide arriving in the lungs was reduced to zero (*Journal of Applied Physiology* vol. 50: 45-54, 1981) may be taking an overly simplistic view of the control of breathing, but it serves to emphasize the primacy of CO_2. Of course, when we take control a few steps further, to understand how CO_2 exerts its effect, it all gets much more complicated, as may be judged from the number of books devoted to the topic. Haldane and Priestley provide a review of the early history in their book *Respiration*. The Haldane Centenary Symposium *The Regulation of Respiration* contains chapters by several experts of the 1950s and 60s, and the history of chemoreflexes is a prominent part of *Respiratory Physiology: People and Ideas*, mentioned above. The book *Control of Breathing in Health and Disease*, edited by Murray Altose and Yoshikasu Kawakami serves to bring the topic up to date (and has on its cover an illustration of the Read-Campbell method!). Corneille Heymans' 1945 acceptance speech is available on the Nobel Prize web site.

An account of Hering and Breuer's research and their lives, and a translation of their two papers, was provided by Elizabeth Ullmann in the Ciba Foundation Symposium *Breathing: Hering-Breuer Centenary Symposium* (1970). Ondine's curse is the topic of a chapter in Julius Comroe's *Retro Specto Scope* (Van Gehr Press, Menlo Park, CA, 1970).

Chapter 8.

The comparative physiology of respiration is a fascinating topic, not least because the mechanisms employed by different animal species are more varied than for any other system, be it the heart and circulation, kidneys, or whatever. The ultimate authority in the topic, as for others to do with gas exchange, is the Danish Nobel Prize recipient August Krogh. In 1940, at the age of 66, he wrote the perfect monograph *The Comparative Physiology of Respiratory Mechanisms* (University of Pennsylvania Press). At only 170 pages in length it is a model of conciseness and full of insights into how animals cope with their metabolic needs. His compatriot and former student, Knut Schmidt-Nielsen, exhibited many of his mentor's admirable traits in his seminal textbook *Animal Physiology* (Cambridge U.P., 1975), which brought the subject up to date through nine editions. Comparative respiratory physiology is a notable feature of Ewald Weibel's *The Pathway for Oxygen* (Harvard University Press). For insect physiology Sir Vincent Wigglesworth's massive work *The Principles of Insect Physiology* (Chapman and Hall, 1972) remains the standard reference. Finally, G.M. Hughes' *Comparative Physiology of Vertebrate Respiration* (Heinemann, 1963) provides an admirably concise and well illustrated account.

The figures reflect the importance of these authors; Figure 24 is from Schmidt-Nielsen and Hughes, Figure 25 from Wigglesworth, and Figure 26 is modified from Weibel and Schmidt-Nielsen.

I was drawn to the literature of scaling physiological systems in animals of varying size when attempting to provide logic-based equations to calculate normal standards for lung volumes and exercise variables. The earliest thoughts on the subject were delightfully presented by Galileo Galilei in his *Two New Sciences* of 1637 (translated by Crew and De Salvio, Northwestern University, 1939). More than two centuries passed before the importance of scaling was set out beautifully by D'Arcy Wentworth Thompson in his *On Growth and Form* (Cambridge University Press, 1942). My attention was drawn to this classic by Marsh Tenney when he wrote an insightful article for the Canadian Respiratory Journal (Vol. 1, 241-247,1994; accessible on-line at pulsus.com) entitled "Art and science: where numerology and mathematics touch the lung". A readable and comprehensive view is provided by Knut Schmidt-Nielsen in his *Scaling. Why is animal size so important?* (Cambridge University Press, 1984). The extraordinary collaboration between Ewald Weibel and C. Richard Taylor is described in a series of articles in volume 44 (1981) of Respiration Physiology. Figures 27 and 28 are adapted from Tenney's paper.

The application of scaling principles to exercise in humans is provided in my book *Clinical Exercise Testing* (4th Ed., W.B. Saunders Co., 1997)

Chapter 9.

The *Gaia* to which the title refers, is the concept of our planet existing as a self regulating organism put forward by the independent British scientist, James Lovelock, in a book of the same title (Oxford U.P., 1979). The book provides a readable account of the evolution of the atmosphere. The linkage between the evolution of life and of the atmosphere is emphasized by Richard Fortey in *Life* (Knopf, 1997). Spencer Weart's *The Discovery of Global Warming* (Harvard U. P., 2003) and Tim Flannery's *The Weather Makers* (Harper Collins, 2005) are also readable accounts of the factors acting on the environment, and in the latter an emphasis on the influence of the oceans. The experiments of Miler and Urey are recounted in an article "Chemical Evolution and the Origin of Life" by Richard Dickerson in an issue of the *Scientific American* devoted to evolution (vol. 239: 70-86, 1978).

Dave Keeling's studies on Mauna Loa have been continued and expanded by his son Ralph, who graciously checked my inferences from their work. Their data are available on the Scripps Institute web site (scripps.co2.ucsd.edu), from which Figure 29 is taken. An article by Ralph Keeling appeared in *Nature* (vol.358:723-727, 1992)

The great importance of the oceans in buffering increases in atmospheric CO_2 is a feature of Tom Flannery's book, with more detailed coverage being provided by C.L. Sabine et al in their paper "The ocean sink for atmospheric CO_2" (*Science* 305: 367-371, 2004). Lawrence Henderson's *The Fitness of the Environment* remains the classic in this field, in spite of being almost a century old.

Primo Levi's quote is from his *Periodic Table* (Penguin, 1986).

Chapter 10.

The quotations and photo of Roger Bannister are from his *First Four Minutes* (Sportsman's Book Club, 1956). His physiological data were obtained from his paper with D.J.C. Cunningham and C.G. Douglas ("The carbon dioxide stimulus to breathing in severe exercise", *Journal of Physiology*, vol. 125: 90-117, 1954).

Elsbeth Heaman has written the wonderful *St Mary's. The History of a London Teaching Hospital* (McGill-Queen's U.P., 2003).

The sources for much of the early biochemistry of exercise are those noted in Chapter 2. The history of the biochemistry of exercise is meticulously described by Dorothy M. Needham in *Machina Carnis* (Cambridge U. P., 1971). A. V. Hill's *Living Machinery* (G. Bell, 1939) remains well worth reading, as does Grace Eggleton's *Muscular Exercise* (Keegan Paul, 1936). For the integrated responses to exercise it would be hard to beat *Textbook of Work Physiology* by P.-O. Åstrand and K. Rodahl (McGraw Hill, 1977). A shorter account is available in my book *Clinical Exercise Testing* (4th Ed, Saunders, 1998). Eric Newsholme's *The Runner* (with Tony Leech; Fitness Books) is perhaps more readable and no less authoritative.

It seems extraordinary that the two Huxleys, who solved the mechanism of muscular contraction, were not related. The Croonian Lecture of 1967 by Andrew F. Huxley (*Proceedings of the Royal Society, Series B*, vol. 178: 1-27) and "The contraction of muscle" by Hugh Esmor Huxley (*Scientific American*, Nov 1958) remain worth reading to this day.

The controversies around "oxygen debt" ("lactacid and alactacid"), the "anaerobic threshold" , centre around the question "is lactate produced because not enough oxygen is being delivered to muscle, or because the muscle metabolic processes are unable to use all the oxygen presented to muscle?" The classical view is well presented by one of its early protagonists, Rodolfo Margaria in *Biomechanics and Energetics of Muscular Exercise* (Oxford U.P., 1976). The concepts were criticized, almost to the point of ridicule, by Peter Harris, in his paper "Lactic acid and the phlogiston debt" (*Cardiovascular Research*, vol. 3: 381-390, 1969). A modern perspective on the question is provided by my colleagues Lawrence Spriet and George Heigenhauser in their paper with R.A. Howlett ("An enzymatic approach to lactate production in human skeletal muscle during exercise"; *Medicine and Science in Sports and Exercise* vol. 32: 756-763, 2000). My paper "An obsession with CO_2," (*Applied Physiology of Nutrition and Metabolism* vol. 33: 1-10, 2008) provides a summary of our work in this area.

Chapter 11.

The Wordsworth quotation was used by Moran Campbell for the title of his paper ("A Being Breathing Thoughtful Breaths") in the "How it *Really* Happened" series in the *American Journal of Respiratory and Critical Care Medicine* (vol.162: 2027-2028, 2000). The paper describes his earliest ventures into the domain of respiratory sensations, and includes his famous assertion "A respiratory physiologist offering a unitary explanation for breathlessness should arouse the same suspicions as a tattooed archbishop offering a free ticket to Heaven".

The "enigma" editorial is in *The Lancet* vol. i:891-892, 1986.

The 1821 translation by John Forbes of Laënnec's classic *Treatise* was produced in facsimile in The Classics of Medicine Library (Gryphon Editions, 1979).

Christies' massive review is in the *Quarterly Journal of Medicine* vol. 7: 421-454, 1938. His colleague Jonathan Meakins (the two are immortalized in the Meakins-Christie Institute at McGill University) also provided an early review of "The cause and treatment of dyspnea in cardiovascular disease" (*British Medical Journal* vol.2 of 1923, p. 1043-1045). The monograph *Dyspnea* by John Howard Means appeared in 1924 (Williams and Wilkins Co.).

The development of measurements applied to sensory physiology was provided by S.S. Stevens in his truly seminal masterpiece *Psychophysics* (Wiley, 1975). Gunnar Borg's category scale is described by him in the *Proceedings of the 22nd International Congress of Psychology* (North-Holland, 1980). The history of psychophysical methods applied to breathing is reviewed by Kieran Killian in *Breathlessness. The Campbell Symposium* (1992). References are also available in my book *Clinical Exercise Testing*.

Chapter 12.

Lt. Col. Norton's words are from his *The Fight for Everest,1924* (Edward Arnold, 1925), and the Messner quotation is from *Everest: Expedition to the Ultimate* (Bâton Wicks, 1999).

Figure 35 is from Haldane and Priestley's *Respiration* (Oxford U.P., 1935)

The account of the ascent of the *Zenith*, and figure 36 are from Paul Bert's *La Pression Barométrique* (1878, ©).

Mabel FitzGerald's studies are described in her paper "Changes in the breathing and the blood at various high altitudes" (*Philosophical Transactions of the Royal Society of London, Series B,* vol. 203: 351-371, 1913). They also feature prominently in Haldane and Priestley's *Respiration*.

The story of the Rochester Group appears in Peter Macklem's chapter, "Modern History of Respiratory Muscle Physiology", in *Respiratory Physiology: People and Ideas* (Oxford U.P., 1996).

There are three chapters in *Hypoxia: Man at Altitude* which was edited by John Sutton, Charles Houston and myself (Thieme-Stratton, 1982), by Griff Pugh, Jim Milledge and John West, which describe physiological studies at high altitudes, and from which Figures 37 and 38 are taken. Operation Everest II led to a large number of publications in the *Journal of Applied Physiology*, mainly in 1987, summarized by John Sutton in *Breathlessness: The Campbell Symposium* (1992) .

Frances Ashcroft includes a very readable account of the problems encountered at extreme altitude in her book *Life at the Extremes* (Flamingo, 2001)

Angelo Mosso was an outstanding experimental physiologist; in addition to *Life of Man in the High Alps* he wrote *Fatigue* (1902) in which he makes many observations regarding breathing under stress.

The early history of the effects of altitude on red blood cells, leading to the discovery of erythropoietin, is exhaustively reviewed (the paper contains almost 400 references) by Wolfgang Jelkmann (Erythropoietin after a century of research: younger than ever, *European Journal of Haematology* vol. 78: 183-205, 2007).

The research into the problems of supplying oxygen and the effects of G forces in aviators is recounted in *Into Thin Air: A History of Aviation Medicine in the RAF* by T.H. Gibson and M.H. Harrison (Robert Hall, 1984).

Chapter 13.

Several of the early sources of diving physiology are the same as those for altitude- such as Paul Bert, Haldane and Priestley and Frances Ashcroft. The research on the diving Ama by S.K. Hong and Hermann Rahn is provided in an article in *Scientific American* (vol. 216: 34-43, 1967). Tanya Streeter and HMS Thetis are the subjects of informative entries in Wikipedia.

J.B.S. Haldane's experiences of "Life at High Pressures" are in his book *What is Life?* (Lindsey Drummond, 1949).

Figure 39 is from Haldane and Priestley's *Respiration*.

Chapter 14.

The quotation of von Neergaard is from the English translation of his paper in *Zeitschrift Gesamte Exp. Med.* (vol. 66:373-394, 1929) by Rainer Arnhold and Hans Hahn, contained in volume 5 of *Benchmark papers in Human Physiology. Pulmonary and Respiratory Physiology* , edited by Julius Comroe (Dowden, Hutchinson and Ross, 1976).

Geoffrey Dawes contributed a notable chapter, "Physiological Changes in the Circulation after Birth", in *Circulation of the blood: Men and Ideas* (Edited by A.P. Fishman and D.W. Richards, Oxford U.P., 1964).

Benjamin Franklin experiments with oil on water were published as letters in the *Philosophical Transactions* of the Royal Society (vol. 64:445-461, 1774). They are cited in a wonderful chapter on the discovery of surfactant by John Clements in *Respiratory Physiology: People and Ideas*. Mary Ellen Avery has provided her own account in "Surfactant Deficiency in Hyaline Membrane Disease" in the *American Journal of Respiratory and Critical Care Medicine* (vol.161:1074-1075, 2000). Her studies with Jere Mead are published in the *American Journal of Diseases in Childhood* (vol.97: 517-523, 1959). The studies on excised lungs, including Figure 40, are published in *The Journal of Clinical Investigation*, vol. 38: 2168-2173, 1959.

R.E. Pattle first published his studies on the surface active properties of the alveolar lining layer in a letter to *Nature* (vol. 175:1125-1126, 1955), followed by a fuller paper in the *Proceedings of the Royal Society of London, Series B* (vol. 148:217-240, 1958). John Clements provided a complete review of his work in "Surface phenomena in relation to pulmonary function" (*Physiologist*, vol.5:12-28, 1962).

Chapter 15.

The initial quotation is from Dickinson Richards' Lewis A. Conner Memorial Lecture; The Nature of Cardiac and Pulmonary Dyspnea (*Circulation* vol. 7: 15-29, 1953).

The history of the autonomic nervous system features prominently in *Circulation of the Blood: Men and Ideas*, mentioned above. Corneille Heymans' Nobel Lecture (1945)- "The part played by vascular presso- and chemo-receptors in respiratory control"- describes the early experiments carried out with his father, and is available on-line (nobelprize.org).

Neil Oldridge's studies on the effects of facial immersion on heart rate are in the *Journal of Applied Physiology*, vol.45: 875-879, 1978.

There is a large literature on yogic breathing, and breathing control is prominent in most texts on Yoga, such as Harvey Day's *About Yoga* (British Book Centre, 1951), *Yoga and Medicine* by Steven Brena (Penguin, 1972), and Frtjof Capra's *Uncommon Wisdom* (Bantam, 1988), and a chapter in *Progress in Brain Research* vol. 122 (Elsevier Science, 2000) by Rolf Sovik- "The science of breathing- the yogic view".

The effect of yogic breathing in asthma was studied by Anne Tattersfield and her colleagues (*Lancet* vol. 335: 1381-1383, 1990).

The links between the autonomic nervous system and the immune system are explored by F.E. Blalock in "The immune system as the sixth sense" (*Journal of Internal Medicine* (vol. 257: 126-138, 2000) and by Paul Martin in *The sickening mind* (Harper Collins, 1997)

Chapter 16.

The reference to "le syndrome de Pickwick" by Gastaut et al is in the proceedings of *Société Française de Neurologie* (Séance du 3 Juin 1965) published in *Revue Neurologique*, vol. 112: 568-579, 1965.

Hans Berger's story was gained mainly from the article published by K. Karbowski in *The Journal of Neurology*, vol. 249: 1130-1131, 2002.

The full scale of the impact sleep medicine may be gauged by an issue (vol. 19, number 1, 1998) of *Clinics in Chest Medicine* that is devoted to Sleep Disorders.

John Remmer's early studies are presented in his paper in the *Journal of Applied Physiology* Vol. 44: 931-938, 1978. Colin Sullivan's breakthrough in the management of obstructive sleep apnoea was published in the *Lancet* vol.317: 862-865, 1981.

A review of Cheyne-Stokes breathing is provided by Neil Cherniack in the *New England Journal of Medicine* (vol. 288: 952-957, 1973). Angelo Mosso's description of Cheyne-Stokes breathing at altitude appears in his book *Life of Man in the High Alps* (1898), now available in a modern edition (Pranava Books, 2008). The studies of Douglas and Haldane appear in the *Journal of Physiology* vol. 38: 401-419, 1909.

Chapter 17.

The initial quotation and subsequent account of Farinelli is from *Prima Donna: a History* by Rupert Christiansen (Penguin, 1986).

Readers may wonder why I wrote this chapter; the reason was a feeling that there were many misconceptions regarding the control of the breath in singing. I was helped by Ian Johnston's *Measured Tones: The Interplay of Physics and Music* (Adam Hilger, 1989), and more importantly by the late Donald F. Proctor, who applied to medical school whilst learning to be an opera singer at the Juilliard, and went on to become a respiratory physiologist at Harvard, working with Jere Mead. His book *Breathing, Speech and Song* (Springer-Verlag, 1980) remains the Bible on this topic. Figure 43 is from this work. Figure 41 is from Charles Singer's *A Short History of Anatomy and Physiology from the Greeks to Harvey* (Dover Edition, 1957).

Chapter 18.

Then initial quotation from Agricola is taken from Keith Morgan and Anthony Seaton's *Occupational Lung Diseases* (2nd Ed, W.B. Saunders Co., 1984). The quotation from the beginning of Dickens' *Bleak House* also appears at the beginning of *Air Pollution and Health*, the Report for the Royal College of Physicians (Pitman Medical, 1970). Figure 44 is adapted from a figure in this report and Figure 45 is reproduced from it.

David Bates, right up to his death in 2006, was the doyen of researchers of air pollution. His books *A Citizen's Guide to Air Pollution* (McGill-Queen's U.P., 1972) and *Environmental Health Risks and Public Policy* (UBC Press, 1994) remain perfect introductions to the topic. David also contributed an article to the *Canadian Respiratory Journal*—"Ozone — 42 years later" (vol. 13:261-265, 2006).

The effects of pollution on children's lung health are reviewed by James Gunderman in an editorial—"Air Pollution and Children – an Unhealthy Mix" in *The New England Journal of Medicine* (vol. 355:78-79, 2006. His major study (David Bates was a co-author) appears in the same journal (vol.351:1057-1067, 2004). The pollution indices in Ontario were obtained from a report to the Ontario Ministry of the Environment (June, 2005) which is available on the Ministry's web site (www.ene.gov.on.ca). Professor Grigg's study is published in *The New England Journal of Medicine* (vol. 355:21-30, 2006).

Ramazzini's classic text is available in translation in the *Classics of Medicine Library* (Gryphon Editions, 1983). There is also the web site of the Collegium Ramazzini (ramazzini.it). A modern approach to occupational lung diseases is presented by Keith Morgan and Anthony Seaton in their textbook of that title (W.B. Saunders, 1984), and there is an excellent review of asbestosis by Raymond Bégin and colleagues in *Canadian Respiratory Journal* (vol. 1:167-186, 1994), from which Figure 46 is taken.

Chapter 19.

Whilst I was able to read Floyer's book at the R.C.P., Alex Sakula has published a long and informative article on it, with many quotations, in *Thorax* (vol. 39:254-284, 1984). Sakula is also the author of "A History of Asthma" (*Journal of the Royal College of Physicians of London, vol.22:36-44, 1988). The Genuine Works of Hippocrates* is in the *Classics of Medicine Library* (Gryphon Editions, 1985). Another work in this series is Osler's 1892 edition of *Principles and Practice of Medicine* (Gryphon Editions,1978). My sources on Maimonides were *Maimonides: a Biography* by Abraham J. Heschel (Doubleday, 1995) and the article by Sidney Bloch in *The Lancet* (vol.358:829-832, 2001). Salter's *On Asthma* is in the R.C.P. Library; excerpts from this, and many other classic papers on asthma, are contained in R.S.L. Brewis' two volume *Classic Papers in Asthma* (Science Press, 1990). His book provides a much more detailed account and bibliography than I have given.

Figure 47 was obtained from the R.C.P. Library copy of Charles Backley's book *Experimental Researches on the Causes and Nature of Catarrhus Aestevus* (1873) ©.

Von Pirquet's first use of the term allergy is recounted in the review "Allergy and Immunology" of D.W. Talmage in *Annual Review of Medicine* (vol.8:239-256, 1957). Jodassohn's use of skin patch tests is viewed in a modern light by J.R. Nethercott in *Current Problems in Dermatology* (vol. 2:87-123, 1990).

The papers by Noon and Freeman are in *The Lancet* (vol. i: 1572-1573, 1911, and vol.ii: 814-817, 1911, respectively).

Prausnitz and Küstner's paper is reproduced in Alastair Brewis' book.

The Ishizakas' paper "Identification of E-antibodies as a carrier of reaginic activity" is in *The Journal of Immunology* (vol. 99:1187-1198, 1967).

Virchow's *Cellular Pathology* is in the *Classics of Medicine Library* (Gryphon Editions, 1978).

Huber and Koessler's paper on the pathology of asthma is in the *Archives of Internal Medicine* (vol. 30: 689-760, 1922).

Stephen Holgate's wide-ranging work in asthma extends from its clinical aspects through to the cellular response in the bronchial wall (in *Trends in Immunology* vol. 28:246-248,2007), the role of viral infections in children (*British Medical Journal* vol. 310:1225-1229, 1995) , to the genetics of asthma (*Thorax* vol. 60:263-264, 2005).

Ben Burrows' study of IgE in the population is in *The New England Journal of Medicine* (vol. 320:271-277, 1989).

Sir Henry Dale's career is described in a lecture by H.O. Schild (*British Journal of Pharmacology* vol. 56:3-7, 1976) and his work is extensively described in *Circulati0on of the Blood: Men and Ideas*. The reference to Kellaway and Trethewie is the *Journal of Physiology* vol. 30:121-146, 1940. Sir John Vane reviews his work in the Croonian Lecture, published in the *Proceedings of the Royal Society, Series B,* vol. 343:225-246, 1994. Bengt Samuelsson's Nobel Prize Lecture is available in the Nobel web site, and contains references to the work of Borgeat and Piper.

The study of Don Cockcroft and Freddy Hargreaves on allergy and airway responsiveness was published in the *American Review of Respiratory Disease*, vol. 136:264-267, 1987.

Noe Zamel's expedition to Tristan da Cunha was published in the *Canadian Respiratory Journal* (vol.2:18-22, 1995). The research of Citron and Pepys on the evacuated islanders is published in the *British Journal of Diseases of the Chest*, vol. 58:119-123, 1964.

Dr Camps' report was published in the *Guy's Hospital Reports vol.* 79:496-498, 1929.

A well-illustrated history of spirometry was provided by E.A. Spriggs in the *British Journal of Diseases of the Chest*, vol. 72:165-180, 1978.

Malcolm Sears' studies of asthma mortality were published in *Chest*, vol. 94:914-918, 1988.

For a comprehensive account of asthma treatment, the *Manual of Asthma Management* (W.B. Saunders, 1995), edited by Paul O'Byrne and Neil Thomson may be recommended. Several editions of the Canadian Guidelines for asthma management have been published in the *Canadian Respiratory Journal* (accessible on the journal's web site at www.pulsus.com) and the *Canadian Medical Association Journal* (vol.173, supp 6:S1-S56, 2003).

Other references-

Ahlquist, *American Journal of Physiology*, vol. 153:586-600, 1948.
Bordley, *Bulletin of the Johns Hopkins Hospital*, vol. 85:396, 1949.
Bullowa and Kaplan, *Medical News (N.Y.)*, vol. 83:787-790, 1903.
Chen and Schmidt, *Journal of Pharmacology and Experimental Therapeutics*, vol. 24:339-357, 1924.
Fineman, *Journal of Allergy*, vol. 4:182-190, 1932.
Howell and Altounyan, *Lancet*, vol. ii:539-542, 1967.
Lands, *Nature*, vol. 214:597, 1967.
Oliver and Sharpey-Schafer, *Journal of Physiology*, vol. 18:277-279, 1895.

Chapter 20.

My colleague Watson Buchanan provided an entertaining account of King James' "counterblaste" in the *Proceedings of the Royal College of Physicians of Edinburgh*, vol.30:154-157, 2000.

The landmark publications of the Royal College of Physicians , *Smoking and Health* (Pitman Medical, 1962), and *Smoking and Health Now* (1971) remain among the best to this day: a biased view perhaps, because Charles Fletcher was the secretary to the committee that produced it- he wanted the title to be Smoking or Health! There have been many reports since then, notably by the United States Public Health Service, which has published a series *The Health Consequences of Smoking* (Department of Health, Education and Welfare, 1967, 1968, 1969, 1973 and 1974). Another, titled *Women and Smoking* came out in 2001. Kahn's study of U.S. veterans (containing Figure 48) was published as monograph 19 of the *National Cancer Institute* (1966).

Richard Doll and Richard Peto review the initial and extended results of the study of British doctors in the *British Medical Journal*, vol. 2:1525-1536, 1976. An "Update in Lung Cancer" is provided by Dubey and Powell (*American Journal of Respiratory and Critical Care*, vol. 177:941-946, 2008).

I was able to read Charles Badham's book in the R.C.P. Library. Lynne Reid's index is described in *Thorax*, vol. 10:199-204, 1955.

The pathology of emphysema is reviewed by William (Whitey) Thurlbeck in the *Canadian Respiratory Journal* (vol. 1:21-39, 1994).

Laurell and Eriksson's landmark paper is in the *Scandinavian Journal of Clinical Investigation*, vol. 15:132-140, 1963.

Charles Fletcher's book *The Natural History of Chronic Bronchitis and Emphysema* (Oxford U.P., 1976) is hard to find; there is a summary of the highlights of his 8-yr study of British postal workers in the *British Medical Journal*, vol.1:1645-1648, 1977, and it contains Figure 51. The Hammersmith-Chicago comparison study was published in *The American Review of Respiratory Diseases*, vol. 90:1-13 and 14-27, 1964, and *Lancet*, vol.1:830-835, 1966.

Kieran Killian's research into the factors that limited exercise in COPD led to the recognition that skeletal muscle fatigue and weakness, paved the way for exercise rehabilitation in the management of patients. We contributed a chapter to Neil Cherniack's book, *Chronic Obstructive Pulmonary Disease* (W.B. Saunders, 1991) on the topic.

Chapter 21.

The history of tuberculosis, and many other aspects of respiratory health , is a feature of *Colleagues in Discovery – One Hundred Years of Improving Respiratory Health* which Joseph Wallace wrote to commemorate the Centenary of the American Thoracic Society (Tehabi Books, 2005). It, too, contains Chopin's lament that begins the chapter.

The importance of Robert Koch, and his great admirer William Osler, is well covered in Roy Porter's *The Greatest Benefit to Mankind* (W.W. Norton, 1997), and also comes through in Michael Bliss' *William Osler: A Life in Medicine* (University of Toronto Press, 1999).

Röntgen's radiograph is in the Deutches Museum, Munich.

As may be gathered, there are many reports of clinical trials in tuberculosis; reviews can be found in standard textbooks, such as *Respiratory Medicine*, edited by R.A.L. Brewis et al (W.B. Saunders, 1995).

Chapter 22.

Vesalius is credited with the seminal concept of the artificial airway by Federico Vallejo-Manzur et al (*Resuscitation* vol. 56:3-7, 2003). The history of artificial ventilation is comprehensively covered by Mushin and Rendell-Baker in *The Origins of Thoracic Anaesthesia* (Wood Library – Museum of Anesthesiology, 1953, 1991). Drinker and McKhann's original (1929) paper is revisited in the *Journal of the American Medical Association* vol. 255:1473-1480, 1986, in which Figure 54 appears.

The Copenhagen polio epidemic is described in a "preliminary report" by Lassen in *The Lancet* (vol. i:37-41, 1953) and also features in Poul Astrup and John W. Severinghaus- *The History of Blood Gases, Acids and Bases* (Munksgaard, 1986).

Moran Campbell's quotation is from Sykes, McNicol and Campbell *Respiratory Failure* (Blackwell, 2nd Ed., 1977)

Index

259

261

265